CONTENTS

Color Illustration Section (16 pages) between pages 416 and 417

SECTION III   TOP-RATED REVIEW RESOURCES   419

FIRST AID

FOR THE®

U
S

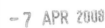
Fifth Edition

TAO LE,
Assistant Prof
Division of All
Department o
University of L

Assistant in M
Division of All
Department o
Johns Hopkin

VIKAS B
Diagnostic Ra

KERRY D
Johns Hopkin
School of Me
Editor, Introdu

ROBERT
Resident
Department of Emergency Medicine
Mayo Clinic
Editor, Emergency Medicine

McGraw-Hill

MEDICAL PUBLISHING DIVISION

New York / Chicago / San Francisco / Lisbon / London / Madrid / Mexico City
Milan / New Delhi / San Juan / Seoul / Singapore / Sydney / Toronto

First Aid for the® USMLE Step 2 CK, Fifth Edition

1 2 3 4 5 6 7 8 9 0   QPD/QPD   0 9 8 7 6 5

ISBN 0-07-144336-3
ISSN 1532-320X

NOTICE

This book was set in Electra LH by Rainbow Graphics.
The editor was Catherine A. Johnson.
The production supervisor was Phil Galea.
Project management was provided by Rainbow Graphics.
Quebecor Dubuque was printer and binder.

This book is printed on acid-free paper.

To our families, friends, and loved ones, who endured and assisted in the task of assembling this guide.

and

To the contributors to this and future editions, who took time to share their knowledge, insight, and humor for the benefit of students.

CONTRIBUTING AUTHORS

Gbemisola Adeseun, MD, MPH

Johns Hopkins University School of Medicine
Class of 2005
Musculoskeletal, Ethics, Epidemiology, Book Reviews

Emilie J. B. Calvello, MPH

Johns Hopkins University School of Medicine
Class of 2006
Gastrointestinal, Pediatrics, Renal, Obstetrics

Amy E. DeZern, MD

Johns Hopkins University School of Medicine
Class of 2005
Endocrine, Neurology, Pulmonology, Psychiatry

Anne Mani, MD

Johns Hopkins University School of Medicine
Class of 2005
Cardiovascular, Dermatology

Hansie Marie Mathelier, MD

Johns Hopkins University School of Medicine
Class of 2005
Hematology/Oncology, Gynecology

FACULTY REVIEWERS

Carolyn Joy Alexander, MD
Fellow in Reproductive Endocrinology and Infertility
Department of Gynecology and Obstetrics
Johns Hopkins University

Dickson Cheung, MD
Clinical Instructor
Assistant Residency Director
Department of Emergency Medicine
Johns Hopkins University

Rachel Chong, MD
Fellow in Endocrinology
Department of Medicine
Johns Hopkins University

Niccolo D. Della Penna, MD
Chief Resident
Department of Psychiatry and Behavioral Sciences
Johns Hopkins University

Michelle Estrella, MD
Fellow in Nephrology
Department of Medicine
Johns Hopkins University

Rosalyn Juergens, MD
Fellow in Medical Oncology
Department of Medicine
Johns Hopkins University

Lynda Kauls, MD
Assistant Professor
Department of Dermatology
University of Maryland

Geoffrey Nguyen, MD
Fellow in Gastroenterology
Department of Medicine
Johns Hopkins University

Patrick O'Connell, MD
Clinician-Educator
York Hospital
York, Pennsylvania

Michael S. Rafii, MD, PhD
Senior Resident
Department of Neurology
Johns Hopkins University

Gita Sinha, MD
Fellow in Infectious Diseases
Department of Medicine
Johns Hopkins University

Karen Schneider, RSM, MD
Faculty in Pediatric Emergency Medicine
Johns Hopkins University

Patrick Sosnay, MD
Fellow in Pulmonary Critical Care Medicine
Department of Medicine
Johns Hopkins University

Véronique Taché, MD
Resident
Department of Obstetrics and Gynecology
University of California, Davis

PREFACE

With the fifth edition of *First Aid for the USMLE Step 2 CK*, we continue our commitment to providing students with the most useful and up-to-date preparation guide for the USMLE Step 2 CK. The fifth edition represents a thorough revision in many ways and includes:

- A revised and updated exam preparation guide for the USMLE Step 2 CK. Includes updated study and test-taking strategies for the new FRED computer-based testing (CBT) format.
- Revisions and new material based on student experience with the 2004 and 2005 administrations of the USMLE Step 2 CK.
- Concise summaries of over 300 heavily tested clinical topics. Most topics rewritten for fast, high-yield studying.
- Topics integrate clinically relevant high-yield basic science facts from *First Aid for the USMLE Step 1*.
- A "rapid review" that tests your knowledge of each topic.
- A high-yield collection of over 120 glossy photos similar to those appearing on the USMLE Step 2 CK exam.
- A completely revised, in-depth guide to clinical science review and sample examination books.

The fifth edition would not have been possible without the help of the many students and faculty members who contributed their feedback and suggestions. We invite students and faculty to continue sharing their thoughts and ideas to help us improve *First Aid for the USMLE Step 2 CK*. (See How to Contribute, p. xv.)

Louisville	Tao Le
Los Angeles	Vikas Bhushan
Baltimore	Kerry Dierberg
Rochester	Robert W. Grow

ACKNOWLEDGMENTS

This has been a collaborative project from the start. We gratefully acknowledge the thoughtful comments, corrections, and advice of the many medical students, international medical graduates, and faculty who have supported the authors in the continuing development of *First Aid for the USMLE Step 2 CK*.

For support and encouragement throughout the process, we are grateful to Thao Pham and Selina Bush. Thanks also to those who supported the authors including Matthew Provenzano, Hari Nathan, Douglas Ramsey, and Jamie Rand.

Thanks to our publisher, McGraw-Hill, for the valuable assistance of their staff. For enthusiasm, support, and commitment for this challenging project, thanks to our editor, Catherine Johnson. For outstanding editorial work, we thank Andrea Fellows. A special thanks to David Hommel (Rainbow Graphics) for remarkable production work, and Silas Wang for creating the Web survey. Thanks to Elizabeth Sanders and Ashley Pound for the interior design.

For contributions, corrections, and surveys we thank Elena Gimenez, George Apergis, Chinyere Azuogu, Karthik Balakrishnan, Joel Balcom, Richard Chung, Jay Cowdry, Prabhjot Singh Dhadialla, Jason Dean Eidahl, Rashiah Elam, Jing Feng, Jessie Glasser, Allison Hunt, Ryan Thomas Hurt, Michael Johnson, Mandy Krauthamer, Mara Lagzdins, Alexander Langerman, Aimee Lee, Deanne Nakamoto, Minal Patel, Sateesh R. Prakash, Ron Reilkoff, Sarah L. Schatz, Jonathan Shapiro, Grace Smith, Natasha Srb, and William Ward. Our apologies in advance if we accidentally omitted or misspelled your name.

Louisville	Tao Le
Los Angeles	Vikas Bhushan
Baltimore	Kerry Dierberg
Rochester	Robert W. Grow

HOW TO CONTRIBUTE

To continue to produce a high-yield review source for the Step 2 CK exam, you are invited to submit any suggestions or corrections. We also offer **paid internships** in medical education and publishing ranging from three months to one year (see below for details). Please send us your suggestions for

- Study and test-taking strategies for the Step 2 CK exam.
- New facts, mnemonics, diagrams, and illustrations.
- Low-yield topics to remove.

For each entry incorporated into the next edition, you will receive a $10 gift certificate, as well as personal acknowledgment in the next edition. Diagrams, tables, partial entries, updates, corrections, and study hints are also appreciated, and significant contributions will be compensated at the discretion of the authors. Also let us know about material in this edition that you feel is low yield and should be deleted.

The **preferred way** to submit entries, suggestions, or corrections is via electronic mail. Please include name, address, school affiliation, phone number, and e-mail address (if different from the address of origin). If there are multiple entries, please consolidate into a single e-mail or file attachment. Please send submissions to:

firstaidteam@yahoo.com

Otherwise, please send entries, neatly written or typed or on disk (Microsoft Word), to:

First Aid for the USMLE Step 2 CK
P.O. Box 27
Woodstock, MD 21163-9982
Attention: Contributions

NOTE TO CONTRIBUTORS

All entries become property of the authors and are subject to editing and reviewing. Please verify all data and spellings carefully. In the event that similar or duplicate entries are received, only the first entry received will be used. Include a reference to a standard textbook to facilitate verification of the fact. Please follow the style, punctuation, and format of this edition if possible.

INTERNSHIP OPPORTUNITIES

The author team is pleased to offer part-time and full-time paid internships in medical education and publishing to motivated physicians. Internships may range from three months (e.g., a summer) up to a full year. Participants will have an opportunity to author, edit, and earn academic credit on a wide variety of projects, including the popular First Aid series. Writing/editing experience, familiarity with Microsoft Word, and Internet access are desired. For more information, e-mail a résumé or a short description of your experience along with a cover letter to the authors at their e-mail address above.

Guide to Efficient Exam Preparation

INTRODUCTION

The United States Medical Licensing Examination (USMLE) Step 2 allows you to pull together your clinical experience on the wards with the numerous "factoids" and classical disease presentations that you have memorized over the years. Whereas Step 1 stresses basic disease mechanisms and principles, Step 2 places more emphasis on clinical diagnosis and management, disease pathogenesis, and preventive medicine.

The Step 2 exam is now composed of two parts:

- The Step 2 Clinical Knowledge examination (Step 2 CK)
- The Step 2 Clinical Skills examination (Step 2 CS)

The USMLE Step 2 CK is the second of three examinations that you must pass in order to become a licensed physician in the United States. The computerized Step 2 CK is a one-day (nine-hour) multiple-choice exam.

Students are also required to take the Step 2 CS, which is a one-day live exam in which students examine 12 standardized patients. The goal of the Step 2 CS is to ensure that students from more than 1600 medical schools worldwide, with varying curricula and educational standards, can collect and interpret a history, perform a physical exam, and communicate with patients at a comparable level. For more information on this examination, please refer to *First Aid for the USMLE Step 2 CS*. Information about the Step 2 CS format and about eligibility, registration, and scoring can be found at www.nbme.org.

The information found in this section as well as in the remainder of the book will address only the Step 2 CK.

USMLE STEP 2 CK—COMPUTER-BASED TESTING BASICS

How Will the CBT Be Structured?

The goal of the Step 2 CK is to apply your knowledge of medical facts to clinical scenarios you may encounter as a resident.

The Step 2 CK is a computer-based test (CBT) administered by Prometric, Inc. It is a one-day exam with 368 questions divided into eight 60-minute blocks of 46 questions each. A new form of testing software called **FRED** is now being used by the USMLE. FRED is different from the Step 1 exam you took in that you can now **highlight** and **strike out** test choices as well as make **brief notes** to yourself. During the time allotted for each block, the examinee can answer test questions in any order as well as review responses and change answers just as in the Step 1 exam—but examinees cannot go back and change answers from previous blocks. Once an examinee finishes a block, he or she must click on a screen icon to continue to the next block. Time not used during a testing block will be added to your overall break time, but it cannot be used to complete other testing blocks. Expect to spend up to nine hours at the test center.

Testing Conditions: What Will the CBT Be Like?

Even if you're familiar with CBT and the Prometric test centers, FRED is a new testing format that you should access from the USMLE CD-ROM or Web site (www.usmle.org) and try out prior to the exam.

If you familiarize yourself with the FRED testing interface ahead of time, you can skip the 15-minute tutorial offered on exam day and add those minutes to your allotted break time of 45 minutes.

For security reasons, examinees are not allowed to bring personal electronic equipment into the testing area—which means that digital watches, watches with computer communication and/or memory capability, cellular telephones, and electronic paging devices are all prohibited. Food and beverages are prohibited as well. Examinees are given laminated writing surfaces for note taking, but these must be returned after the examination. The testing centers are monitored by audio and video surveillance equipment.

You should become familiar with a typical question screen (see Figure 1-1). A window to the left displays all the questions in the block and shows you the unanswered questions (marked with an "i"). Some questions will contain figures or color illustrations adjacent to the question. Although the contrast and brightness of the screen can be adjusted, there are no other ways to manipulate the picture (e.g., zooming, panning). Larger images are accessed with an "**exhibit**" button. The examinee can also call up a window displaying normal **lab values**. You may **mark** questions to review at a later time by clicking the check mark at the top of the screen. The **annotation** feature functions like the provided erasable dry boards and allows you to jot down notes during

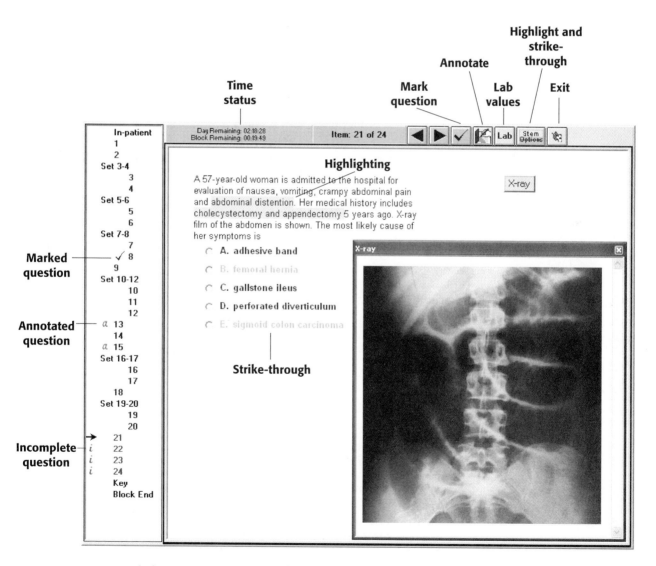

FIGURE 1-1. Typical FRED Question Screen

Keyboard shortcuts:
A–E–Letter choices.
Enter or Spacebar–Move to
next question.
Esc–Exit pop-up Lab and
Exhibit windows.
Alt-T–Countdown timers
for current session and
overall test.

the exam. Play with the **highlighting/strike-out** and annotation feature with the vignettes and multiple answers.

You should also do a few practice blocks to get a feel for which tools actually help you process questions more efficiently and accurately. If you find that you are not using the marking, annotation, or highlighting tools, then **keyboard shortcuts** can save you time over using a mouse.

What Does the CBT Format Mean for Me?

The CBT format is the same format as that of the USMLE Step 1. If you are uncomfortable with this testing format, spend some time playing with a Windows-based system and pointing and clicking icons or buttons with a mouse.

The USMLE also offers an opportunity to take a simulated test, or practice session, at a Prometric center. The session is divided into three one-hour blocks of 50 test items each. The USMLE Step 2 CK sample test items (150 questions) that are available on the CD-ROM or on the USMLE Web site (www.usmle.org) are the same as those used at CBT practice sessions. **No new items will be presented.** The cost is about $42 for U.S. and Canadian students but is higher for international students. The student receives a printed percent-correct score after completing the session. No explanations of questions are provided. You may register for a practice session online at www.usmle.org.

How Do I Register to Take the Exam?

Information on Step 2 CK format, content, and registration requirements can be found on the USMLE Web site. To register for the exam in the United States and Canada, apply online at the National Board of Medical Examiners (NBME) Web site (www.nbme.org). A printable version of the application is also available on this site.

The preliminary registration process for the USMLE Step 2 CK is as follows:

- Complete a registration form and send examination fees to the NBME (online).
- Select a three-month block in which you wish to be tested (e.g., June/July/August).
- Attach a passport-type photo to your completed application form.
- Complete a Certification of Identification and Authorization Form. This must be signed by an official at your medical school (e.g., the registrar's office) to verify your identity. This is a new form and is valid for five years, allowing you to use only your USMLE identification number for future transactions.
- Send your certified application form to the NMBE for processing. (Applications may be submitted more than six months before the test date, but examinees will not receive their scheduling permits until six months prior to the eligibility period.)
- The NBME will process your application within four to six weeks and will send you a fluorescent orange slip of paper that will serve as your scheduling permit.
- Once you have received your orange scheduling permit, decide when and where you would like to take the exam. For a list of Prometric locations nearest you, visit www.prometric.com.

- Call Prometric's toll-free number or visit www.prometric.com to arrange a time to take the exam.
- The Step 2 CK is offered on a year-round basis except for the first two weeks in January. For the most up-to-date information on available testing days at your preferred testing location, refer to www.usmle.org.

Your orange scheduling permit will contain the following important information:

- Your USMLE identification number
- The eligibility period in which you may take the exam
- Your "scheduling number," which you will need to make your exam appointment with Prometric
- Your candidate identification number, or CIN, which you must enter at your Prometric workstation in order to access the exam

Prometric has no access to the codes and will not be able to supply these numbers. **Do not lose your permit!** You will not be allowed to take the Step 2 CK unless you present your permit along with an unexpired, government-issued photo identification that contains your signature (e.g., driver's license, passport). Make sure the name on your photo ID exactly matches the name that appears on your scheduling permit.

Because the exam is scheduled on a "first-come, first-served" basis, you should be sure to call Prometric as soon as you receive your scheduling permit!

What If I Need to Reschedule the Exam?

You can change your date and/or center within your three-month period without charge by contacting Prometric. If space is available, you may reschedule up to five days before your test date. If you need to reschedule outside your initial three-month period, you can apply for a single three-month extension (e.g., April/May/June can be extended through July/August/September) after your eligibility period has begun (visit www.nbme.org for more information). This extension currently costs $50. For other rescheduling needs, you must submit a new application along with another application fee.

What About Time?

Time is of special interest on the CBT exam. Here is a breakdown of the exam schedule:

Tutorial	15 minutes
60-minute question blocks (46 questions per block)	8 hours
Break time (includes time for lunch)	45 minutes
Total test time	9 hours

The computer will keep track of how much time has elapsed during the exam. However, the computer will show you only how much time you have remaining in a given block. Therefore, it is up to you to determine if you are pacing yourself properly.

The computer will not warn you if you are spending more than the 45 minutes allotted for break time. However, you can elect not to use all of your break time, or you can gain extra break time either by skipping the tutorial or by finishing a block ahead of the allotted time.

If I Leave During the Exam, What Happens to My Score?

You are considered to have started the exam once you have entered your CIN onto the computer screen. In order to receive an official score, you must finish the entire exam. This means that you must start and either finish or run out of time for each block of the exam. If you do not complete all the blocks, your exam will be documented on your USMLE score transcript as an incomplete attempt, but no actual score will be reported.

The exam ends when all blocks have been completed or time has expired. As you leave the testing center, you will receive a written test-completion notice to document your completion of the exam.

What Types of Questions Are Asked?

- Almost all questions on the Step 2 CK are case based. A substantial amount of extraneous information may be given, or a clinical scenario may be followed by a question that could be answered without actually requiring that you read the case. It is your job to determine which information is superfluous and which is pertinent to the case at hand.
- Subject areas vary randomly from question to question.
- Most questions have a **single best answer**, but some **matching sets** call for multiple responses (the number to select will be specified). The part of the vignette that actually asks the question—the stem—is usually found at the end of the scenario. From student experience, there are a few stems that are consistently addressed throughout the exam:
  - What is the most likely diagnosis? (40%)
  - Which of the following is the most appropriate initial step in management? (20%)
  - Which of the following is the most appropriate next step in management? (20%)
  - Which of the following is the most likely cause of . . . ? (5%)
  - Which of the following is the most likely pathogen . . . ? (3%)
  - Which of the following would most likely prevent . . . ? (2%)
  - Other (10%)
- Note the age and race of the patient in each clinical scenario. When ethnicity is given, it is often relevant. Know these well (see high-yield facts), especially for more common diagnoses.
- Be able to recognize key facts that distinguish major diagnoses.
- Questions often describe clinical findings instead of naming eponyms (e.g., they cite "audible hip click" instead of "positive Ortolani's sign").
- Questions about acute patient management (e.g., trauma) in an emergency setting are common.

The cruel reality of the Step 2 CK is that no matter how much you study, there will still be questions you will not be able to answer with confidence. If you recognize that a question is not solvable in a reasonable period of time, make an educated guess and move on; you will not be penalized for guessing. Also keep in mind that 10–20% of the USMLE exam questions are "experimental" and will not count toward your score.

How Long Will I Have to Wait Before I Get My Scores?

The USMLE reports scores three to four weeks after the examinee's test date. During peak times, however, reports may take up to six weeks to be scored.

Official information concerning the time required for score reporting is posted on the USMLE Web site, www.usmle.org.

How Are the Scores Reported?

Like the Step 1 score report, your Step 2 CK report includes your pass/fail status, two numeric scores, and a performance profile organized by discipline and disease process (see Figures 1-2A and 1-2B). The first score is a three-digit scaled score based on a predefined proficiency standard. In 2002, the required passing score was increased from 170 to 174. The second score scale, the two-digit score, defines 75 as the minimum passing score (equivalent to a score of 174 on the first scale). This score is not a percentile. A score of 82 is equivalent to a score of 200 on the first scale. Any adjustments in the required passing score will be available on the USMLE Web site.

US·MLE
United States
Medical
Licensing
Examination

UNITED STATES MEDICAL LICENSING EXAMINATION™

USMLE Step 2 is administered to students and graduates of U.S. and Canadian medical schools by the
NATIONAL BOARD OF MEDICAL EXAMINERS® (NBME®)
3750 Market Street, Philadelphia, Pennsylvania 19104-3190.
Telephone: (215) 590-9700

STEP 2 SCORE REPORT

Schmoe, Joe T   USMLE ID: 1-234-567-8
Anytown, CA 12345   Test Date: August 1998

The USMLE is a single examination program for all applicants for medical licensure in the United States; it has replaced the Federation Licensing Examination (FLEX) and the certifying examinations of the National Board of Medical Examiners (NBME Parts I, II and III). The program consists of three Steps designed to assess an examinee's understanding of and ability to apply concepts and principles that are important in health and disease and that constitute the basis of safe and effective patient care. **Step 2** is designed to assess whether an examinee possesses the medical knowledge and understanding of clinical science considered essential for the provision of patient care under supervision, including emphasis on health promotion and disease prevention. The inclusion of Step 2 in the USMLE sequence ensures that attention is devoted to principles of clinical science that undergird the safe and competent practice of medicine. Results of the examination are reported to medical licensing authorities in the United States and its territories for use in granting an initial license to practice medicine. The two numeric scores shown below are equivalent; each state or territory may use either score in making licensing decisions. These scores represent your results for the administration of Step 2 on the test date shown above.

PASS	This result is based on the minimum passing score set by USMLE for Step 2. Individual licensing authorities may accept the USMLE-recommended pass/fail result or may establish a different passing score for their own jurisdictions.

200	This score is determined by your overall performance on Step 2. For recent administrations, the mean and standard deviation for first-time examinees from U.S. and Canadian medical schools are approximately 208 and 23, respectively, with most scores falling between 140 and 260. A score of 170 is set by USMLE to pass Step 2. The standard error of measurement (SEM)‡ for this scale is approximately six points.

82	This score is also determined by your overall performance on the examination. A score of 82 on this scale is equivalent to a score of 200 on the scale described above. A score of 75 on this scale, which is equivalent to a score of 170 on the scale described above, is set by USMLE to pass Step 2. The SEM‡ for this scale is one point.

‡Your score is influenced both by your general understanding of clinical science and the specific set of items selected for this Step 2 examination. The standard error of measurement (SEM) provides an estimate of the range within which your scores might be expected to vary by chance if you were tested repeatedly using similar tests.

267PU007

NOTE: Original score report has copy-resistant watermark.

FIGURE 1-2A.   Sample Score Report—Front Page

INFORMATION PROVIDED FOR EXAMINEE USE ONLY

The Performance Profile below is provided solely for the benefit of the examinee.
These profiles are developed as assessment tools for examinees only and will not be reported or verified to any third party.

USMLE STEP 2 PERFORMANCE PROFILES

PHYSICIAN TASK PROFILE	Lower Performance	Borderline Performance	Higher Performance
Preventive Medicine & Health Maintenance			xxxxxxxxxxx*
Understanding Mechanisms of Disease			xxxx*
Diagnosis			xxxxx*
Principles of Management			xxxxxxxxx*

NORMAL CONDITIONS & DISEASE CATEGORY PROFILE

	Lower Performance	Borderline Performance	Higher Performance
Normal Growth & Development; Principles of Care			xxxxxxxxxxxxxxx*
Immunologic Disorders			xxxxxxxxxxxx*
Diseases of Blood & Blood Forming Organs			xxxxxxxxxx*
Mental Disorders			xxxxxxxxxxx*
Diseases of the Nervous System & Special Senses			xxxxxxxxxx*
Cardiovascular Disorders		xxxxxxxxxxxxxxx	
Diseases of the Respiratory System			xxxxxxxxxxxx*
Nutritional & Digestive Disorders			xxxxxxxxxx*
Gynecologic Disorders			xxxxxxxxxxxx*
Renal, Urinary & Male Reproductive Systems			xxxxxxxxxx*
Disorders of Pregnancy, Childbirth & Puerperium			xxxxxxxxxxxxxxxxxx
Musculoskeletal, Skin & Connective Tissue Diseases			xxxxxxxxx*
Endocrine & Metabolic Disorders			xxxxxxxxxxx*

DISCIPLINE PROFILE

	Lower Performance	Borderline Performance	Higher Performance
Medicine			xxx*
Obstetrics & Gynecology			xxxxxxxxxx*
Pediatrics			xxxxxxxx*
Psychiatry			xxxxxxxxxxxx*
Surgery			xx*

The above Performance Profile is provided to aid in self-assessment. The shaded area defines a borderline level of performance for each content area; borderline performance is comparable to a HIGH FAIL / LOW PASS on the total test.

Performance bands indicate areas of relative strength and weakness. Some performance bands are wider than others. The width of a performance band reflects the precision of measurement: narrower bands indicate greater precision. An asterisk indicates that your performance band extends beyond the displayed portion of the scale. Small differences in the location of bands should not be over interpreted. If two bands overlap, the performance in the associated areas should not be interpreted as significantly different.

This profile should not be compared to those from other Step 2 administrations.

Additional information concerning the topics covered in each content area can be found in the *USMLE Step 2 General Instructions, Content Description, and Sample Items.*

007PU267

FIGURE 1-2B. Sample Score Report—Back Page

DEFINING YOUR GOAL

The first and most important thing to do in your Step 2 CK preparation is define how well you want to do on the exam, as this will ultimately determine the extent of preparation that will be necessary. The amount of time spent in preparation for this exam varies widely among medical students. Possible goals include the following:

- **"Simply passing."** This goal may be sufficient for the majority of U.S. medical students, especially if you are entering a less competitive specialty.
- **Beating the mean.** This signifies an ability to integrate your clinical and factual knowledge to an extent that is superior to that of your peers (213 for recent exam administrations). Others redefine this goal as achieving a score one SD above the mean (237). Highly competitive residency programs may use your Step 1 and Step 2 (if available) scores as a screening

tool or as selection criteria (see Figure 1-3). International medical graduates (IMGs) should aim to beat the mean, as USMLE scores are likely to be a selection factor even for less competitive U.S. residency programs.

- **Acing the exam.** Perhaps you are one of those individuals for whom nothing less than the best will do—and for whom excelling on standardized exams is a source of pride and satisfaction. A high score on the Step 2 CK might also represent a way to strengthen your application and "make up" for a less-than-satisfactory score on Step 1, especially if you are taking the exam in the fall before applying for residency.
- **Evaluating your clinical knowledge.** In many ways, this goal should serve as the ultimate rationale for taking the exam, since it is technically the reason the exam was initially designed. The case-based nature of the Step 2 CK differs significantly from the more fact-based Step 1 exam in that it more thoroughly examines your ability to recognize classic clinical presentations, deal with acute emergent situations, and follow the step-by-step thought processes involved in the treatment of particular diseases.
- **Preparing for internship.** Studying for the USMLE Step 2 CK is an excellent way to review and consolidate all of the information you have learned in preparation for internship, especially if the exam is taken in the spring.

When to Take the Exam

With the CBT, you now have a wide variety of options regarding when to take the Step 2 CK. Here are a few factors to consider:

- **The nature of your objectives,** as defined above.

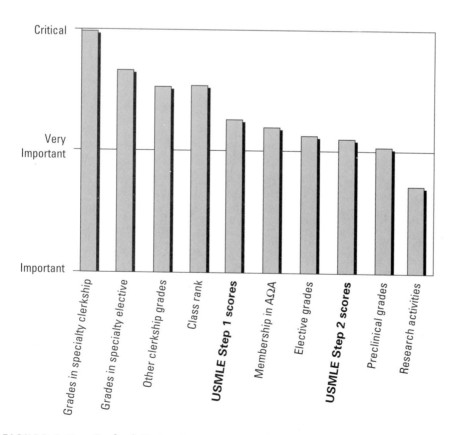

FIGURE 1-3. Academic Factors Important to Residency Directors

The Step 2 CK is an opportunity to consolidate your clinical knowledge and prepare for internship.

- **The specialty to which you are applying.** Some competitive residency programs may request your Step 2 CK scores, so you should consider taking the exam in the fall. If you already have a strong application and do not need Step 2 CK scores for residency applications, taking the exam in the fall could potentially hurt your application if you do poorly.
- **Prerequisite to graduation.** If passing the USMLE Step 2 CK is a prerequisite to graduation at your medical school, you will need to take the exam in the fall or winter.
- **Proximity to clerkships.** Many students feel that the core clerkship material is fresher in their minds early in the fourth year, making a good argument for taking the Step 2 CK earlier in the fall.
- **The nature of your schedule.**

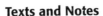

STUDY RESOURCES

Quality Considerations

Although an ever-increasing number of USMLE Step 2 review books and software packages are available on the market, the quality of this material is highly variable (see Section 3). Some common problems include the following:

- Some review books are too detailed to be reviewed in a reasonable amount of time or cover subtopics that are not emphasized on the exam (e.g., a 400-page anesthesiology book).
- Many sample question books have not been updated to reflect current trends on the Step 2 CK.
- Many sample question books use poorly written questions, contain factual errors in their explanations, give overly detailed explanations, or offer no explanations at all.
- Software for boards review is of highly variable quality, may be difficult to install, and may be fraught with bugs.

Clinical Review Books

The best review book for you reflects the way you like to learn. If a given review book is not working for you, stop using it no matter how highly rated it may be.

Many review books are available, so you must decide which ones to buy by evaluating their relative merits. Toward this goal, you should weigh different opinions from other medical students against each other; read the reviews and ratings in Section 3 of this guide; and examine the various books closely in the bookstore. Do not worry about finding the "perfect" book, as many subjects simply do not have one.

There are two types of review books: those that are stand-alone titles and those that are part of a series. Books in a series generally have the same style, and you must decide if that style is helpful for you and optimal for a given subject.

Texts and Notes

Most textbooks are too detailed for high-yield boards review and should be avoided. When using texts or notes, engage in active learning by making tables, diagrams, new mnemonics, and conceptual associations whenever possible. If you already have your own mnemonics, do not bother trying to memorize someone else's. Textbooks are useful, however, to supplement incomplete or unclear material.

Commercial Courses

Commercial preparation courses can be helpful for some students, as they offer an effective way to organize study material. However, multiweek courses are costly and require significant time commitment, leaving limited time for independent study. Also note that some commercial courses are designed for first-time test takers, students who are repeating the examination, or IMGs.

Practice Tests

Taking practice tests can serve multiple functions for examinees, including the following:

- Provide information about strengths and weaknesses in your fund of knowledge
- Add variety to your study schedule
- Serve as the main form of study
- Improve test-taking skills
- Familiarize examinees with the style of the USMLE Step 2 CK exam

Students report that many practice tests have questions that are, on average, shorter and less clinically oriented than those on the current Step 2 CK. Step 2 CK questions demand fast reading skills and application of clinical facts in a problem-solving format. Approach sample examinations critically, and do not waste time with low-quality questions until you have exhausted better sources.

After you have taken a practice test, try to identify concepts and areas of weakness, not just the facts that you missed. Use this experience to motivate your study and to prioritize the areas in which you need the most work. Analyze the pattern of your responses to questions to determine if you have made systematic errors in answering questions. Common mistakes include reading too much into the question, second-guessing your initial impression, and misinterpreting the question.

NBME/USMLE Publications

We strongly encourage students to use the free materials provided by the testing agencies and to study the following NBME publications:

- **USMLE *Bulletin of Information*.** This publication provides you with nuts-and-bolts details about the exam (included on the Web site www.usmle.org; free to all examinees).
- **USMLE *Step 2 Computer-Based Content and Sample Test Questions*.** This is a hard copy of test questions and test content also found on the CD-ROM.
- **NBME Test Delivery Software (FRED) and Tutorial.** This includes 168 valuable practice questions. The questions are available on the USMLE CD-ROM and on the USMLE Web site. Make sure you are using the new FRED version and not the older Prometric version.
- **USMLE Web site (www.usmle.org).** In addition to allowing you to become familiar with the CBT format, the sample items on the USMLE Web site provide the only questions that are available directly from the test makers. Student feedback varies as to the similarity of these questions to those on the actual exam, but they are nonetheless worthwhile to know.

Use practice tests to identify concepts and areas of weakness, not just facts that you missed.

TEST-DAY CHECKLIST

Things to Bring with You to the Exam

- Be sure to bring your orange scheduling permit and a photo ID with signature. (You will not be admitted to the exam if you fail to bring your permit, and Prometric will charge a rescheduling fee.)
- A watch can help you pace yourself (but do not bring a digital watch).
- Remember to bring lunch, snacks (for a little "sugar rush" on breaks), and fluids.
- Bring clothes to layer to accommodate temperature variations at the testing center.
- Earplugs will be provided at the Prometric center.

TESTING AGENCIES

National Board of Medical Examiners (NBME)
Department of Licensing Examination Services
3750 Market Street
Philadelphia, PA 19104-3102
(215) 590-9500
www.nbme.org

USMLE Secretariat
3750 Market Street
Philadelphia, PA 19104-3190
(215) 590-9700
www.usmle.org

Educational Commission for Foreign Medical Graduates (ECFMG)
3624 Market Street
Philadelphia, PA 19104-2685
(215) 386-5900
Fax: (215) 386-9196
www.ecfmg.org

Federation of State Medical Boards (FSMB)
P.O. Box 619850
Dallas, TX 75261-9850
(817) 868-4000
Fax: (817) 868-4099
www.fsmb.org

Special Situations

▶ First Aid for the International Medical Graduate

▶ First Aid for the Student with a Disability

"International medical graduate" (IMG) is the term now used to describe any student or graduate of a non-U.S., non-Canadian, non–Puerto Rican medical school, regardless of whether he or she is a U.S. citizen. The old term "foreign medical graduate" (FMG) was replaced because it was misleading when applied to U.S. citizens attending medical schools outside the United States.

The IMG's Steps to Licensure in the United States

If you are an IMG, you must go through the following steps (not necessarily in this order) to become licensed to practice in the United States. You must complete these steps even if you are already a practicing physician and have completed a residency program in your own country.

- Complete the basic sciences program of your medical school (equivalent to the first two years of U.S. medical school).
- Take the USMLE Step 1. You can do this while still in school or after graduating, but in either case your medical school must certify that you completed the basic sciences part of your school's curriculum before taking the USMLE Step 1.
- Complete the clinical clerkship program of your medical school (equivalent to the third and fourth years of U.S. medical school).
- Take the USMLE Step 2 Clinical Knowledge (CK) exam. If you are still in medical school, you must have completed two years of school.
- Take the Step 2 Clinical Skills (CS) exam.
- Graduate with your medical degree.
- Then, send the ECFMG a copy of your degree and transcript, which they will verify with your medical school.
- Obtain an ECFMG certificate. To do this, candidates must accomplish the following:
  - Graduate from a medical school that is listed in the International Medical Education Directory (IMED). The list can be accessed at www.ecfmg.org.
  - Pass Step 1, the Step 2 CK, and the Step 2 CS within a seven-year period.
  - Have their medical credentials verified by the ECFMG.
- The standard certificate is usually sent two weeks after all the above requirements have been fulfilled. You must have a valid certificate before entering an accredited residency program, although you may begin the application process before you receive your certification.
- Apply for residency positions in your field of interest, either directly or through the Electronic Residency Application Service (ERAS) and the National Residency Matching Program ("the Match"). To be entered into the Match, you need to have passed all the examinations necessary for ECFMG certification (i.e., Step 1, the Step 2 CK, and the Step 2 CS) by a certain deadline (January 31, 2006, for the 2006 Match). If you do not pass these exams by the deadline, you will be withdrawn from the Match.
- Obtain a visa that will allow you to enter and work in the United States if you are not already a U.S. citizen or a green-card holder (permanent resident).
- If required for IMGs by the state in which your residency is located, obtain an educational/training/limited medical license. Your residency program may assist you with this application. Note that medical licensing is

More detailed information can be found in the 2005 edition of the ECFMG Information Booklet, available at www.ecfmg.org/pubshome.html.

Applicants may apply online for the USMLE Step 2 CK or Step 2 CS, or request an extension of the USMLE eligibility period, at http://iwa.ecfmg.org.

the prerogative of each individual state, not of the federal government, and that states vary with respect to their laws about licensing (although all 50 states recognize the USMLE).

- In order to begin your residency program, make sure your scores are valid.
- Once you have the ECFMG certification, take the USMLE Step 3 during your residency, and then obtain a full medical license. Once you have a license in any state, you are permitted to practice in federal institutions such as VA hospitals and Indian Health Service facilities in any state. This can open the door to "moonlighting" opportunities and possibilities for an H1B visa application. For details on individual state rules, write to the licensing board in the state in question or contact the FSMB.
- Complete your residency and then take the appropriate specialty board exams in order to become board certified (e.g., in internal medicine or surgery). If you already have a specialty certification in your home country (e.g., in surgery or cardiology), some specialty boards may grant you six months' or one year's credit toward your total residency time.
- Currently, many residency programs are accepting applications through ERAS. For more information, see *First Aid for the Match* or contact:

ECFMG/ERAS Program
P.O. Box 11746
Philadelphia, PA 19101-1746
(215) 386-5900
Fax: (215) 222-5641
e-mail: eras-support@ecfmg.org
www.ecfmg.org/eras

The USMLE and the IMG

The USMLE is a series of standardized exams that give IMGs a level playing field. It is the same exam series taken by U.S. graduates even though it is administered by the ECFMG rather than by the NBME. This means that passing marks for IMGs for Step 1, the Step 2 CK, and the Step 2 CS are determined by a statistical process that is based on the scores of U.S. medical students. For example, to pass Step 1, you will probably have to score higher than the bottom 8–10% of U.S. and Canadian graduates.

Timing of the USMLE

For an IMG, the timing of a complete application is critical. It is extremely important that you send in your application early if you are to garner the maximum number of interview calls. A rough guide would be to complete all exam requirements by August of the year in which you wish to apply. This would translate into sending both your score sheets and your ECFMG certificate with your application.

In terms of USMLE exam order, arguments can be made for taking the Step 1 or the Step 2 CK exam first. For example, you may consider taking the Step 2 CK exam first if you have just graduated from medical school and the clinical topics are still fresh in your mind. However, keep in mind that there is a large overlap between Step 1 and Step 2 CK topics in areas such as pharmacology, pathophysiology, and biostatistics. You might therefore consider taking the Step 1 and Step 2 CK exams close together to take advantage of this overlap in your test preparation.

USMLE Step 1 and the IMG

What Is the USMLE Step 1? It is a computerized test of the basic medical sciences that consists of 350 multiple-choice questions and is divided into seven blocks.

Significance of the Test. Step 1 is required for the ECFMG certificate as well as for registration for the Step 2 CS. Since most U.S. graduates apply to residency with their Step 1 scores only, it may be the only objective tool available with which to compare IMGs with U.S. graduates.

Official Web Sites. www.usmle.org and www.ecfmg.org/usmle.

Eligibility. Both students and graduates from medical schools that are listed in IMED are eligible to take the test. Students must have completed at least two years of medical school by the beginning of the eligibility period selected.

Eligibility Period. A three-month period of your choice.

Fee. The fee for Step 1 is $685 plus an international test delivery surcharge (if you choose a testing region other than the United States or Canada).

Retaking the Exam. In the event that you failed the test, you can reapply and select an eligibility period that begins at least 60 days after the last attempt. You cannot take the same Step more than three times in any 12-month period. You cannot retake the exam if you passed. The minimum score to pass the exam is 75 on a two-digit scale. To pass, you must answer roughly 60–65% of the questions correctly.

Statistics. In 2001, only 66% of ECFMG candidates passed Step 1 on their first attempt, compared with 91% of U.S. and Canadian medical students and graduates. Of note, 1994–1995 data showed that USFMGs (U.S. citizens attending non-U.S. medical schools) performed 0.4 SD lower than IMGs (non-U.S. citizens attending non-U.S. medical schools). Although their overall scores were lower, USFMGs performed better than IMGs on behavioral sciences. In general, students from non-U.S. medical schools perform worst in behavioral science and biochemistry (1.9 and 1.5 SDs below U.S. students) and comparatively better in gross anatomy and pathology (0.7 and 0.9 SD below U.S. students). Although derived from data collected in 1994–1995, these data may help you focus your studying efforts.

Tips. Although few if any students feel totally prepared to take Step 1, IMGs in particular require serious study and preparation to reach their full potential on this exam. It is also imperative that IMGs do their best on Step 1, as a poor score on Step 1 is a distinct disadvantage in applying for most residencies. Remember that if you pass Step 1, you cannot retake it to try to improve your score. Your goal should thus be to beat the mean, because you can then confidently assert that you have done better than average for U.S. students. Good Step 1 scores will also lend credibility to your residency application and help you get into highly competitive specialties such as radiology, orthopedics, and dermatology.

Commercial Review Courses. Do commercial review courses help improve your scores? Reports vary, and such courses can be expensive. Many IMGs decide to try the USMLE on their own and then consider a review course only if they fail. Just keep in mind that many states require that you pass the USMLE within three attempts. (For more information on review courses, see Section 3.)

USMLE Step 2 CK and the IMG

What Is the Step 2 CK? It is a computerized test of the clinical sciences consisting of 370 multiple-choice questions and divided into eight blocks. It can be taken at Prometric centers in the United States and several other countries.

Significance of the Test. The Step 2 CK is required for the ECFMG certificate. It reflects the level of clinical knowledge of the applicant. It tests clinical subjects, primarily internal medicine. Other areas that are tested are surgery, obstetrics and gynecology, pediatrics, orthopedics, psychiatry, ENT, ophthalmology, and medical ethics.

Official Web Sites. www.usmle.org and www.ecfmg.org/usmle.

Eligibility. Students and graduates from medical schools that are listed in IMED are eligible to take the Step 2 CK. Students must have completed at least two years of medical school. This means that students must have completed the basic medical science component of the medical school curriculum by the beginning of the eligibility period selected.

Eligibility Period. A three-month period of your choice.

Fee. The fee for the Step 2 CK is $685 plus an international test delivery surcharge (if you choose a testing region other than the United States or Canada).

Retaking the Exam. In the event that you fail the Step 2 CK, you can reapply and select an eligibility period that begins at least 60 days after the last attempt. You cannot take the same Step more than three times in any 12-month period. You cannot retake the exam if you passed.

Statistics. In 2000–2001, 75% of ECFMG candidates passed the Step 2 CK on their first attempt, compared with 95% of U.S. and Canadian candidates.

Tips. It's better to take the Step 2 CK after you have completed your internal medicine rotation because most of the questions give clinical scenarios and ask you to make medical diagnoses and clinical decisions. In addition, because this is a clinical sciences exam, cultural and geographic considerations play a greater role than is the case with Step 1. For example, if your medical education gave you ample exposure to malaria, brucellosis, and malnutrition but little to alcohol withdrawal, child abuse, and cholesterol screening, you must work to familiarize yourself with topics that are more heavily emphasized in U.S. medicine. You must also have a basic understanding of the legal and social aspects of U.S. medicine, because you will be asked questions about communicating with and advising patients.

USMLE Step 2 CS and the IMG

What Is the Step 2 CS? The Step 2 CS is a test of clinical and communication skills administered as a one-day, eight-hour exam. It includes 10 to 12 encounters with standardized patients (15 minutes each, with 10 minutes to write a note after each encounter). Test results are valid indefinitely.

Topics Covered by This Exam. The Step 2 CS tests the ability to communicate in English as well as interpersonal skills, data-gathering skills, the ability to perform a physical exam, and the ability to formulate a brief note, a differential diagnosis, and a list of diagnostic tests. The areas that are covered in the exam are as follows:

- Internal medicine
- Surgery
- Obstetrics and gynecology
- Pediatrics
- Psychiatry
- Family medicine

Significance of the Test. The Step 2 CS is required for the ECFMG certificate. It has eliminated the Test of English as a Foreign Language (TOEFL) as a requirement for ECFMG certification.

Official Web Site. www.ecfmg.org/usmle/step2cs.

Eligibility. Students must have completed at least two years of medical school in order to take the test. That means students must have completed the basic medical science component of the medical school curriculum at the time they apply for the exam.

Fee. The fee for the Step 2 CS is $1200.

Scheduling. You must schedule the Step 2 CS within **four months** of the date indicated on your notification of registration. You must take the exam within 12 months of the date indicated on your notification of registration.

Retaking the Exam. There is no limit to the number of attempts you can make to pass the Step 2 CS. However, you cannot retake the exam within 60 days of a failed attempt, and you cannot take it more than three times in a 12-month period.

Test Site Locations. The Step 2 CS is currently administered at the following five locations:

- Philadelphia, PA
- Atlanta, GA
- Los Angeles, CA
- Chicago, IL
- Houston, TX

For more information about the Step 2 CS exam, please refer to *First Aid for the Step 2 CS.*

USMLE Step 3 and the IMG

What Is the USMLE Step 3? It is a two-day computerized test in clinical medicine consisting of 480 multiple-choice questions and nine computer-based case simulations (CCS). The exam aims at testing your knowledge and its application to patient care and clinical decision making (i.e., this exam tests if you can safely practice medicine independently and without supervision).

Significance of the Test. Taking Step 3 before residency is critical if an IMG is seeking an H1B visa and is a bonus that can be added to the application for residency. Step 3 is also required to obtain a full medical license in the United States and can be taken during residency for this purpose.

Official Web Site. www.usmle.org.

Fee. The fee for Step 3 is $590 (the total application fee can vary among states).

Eligibility. Most states require that applicants have completed one, two, or three years of postgraduate training (residency) prior to applying for Step 3 and permanent state licensure. The exceptions are the 13 states mentioned below, which allow IMGs to take Step 3 at the beginning of or even before residency. So if you don't fulfill the prerequisites to taking Step 3 in your state of choice, simply use the name of one of the 11 states in your Step 3 application. You can take the exam in any state you choose regardless of the state that you mentioned on your application. Once you pass Step 3, it will be recognized by all states. Basic eligibility requirements for the USMLE Step 3 are as follows:

- Obtaining an MD or DO degree (or its equivalent) by the application deadline.
- Obtaining an ECFMG certificate if you are a graduate of a foreign medical school or are successfully completing a "fifth pathway" program (at a date no later than the application deadline).
- Meeting the requirements imposed by the individual state licensing authority to which you are applying to take Step 3. Please refer to www.fsmb.org for more information.

The following states do not have postgraduate training as an eligibility requirement to apply for Step 3:

- Arkansas
- California
- Connecticut
- Florida
- Louisiana
- Maryland
- Nebraska*
- New York
- South Dakota
- Texas
- Utah*
- Washington
- West Virginia

* Requires that IMGs obtain a "valid indefinite" ECFMG certificate.

The Step 3 exam is not available outside the United States. Applications can be found online at www.fsmb.org and must be submitted to the FSMB.

Residencies and the IMG

It is becoming increasingly difficult for IMGs to obtain residencies in the United States given the rising concern about an oversupply of physicians in the United States. Official bodies such as the Council on Graduate Medical Education (COGME) have recommended that the total number of residency slots be reduced from the current 144% of the number of U.S. graduates to 110%. Furthermore, changes in immigration law are likely to make it much harder for noncitizens or legal residents of the United States to remain in the country after completing a residency.

In the residency Match, the number of U.S.-citizen IMG applications has been stable for the last few years, while the percentage accepted has slowly increased. For non-U.S.-citizen IMGs, applications fell from 7977 in 1999 to 4556 in 2002, while the percentage accepted significantly increased (see Table 1-1). This decrease in the total number of IMGs applying for the Match may be attributed to several factors:

- A decrease in the Step 2 CS passing rate to 80%
- Increased difficulty obtaining U.S. visas
- Increased expenses associated with the USMLE exams, ERAS, and travel to the United States
- An increase in the number of IMGs who are withdrawing from the Match to sign a separate "pre-Match" contract with programs

Visa Options for the IMG

If you are living outside the United States, you will need to apply for a visa that will allow you lawful entry into the United States in order to take the Step 2 CS and/or do your interviews for residency. A B1 or B2 visitor visa may be issued by the U.S. consulate in your country. Citizens of some countries may have to undergo an additional security check that could take up to six months. Upon your entry into the United States, either the B1 or, more commonly, the B2 will be issued on your I-94. Both visas allow you a limited period to stay in the United States (two to six months) in order to take the exam. If the given period is not sufficient, you may apply for an extension before the expiration of your I-94.

Documents that are recommended to facilitate this process include:

- The Step 2 CS admission permit and a letter from the ECFMG (which explains why the applicant must enter the United States)
- Your medical diploma
- Transcripts from your medical school
- Your USMLE score sheets

TABLE 1-1. IMGs in the Match

APPLICANTS	2000	2001	2002
U.S.-citizen IMGs	2169	1999	2029
% U.S. citizens accepted	51	52	54
Non-U.S.-citizen IMGs	7287	5116	4556
% non-U.S. citizens accepted	38	45	51
U.S. graduates (non-IMGs)	14,358	14,455	14,336
% U.S. graduates accepted	94	94	94

- A sponsor letter or affidavit of support stating that you (if you are sponsoring yourself) or your sponsor will bear the expense of your trip and that you have sufficient funds to meet that expense
- An alien status affidavit

Individuals from certain countries may be allowed to enter the United States for up to 90 days without a visa under the Visa Waiver Program. See www.immigration.gov.

As an IMG, you need a visa to work or train in the United States unless you are a U.S. citizen or a permanent resident (i.e., hold a green card). Two types of visas enable you to accept a residency appointment in the United States: Jl and H1B. Most sponsoring residency programs (SRPs) prefer a Jl visa. Above all, this is because SRPs are authorized by the Department of Homeland Security (DHS)—which in 2003 took the place of the U.S. Immigration and Naturalization Service—to issue a Form DS-2019 (which replaced Form IAP-66 as of September 1, 2002) directly to an IMG. By contrast, SRPs must complete considerable paperwork, including an application to the Immigration and Labor Department, to apply to the DHS for an H1B visa on behalf of an IMG.

The J1 Visa

Also known as the Exchange Visitor Program, the J1 visa was introduced to give IMGs in diverse specialties the chance to use their training experience in the United States to improve conditions in their home countries. As mentioned above, the DHS authorizes most SRPs to issue Form DS-2019 in the same manner that I-20s are issued to regular international students in the United States.

To enable an SRP to issue a DS-2019, you must obtain a certificate from the ECFMG indicating that you are eligible to participate in a residency program in the United States. First, however, you must ask the Ministry of Health in your country to issue a statement indicating that your country needs physicians with the skills you propose to acquire from a U.S. residency program. This statement, which must bear the seal of your country's government and must be signed by a duly designated government official, is intended to satisfy the U.S. Secretary of Health and Human Services (HHS) that there is such a need. The Health Ministry in your country should send this statement to the ECFMG (or they may allow you to mail it to the ECFMG).

How can you find out if the government of your country will issue such a statement? In many countries, the Ministry of Health maintains a list of medical specialties in which there is a need for further training abroad. You can also consult seniors in your medical school. A word of caution: If you are applying for a residency in internal medicine and internists are not in short supply in your country, it may help to indicate an intention to pursue a subspecialty after completing your residency training.

The text of your statement of need should read as follows:

> Name of applicant for visa: _____. There currently exists in _____ (your country) a need for qualified medical practitioners in the specialty of _____. (Name of applicant for visa) has filed a written assurance with the government of this country that he/she will return to _____ (your country) upon completion of training in the United States and intends to enter the practice of medicine in the specialty for which training is being sought.
>
> Stamp (or seal and signature) of issuing official of named country. Dated _____

To facilitate the issuing of such a statement by the Ministry of Health in your country, you should submit a certified copy of the agreement or a contract from your SRP in the United States. The agreement or contract must be signed by you and the residency program official responsible for the training.

Armed with Form DS-2019, you should then go to the U.S. consulate closest to the residential address indicated in your passport. As for other nonimmigrant visas, you must show that you have a genuine nonimmigrant intent to return to your home country. You must also show that all your expenses will be paid.

When you enter the United States, bring your Form DS-2019 along with your visa. You are usually admitted to the United States for the length of the Jl program, designated as "D/S," or duration of status. The duration of your program is indicated on the DS-2019.

In the wake of the terrorist attacks of September 11, 2001, a number of new regulations have been introduced to improve the monitoring of exchange visitors during their time in the United States. As of January 30, 2003, all SRPs and students are required to register with the Student and Exchange Visitor Program (SEVP) via the Student and Exchange Visitor Information System (SEVIS). SEVIS allows the DHS to maintain up-to-date information (e.g., enrollment status, current address) on exchange visitors. As of January 30, 2002, SEVIS Form DS-2019 will be used for visa applications, admission, and change of status. Non-SEVIS forms such as Form IAP-66 issued prior to January 30, 2003, have not been accepted since August 1, 2003. Procedural details for this new legislation are still being hammered out, so contact your SRP or check the DHS Web site (www.immigration.gov) for the most current information.

Duration of Participation. The duration of a resident's participation in a program of graduate medical education or training is limited to the time normally required to complete such a program. If you would like to get an idea of the typical training time for the various medical subspecialties, you may consult the *Directory of Medical Specialties*, published by Marquis Who's Who for the American Board of Medical Specialties. The authority charged with determining the duration of time required by an individual IMG is the State Department. The maximum amount of time for participation in a training program is ordinarily limited to seven years unless the IMG has demonstrated to the satisfaction of the ECFMG and the State Department that his or her home country has an exceptional need for the specialty in which he or she will receive further training. An extension of stay may be granted in the event that an IMG needs to repeat a year of clinical medical training or needs time for training or education to take an exam required for board certification.

Requirements After Entry into the United States. Each year, all IMGs participating in a residency program on a Jl visa must furnish the Attorney General of the United States with an affidavit (Form I-644) attesting that they are in good standing in the program of graduate medical education or training in which they are participating and that they will return to their home countries upon completion of the education or training for which they came to the United States.

Restrictions Under the Jl Visa. No later than two years after the date of entry into the United States, an IMG participating in a residency program on a Jl visa is allowed one opportunity to change his or her designated program of graduate medical education or training if his or her director approves that change.

The J1 visa includes a condition called the "two-year foreign residence requirement." The relevant section of the Immigration and Nationality Act states:

> Any exchange visitor physician coming to the United States on or after January 10, 1977, for the purpose of receiving graduate medical education or training is automatically subject to the two-year home-country physical presence requirement of section 212(e) of the Immigration and Nationality Act, as amended. Such physicians are not eligible to be considered for section 212(e) waivers on the basis of "No Objection" statements issued by their governments.

The law thus requires that a J1 visa holder, upon completion of the training program, leave the United States and reside in his or her home country for a period of at least two years. Currently, the American Medical Association (AMA) is advocating that this period be extended to five years.

An IMG on a J1 visa is ordinarily not allowed to change from a J1 to most other types of visas or (in most cases) to change from J1 to permanent residence while in the United States until he or she has fulfilled the "foreign residence requirement." The purpose of the foreign residence requirement is to ensure that an IMG uses the training he or she obtained in the United States for the benefit of his or her home country. The U.S. government may, however, waive the two-year foreign residence requirement under the following circumstances:

- If you as an IMG can prove that returning to your country would result in "exceptional hardship" to you or to members of your immediate family who are U.S. citizens or permanent residents;
- If you as an IMG can demonstrate a "well-founded fear of persecution" due to race, religion, or political opinions if forced to return to your country;
- If you obtain a "no objection" statement from your government; or
- If you are sponsored by an "interested governmental agency" or a designated state Department of Health in the United States.

Applying for a J1 Visa Waiver. IMGs who have sought a waiver on the basis of the last alternative have found it beneficial to approach the following potentially "interested government agencies":

- **The Department of Health and Human Services.** As of 2003, HHS has expanded its role in reviewing J1 waiver applications. HHS's considerations for a waiver have classically been as follows: (1) the program or activity in which the IMG is engaged is "of high priority and of national or international significance in an area of interest" to HHS; (2) the IMG must be an "integral" part of the program or activity "so that the loss of his/her services would necessitate discontinuance of the program or a major phase of it"; and (3) the IMG "must possess outstanding qualifications, training, and experience well beyond the usually expected accomplishments at the graduate, postgraduate, and residency levels and must clearly demonstrate the capability to make original and significant contributions to the program." Under these criteria, HHS waivers are granted to physicians working in high-level biomedical research.

  New rules will also allow HHS to review J1 waiver applications from community health centers, rural hospitals, and other health care providers. In the past, the U.S. Department of Agriculture (USDA) served as the interested federal government agency that reviewed waiver applications to allow foreign doctors to serve in rural underserved communities outside Appalachia, while the Appalachian Regional Commission (ARC) played that role for Appalachian communities. The USDA is no longer handling applications for J1 waivers. HHS will now review waiver applications for primary care practitioners and psychiatrists who have completed residency training within one year of application to practice in designated Health Professional Shortage Areas (HPSAs), Medically Underserved Areas and Populations (MUA/Ps), and Mental Health Professional Shortage Areas (MHPSAs). HHS waiver applications should be mailed to Joyce E. Jones, Executive Secretary, Exchange Visitor Waiver Review Board, Room 639-H, Hubert H. Humphrey Building, Department of Health and Human Services, 200 Independence Avenue, S.W., Washington, D.C. 20201; phone (202) 690-6174; fax (202) 690-7127.

■ **The Department of Veterans Affairs.** With more than 170 health care facilities located in various parts of the United States, the VA is a major employer of physicians in this country. In addition, many VA hospitals are affiliated with university medical centers. The VA sponsors IMGs working in research, patient care (regardless of specialty), and teaching. The waiver applicant may engage in teaching and research in conjunction with clinical duties. The VA's latest guidelines (issued on June 22, 1994) provide that it will act as an interested government agency only when the loss of an IMG's services would necessitate the discontinuance of a program or a major phase of it and when recruitment efforts have failed to locate a U.S. physician to fill the position.

The procedure for obtaining a VA sponsorship for a J1 waiver is as follows: (1) the IMG should deal directly with the Human Resources Department at the local VA facility; and (2) the facility must request that the VA's chief medical director sponsor the IMG for a waiver. The waiver request should include the following documentation: (1) a letter from the director of the local facility describing the program, the IMG's immigration status, the health care needs of the facility, and the facility's recruitment efforts; (2) recruitment efforts, including copies of all job advertisements run within the preceding year; and (3) copies of the IMG's licenses, test results, board certifications, IAP-66 or SEVIS DS-2019 forms, and the like. The VA contact person in Washington, D.C., should be contacted by the local medical facility rather than by IMGs or their attorneys.

■ **The Appalachian Regional Commission.** ARC sponsors physicians in certain places in the eastern and southern United States—namely, in Alabama, Georgia, Kentucky, Maryland, Mississippi, New York, North Carolina, Ohio, Pennsylvania, South Carolina, Tennessee, Virginia, and West Virginia. Since 1992, ARC has sponsored approximately 200 primary care IMGs annually in counties within its jurisdiction that have been designated as HPSAs by HHS.

In accordance with its February 1994 revision of its J1 waiver policies, ARC requires that waiver requests initially be submitted to the ARC contact person in the state of intended employment. Contact information for each state can be found on the ARC Web site (www.arc.gov). If the state concurs, a letter from the state's governor recommending the waiver must be addressed to Anne B. Pope, the federal cochairman of ARC. The waiver request should include the following: (1) a letter from the facility to Ms. Pope stating the proposed dates of employment, the IMG's medical specialty, the address of the practice location, an assertion that the IMG will practice primary care for at least 40 hours per week in the HPSA, and details as to why the facility needs the services of the IMG; (2) a J1 Visa

Data Sheet; (3) the ARC federal cochairman's J1 Visa Waiver Policy and the J1 Visa Waiver Policy Affidavit and Agreement with the notarized signature of the IMG; (4) a contract of at least three years' duration; (5) evidence of the IMG's qualifications, including a résumé, medical diplomas and licenses, and IAP-66 or SEVIS DS-2019 forms; and (6) evidence of unsuccessful attempts to recruit qualified U.S. physicians within the preceding six months. Copies of advertisements, copies of résumés received, and reasons for rejection must also be included. ARC will not sponsor IMGs who have been out of status for six months or longer.

Requests for ARC waivers are then processed in Washington, D.C. (ARC, 1666 Connecticut Avenue, N.W., Washington, D.C. 20009). ARC is usually able to forward a letter confirming that a waiver has been recommended to the requesting facility or attorney within 30 days of the request.

- **The Department of Agriculture.** At the time of publication, the USDA is no longer sponsoring J1 waivers. The scope of the HHS J1 waiver program has been expanded to fill the gap.

- **State Departments of Public Health.** There is no application form for a state-sponsored J1 waiver. However, regulations specify that an application must include the following documents: (1) a letter from the state Department of Public Health identifying the physician and specifying that it would be in the public interest to grant him or her a J1 waiver; (2) an employment contract that is valid for a minimum of three years and that states the name and address of the facility that will employ the physician and the geographic areas in which he or she will practice medicine; (3) evidence that these geographic areas are located within HPSAs; (4) a statement by the physician agreeing to the contractual requirements; (5) copies of all IAP-66 or SEVIS DS-2019 forms; and (6) a completed United States Information Agency (USIA) Data Sheet. Applications are numbered in the order in which they are received, since only 30 physicians per year may be granted waivers in a particular state under the Conrad State 30 program. Individual states may choose to participate or not to participate in this program. At the time of publication, nonparticipating states included Idaho, Oklahoma, and Wyoming, while Texas had suspended its J1 waiver program pending new legislation.

The H1B Visa

Since 1991, the law has allowed medical residency programs to sponsor foreign-born medical residents for H1B visas. There are no restrictions on changing the H1B visa to any other kind of visa, including permanent resident status (green card), through employer sponsorship or through close relatives who are U.S. citizens or permanent residents. It is advisable for SRPs to apply for H1B visas as soon as possible in the official year (beginning October 1) when the new quota officially opens up.

According to the Web site www.immihelp.com, as of October 17, 2000, the following beneficiaries of approved H1B petitions are exempt from the H1B annual cap:

- Beneficiaries who are in J1 nonimmigrant status in order to receive graduate medical education or training, and who have obtained a waiver of the two-year home residency requirement
- Beneficiaries who are employed at, or who have received an offer of employment at, an institution of higher education or a related or affiliated nonprofit entity

- Beneficiaries who are employed by, or who have received an offer of employment from, a nonprofit research organization
- Beneficiaries who are employed by, or who have received an offer of employment from, a governmental research organization
- Beneficiaries who are currently maintaining, or who have held within the last six years, H1B status, and are ineligible for another full six-year stay as an H1B
- Beneficiaries who have been counted once toward the numerical limit and are the beneficiary of multiple petitions

H1B visas are intended for "professionals" in a "specialty occupation." This means that an IMG intending to pursue a residency program in the United States with an H1B visa needs to clear all three USMLE Steps before becoming eligible for the H1B. The ECFMG administers Steps 1 and 2, whereas Step 3 is conducted by the individual states. You will need to contact the FSMB or the medical board of the state where you intend to take Step 3 for details (see p. 19).

H1B Application. An application for an H1B visa is filed not by the IMG but rather by his or her employment sponsor—in your case, by the SRP in the United States. If an SRP is willing to do so, you will be told about it at the time of your interview for the residency program.

Before filing an H1B application with the DHS, an SRP must file an application with the U.S. Department of Labor affirming that the SRP will pay at least the normal salary for your job that a U.S. professional would earn. After receiving approval from the Labor Department, your SRP should be ready to file the H1B application with the DHS. The SRP's supporting letter is the most important part of the H1B application package; it must describe the job duties to make it clear that the physician is needed in a "specialty occupation" (resident) under the prevalent legal definition of that term.

Most SRPs prefer to issue a SEVIS Form DS-2019 for a J1 visa rather than file papers for an H1B visa because of the burden of paperwork and the attorney costs involved in securing approval of an H1B visa application. Even so, a sizable number of SRPs are willing to go through the trouble, particularly if an IMG is an excellent candidate or if the SRP concerned finds it difficult to fill all the available residency slots (although this is becoming rarer with continuing cuts in residency slots). If an SRP is unwilling to file for an H1B visa because of attorney costs, you could suggest that you would be willing to bear the burden of such costs. The entire process of getting an H1B visa can take anywhere from 10 to 20 weeks.

H1B Premium Processing Service. According to the Web site www.myvisa.com, the DHS offers the opportunity to obtain processing of an H1B visa application within 15 calendar days. Within 15 days of receiving Form I-907, the DHS will mail you a notice of approval, request for evidence, intent to deny, or notice of investigation for fraud or misrepresentation. If the notice requires the submission of additional evidence or indicates an intent to deny, a new 15-day period will begin upon delivery to the DHS of a complete response to the request for evidence or notice of intent to deny. The fee for this service is $1000. With this service, the total time needed to obtain an H1B visa has become significantly shorter than that required for the J1.

Although an H1B visa can be stamped by any U.S. consulate abroad, it is advisable that you have it stamped at the U.S. consulate where you first applied for a visitor visa to travel to the United States for interviews.

A Final Word

IMGs should also be aware of a new program called the National Security Entry-Exit Registration System, which aims to tighten up homeland security by keeping closer tabs on nonimmigrants residing in or entering the United States on temporary visas.

Male citizens or nationals of specific countries who are already residing in the United States may be required to report to a designated DHS office for registration, which includes being fingerprinted, photographed, and interviewed under oath. The official list of countries includes Bangladesh, Egypt, Indonesia, Jordan, Kuwait, Pakistan, Saudi Arabia, Afghanistan, Algeria, Bahrain, Eritrea, Lebanon, Morocco, North Korea, Oman, Qatar, Somalia, Tunisia, the United Arab Emirates, Yemen, Iran, Iraq, Libya, Sudan, and Syria. Different registration deadlines and criteria have been assigned to citizens of the above-mentioned countries, so please refer to the DHS Web site for details (www.immigration.gov).

If you are entering the United States, you may be registered at the port of entry if you are (1) a citizen or national of Iran, Iraq, Libya, Sudan, or Syria; (2) a nonimmigrant who has been designated by the State Department; or (3) any other nonimmigrant identified by immigration officers at airports, seaports, and land ports of entry in accordance with new regulation 8 CFR 264.1(f)(2). If you will be staying in the United States for more than 30 days, you will then be required to register in person at a DHS district office within 30 days for an interview and will be required to reregister annually.

Once you are registered, certain special procedures will apply. If you leave the United States for any reason, you must appear in person before a DHS inspecting officer at a preapproved airport, seaport, or land port and leave the United States from that port on the same day. If you change your address, employment, or school, you must report to the DHS in writing within ten days using Form AR-11 SR. If any of these regulations are not followed, you may be considered out of status and subject to arrest, detention, fines, and/or removal from the United States, and any further application for immigration may be affected.

For the most up-to-date information regarding policies and procedures, please consult www.immigration.gov.

Summary

Despite some significant obstacles, a number of viable methods are available to IMGs who seek visas to pursue a residency program or eventually practice medicine in the United States. There is no doubt that the best alternative for an IMG is to obtain an H1B visa to pursue a medical residency. However, in cases where an IMG joins a residency program with a J1 visa, there are some possibilities for obtaining waivers of the two-year foreign residency requirement, particularly for those who are willing to make a commitment to perform primary care medicine in medically underserved areas.

Resources for the IMG

- **ECFMG**
  3624 Market Street
  Philadelphia, PA 19104-2685
  (215) 386-5900 or (215) 375-1913
  Fax: (215) 386-9196
  www.ecfmg.org

The ECFMG telephone number is answered only between 9:00 A.M. and 12:30 P.M. and between 1:30 P.M. and 5:00 P.M. Monday through Friday EST. The ECFMG often takes a long time to answer the phone, which is frequently busy at peak times of the year, and then gives you a long voice-mail message—so it is better to write or fax early than to rely on a last-minute phone call. Do not contact the NBME, as all IMG exam matters are conducted by the ECFMG. The ECFMG also publishes an information booklet on ECFMG certification and the USMLE program, which gives details on the dates and locations of forthcoming USMLE and English tests for IMGs together with application forms. It is free of charge and is also available from the public affairs offices of U.S. embassies and consulates worldwide as well as from Overseas Educational Advisory Centers. You may order single copies of the handbook by calling (215) 386-5900, preferably on weekends or between 6 P.M. and 6 A.M. Philadelphia time, or by faxing to (215) 387-9963. Requests for multiple copies must be made by fax or mail on organizational letterhead. The full text of the booklet is also available on the ECFMG's Web site at www.ecfmg.org.

- **Federation of State Medical Boards**
  P.O. Box 619850
  Dallas, TX 75261-9850
  (817) 868-4000
  Fax: (817) 868-4099
  www.fsmb.org

  The FSMB has a number of publications available, including *The Exchange, Section I*, which gives detailed information on examination and licensing requirements in all U.S. jurisdictions. The cost is $30. (Texas residents must add 8.25% state sales tax.) To obtain these publications, submit the online order form. Payment options include Visa or MasterCard. Alternatively, write to Federation Publications at the above address. All orders must be prepaid with a personal check drawn on a U.S. bank, a cashier's check, or a money order payable to the federation. Foreign orders must be accompanied by an international money order or the equivalent, payable in U.S. dollars through a U.S. bank or a U.S. affiliate of a foreign bank. For Step 3 inquiries, the telephone number is (817) 868-4041. You may e-mail the FSMB at usmle@fsmb.org or write to Examination Services at the address above.

- The Internet newsgroups misc.education.medical and bit.listserv.medforum can be valuable forums through which to exchange information on licensing exams, residency applications, and the like.

- Immigration information for IMGs is available from the site of Siskind, Susser, Haas & Devine, a firm of attorneys specializing in immigration law: www.visalaw.com/IMG/resources.html.

- Another source of immigration information can be found on the Web site of the law offices of Carl Shusterman, a Los Angeles attorney specializing in medical immigration law: www.shusterman.com.

- The AMA has dedicated a portion of its Web site to information on IMG demographics, residencies, immigration, and the like: www.ama-assn.org/ama/pub/category/17.html.

- International Medical Placement Ltd., a U.S. company specializing in recruiting foreign physicians to work in the United States, has a site at www.intlmedicalplacement.com.

- Two more useful Web sites are www.myvisa.com and www.immihelp.com.

- *First Aid for the International Medical Graduate*, 2nd ed., by Keshav Chander (2002; 313 pages; ISBN 0071385320), is an excellent resource written by a successful IMG. The book includes interviews with successful IMGs and students gearing up for the USMLE, complete "getting settled" information for new residents, and tips for dealing with possible social and cultural transition difficulties. The book provides useful advice on the U.S. curriculum, the health care delivery system, and ethical issues—and the differences IMGs should expect. Dr. Chander points out the weaknesses often found in IMG hopefuls and suggests ways to improve their performance on standardized tests as well as on academic and clinical evaluations. As a bonus, the guide contains information on how to get good fellowships after residency. The bottom line is that this is a reassuring guide that can help IMGs boost their confidence and proficiency. A great "first of its kind" that will empower IMGs with information that they need to succeed.

Other books that may be useful and of interest to IMGs are as follows:

- *International Medical Graduates in U.S. Hospitals: A Guide for Directors and Applicants*, by Faroque A. Khan and Lawrence G. Smith (1995; ISBN 094312641x).
- *Insider's Guide for the International Medical Graduate to Obtain a Medical Residency in the U.S.A.*, by Ahmad Hakemi (1999; ISBN 1929803001).

▶ FIRST AID FOR THE STUDENT WITH A DISABILITY

The USMLE provides accommodations for students with documented disabilities. The basis for such accommodations is the Americans with Disabilities Act (ADA) of 1990. The ADA defines a disability as "a significant limitation in one or more major life activities." This includes both "observable/physical" disabilities (e.g., blindness, hearing loss, narcolepsy) and "hidden/mental disabilities" (e.g., attention-deficit hyperactivity disorder, chronic fatigue syndrome, learning disabilities).

To provide appropriate support, the administrators of the USMLE must be informed of both the nature and the severity of an examinee's disability. Such documentation is required for an examinee to receive testing accommodations. Accommodations include extra time on tests, low-stimulation environments, extra or extended breaks, and zoom text.

Who Can Apply for Accommodations?

Students or graduates of a school in the United States or Canada that is accredited by the Liaison Committee on Medical Education (LCME) or the American Osteopathic Association (AOA) may apply for test accommodations directly from the NBME. Requests are granted only if they meet the ADA definition of a disability. If you are a disabled student or a disabled graduate of a foreign medical school, you must contact the ECFMG (see below).

Who Is Not Eligible for Accommodations?

Individuals who do not meet the ADA definition of disabled are not eligible for test accommodations. Difficulties not eligible for test accommodations include test anxiety, slow reading without an identified underlying cognitive deficit, English as a second language, or learning difficulties that have not been diagnosed as a medically recognized disability.

Understanding the Need for Documentation

Although most learning-disabled medical students are all too familiar with the often exhausting process of providing documentation of their disability, you should realize that **applying for USMLE accommodation is different from these previous experiences.** This is because the NBME determines whether an individual is disabled solely on the basis of the guidelines set by the ADA. Previous accommodation does not in itself justify provision of an accommodation, so be sure to review the NBME guidelines carefully.

Getting the Information

The first step in applying for USMLE special accommodations is to contact the NBME and obtain a guidelines-and-questionnaire booklet. This can be obtained by calling or writing to:

Testing Coordinator
Office of Test Accommodations
National Board of Medical Examiners
3750 Market Street
Philadelphia, PA 19104-3102
(215) 590-9500

Internet access to this information is also available at www.nbme.org. This information is also relevant for IMGs, since the information is the same as that sent by the ECFMG.

Foreign graduates should contact the ECFMG to obtain information on special accommodations by calling or writing to:

ECFMG
3624 Market Street
Philadelphia, PA 19104-2685
(215) 386-5900

When you get this information, take some time to read it carefully. The guidelines are clear and explicit about what you need to do to obtain accommodations.

SECTION 2

Database
of High-Yield Facts

The fifth edition of *First Aid for the USMLE Step 2 CK* contains a revised and expanded database of clinical material that student authors and faculty have identified as high yield for boards review. The facts are organized according to subject matter, whether medical specialty (e.g., Cardiovascular, Renal) or high-yield topic (e.g., Ethics) in medicine. Each subject is then divided into smaller subsections of related facts. Individual facts are generally presented in a logical approach, from basic definitions and epidemiology to **History/Physical Exam, Diagnosis,** and **Treatment.** Lists, mnemonics, and tables are used when helpful in forming key associations.

The content is mostly useful for reviewing material already learned. This section is not ideal for learning complex or highly conceptual material for the first time. Black-and-white images appear throughout the text. In some cases, reference is made to the "clinical image" section at the end of Section 2, which contains full-color glossy plates of histology and patient pathology by topic. At the end of Section 2, we also feature a Rapid Review chapter of key facts and classic associations to cram a day or two before the exam.

The Database of High-Yield Facts is not comprehensive. Use it to complement your core study material and not as your primary study source. The facts and notes have been condensed and edited to emphasize the essential material. Work with the material, add your own notes and mnemonics, and recognize that not all memory techniques work for all students.

We update Section 2 biannually to keep current with new trends in boards content as well as to expand our database of high-yield information. However, we must note that inevitably many other very high-yield entries and topics are not yet included in our database.

We actively encourage medical students and faculty to submit entries and mnemonics so that we may enhance the database for future students. We also solicit recommendations of additional tools for study that may be useful in preparing for the examination, such as diagrams, charts, and computer-based tutorials (see How to Contribute, page xiii).

Disclaimer

The entries in this section reflect student opinions of what is high yield. Owing to the diverse sources of material, no attempt has been made to trace or reference the origins of entries individually. We have regarded mnemonics as essentially in the public domain. All errors and omissions will be gladly corrected if brought to the attention of the authors, either through the publisher or directly by e-mail.

Cardiovascular

A normal axis has an upright QRS in leads I and aVF—the "double thumbs-up" sign.

In a patient with COPD, think RBBB.

To evaluate abnormalities of cardiac rhythm, assess the ECG for rate, rhythm, axis, and intervals (see Figure 2.1-1):

- **Rate:** Normal rate is 60–100 bpm. A rate < 60 bpm is bradyarrhythmia; > 100 bpm is tachyarrhythmia.
- **Rhythm:** Look for sinus rhythm (P before every QRS and QRS after every P), irregular rhythms, and junctional or ventricular rhythms (no P before a QRS).
- **Axis:** An upright QRS in leads I and aVF is a normal axis. An upright QRS in lead I and a downward QRS in lead aVF is left-axis deviation. A downward QRS in lead I and an upright QRS in lead aVF is right-axis deviation.
- **Intervals:** Look for heart block (PR interval > 200 msec, or P with no QRS afterward) or bundle branch blocks (QRS > 120 msec).

Bradyarrhythmias and Conduction Abnormalities

Table 2.1-1 outlines the etiologies, clinical presentation, and treatment of common bradyarrhythmias and conduction abnormalities.

Tachyarrhythmias

Tables 2.1-2 and 2.1-3 outline the etiologies, clinical presentation, and treatment of common supraventricular and ventricular tachyarrhythmias.

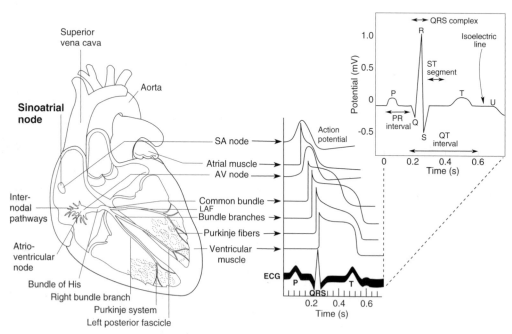

FIGURE 2.1-1. Electrocardiogram measurements.

(Adapted, with permission, from Ganong WF. *Review of Medical Physiology*, 20th ed. New York: McGraw-Hill, 2001.)

TABLE 2.1-1. Bradyarrhythmias and Conduction Abnormalities

Type	Etiology	Signs/Symptoms	ECG Findings	Treatment
Sinus bradycardia	Normal response to cardiovascular conditioning. Can result from sinus node dysfunction or from β-blocker or calcium channel blocker excess.	May be asymptomatic or present with light-headedness, syncope, and hypotension.	Ventricular rate < 60 bpm; normal P waves before every QRS complex.	None necessary if asymptomatic; atropine may be used to ↑ heart rate. Pacemaker placement is the definitive treatment.
Right bundle branch block (RBBB)	Can occur in normal individuals. May result from COPD, valvular disease, or chronic CAD, or may follow the surgical repair of a VSD.	Asymptomatic.	QRS duration > 120 msec; rSR complex with a wide R wave in V_1; QRS pattern with a wide S wave in V_6.	None necessary.
Left bundle branch block (LBBB)	Usually a sign of organic heart disease (hypertension, valvular disease, cardiomyopathy, CAD).	Often asymptomatic.	QRS duration > 120 msec; wide, entirely ⊖ QS complex in V_1; wide, tall R wave with no Q wave in V_6.	Usually none necessary. A ventricular pacemaker is the definitive therapy in post-MI LBBB patients with conduction defects.
First-degree AV block	Can occur in normal individuals; associated with ↑ vagal tone and with β-blockers and calcium channel blockers.	Asymptomatic.	PR interval > 200 msec.	None necessary.
Second-degree AV block (Mobitz I)	Drug effect (digoxin, β-blockers, calcium channel blockers) or a result of ↑ vagal tone.	Usually asymptomatic.	↑ PR interval until a dropped beat occurs (Wenckebach); PR then resets.	Stop the offending drug.
Second-degree AV block (Mobitz II)	Results from fibrotic disease of the conduction system or from a previous septal MI.	Occasionally syncope or progression to third-degree AV block.	Unexpected dropped beat without a change in PR interval.	Pacemaker placement.
Third-degree (complete) AV block	No electrical communication between the atria and ventricles.	Syncope, dizziness, acute heart failure, hypotension, cannon A waves.	No relationship between P waves and QRS complexes.	Pacemaker placement.

TABLE 2.1-2. Supraventricular Tachyarrhythmias

TYPE	ETIOLOGY	SIGNS/SYMPTOMS	ECG FINDINGS	TREATMENT
Sinus tachycardia	Normal physiologic response to fear, pain, and exercise. Can also be due to hyperthyroidism, dehydration, infection, or pulmonary embolism.	Palpitations, shortness of breath.	Ventricular rate > 100 bpm; normal P waves before every QRS complex.	Treat the underlying cause.
Atrial fibrillation	**PIRATES:** **P**ulmonary disease **I**schemia **R**heumatic heart disease **A**nemia/**A**trial myxoma **T**hyrotoxicosis **E**thanol **S**epsis	Often asymptomatic, but may present with shortness of breath, chest pain, or palpitations. Irregularly irregular pulse.	Wavy baseline without discernible P waves, with variable and irregular QRS response (see Figure 2.1-2).	Anticoagulation (to prevent thrombus formation and stroke), rate control (calcium channel blockers, β-blockers, digoxin). Cardioversion only if new onset (< 48 hours), if transesophageal echocardiography (TEE) shows no clot in the left atrium, or after six weeks of warfarin treatment.
Atrial flutter	Circular movement of electrical activity around the atrium at a rate of 300 times per minute.	Asymptomatic or presents with palpitations, syncope, and light-headedness.	Regular rhythm; "sawtooth" appearance of P waves (see Figure 2.1-2).	Anticoagulation and rate control. Cardioversion criteria are the same as those for atrial fibrillation.
Multifocal atrial tachycardia	Multiple atrial pacemakers or reentrant pathways, COPD, hypoxemia.	May be asymptomatic.	Three or more unique P-wave morphologies; rate > 100 bpm.	Treat the underlying disorder; verapamil or β-blockers for rate control and suppression of atrial pacemakers.
Atrioventricular nodal reentry tachycardia (AVNRT)	A reentry circuit in the AV node depolarizes the atrium and ventricle simultaneously.	Palpitations, shortness of breath, angina, syncope, light-headedness.	Rate 150–250 bpm; P wave is often **buried in** QRS or shortly after.	Carotid massage, Valsalva, or adenosine can stop the arrhythmia. Cardioversion if hemodynamically unstable.

TABLE 2.1-2 (continued). **Supraventricular Tachyarrhythmias**

TYPE	ETIOLOGY	SIGNS/SYMPTOMS	ECG FINDINGS	TREATMENT
Atrioventricular reciprocating tachycardia (AVRT)	Circular movement of an impulse down the AV node and back up to the atrium through a bypass tract. Seen in Wolff-Parkinson-White syndrome.	Palpitations, shortness of breath, angina, syncope, light-headedness.	Retrograde P wave is often seen **after** a normal QRS.	Same as that for AVNRT.
Paroxysmal atrial tachycardia	Rapid ectopic pacemaker in the atrium (not sinus node).	Palpitations, shortness of breath, angina, syncope, light-headedness.	Rate > 100 bpm; P wave with an unusual axis **before** each normal QRS.	Adenosine can be used for diagnosis (turns off ventricular response for seconds so that underlying atrial activity can be seen).

TABLE 2.1-3. **Ventricular Tachyarrhythmias**

TYPE	ETIOLOGY	SIGNS/SYMPTOMS	ECG FINDINGS	TREATMENT
Premature ventricular contraction (PVC)	Ectopic beats arise from ventricular foci. Associated with hypoxia, electrolyte abnormalities, and hyperthyroidism.	Usually asymptomatic, but may → palpitations.	Early, wide QRS not preceded by a P wave; PVCs are followed by a compensatory pause.	Treat the underlying cause. If symptomatic, give β-blockers or other antiarrhythmics.
Ventricular tachycardia	Associated with CAD and MI.	Nonsustained ventricular tachycardia is often asymptomatic; sustained ventricular tachycardia can → palpitations, hypotension, angina, and syncope. Can progress to ventricular fibrillation.	Three or more consecutive PVCs; wide QRS complexes in a regular rapid rhythm; AV dissociation (see Figure 2.1-3).	Cardioversion and antiarrhythmics (amiodarone, lidocaine, procainamide).
Ventricular fibrillation	Associated with CAD and MI.	Syncope, hypotension, pulselessness.	Totally erratic tracing (see Figure 2.1-3).	Immediate electrical cardioversion and ACLS protocol.

HIGH-YIELD FACTS

CARDIOVASCULAR

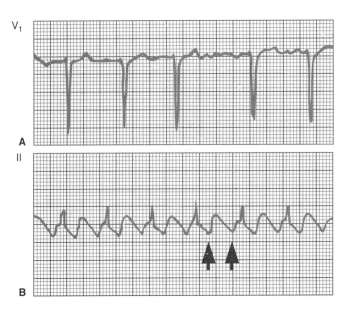

FIGURE 2.1-2. **Atrial fibrillation and atrial flutter.**

(A) Lead V$_1$ demonstrates an irregular ventricular rhythm associated with poorly defined irregular atrial activity consistent with atrial fibrillation. (B) Lead II demonstrates atrial flutter, identified by the regular "sawtooth-like" activity (arrows) at an atrial rate of 300 bpm with 2:1 ventricular response. (Reproduced, with permission, from Kasper DL et al [eds.]. *Harrison's Principles of Internal Medicine*, 16th ed. New York: McGraw-Hill, 2005:1345.)

> ***To distinguish between LBBB and RBBB—***
>
> **WiLLiaM MaR-RoW:**
>
> **W** pattern of QRS in V$_1$–V$_2$ and **M** pattern of QRS in V$_3$–V$_6$ for **L**BBB
> **M** pattern of QRS in V$_1$–V$_2$ and **W** pattern of QRS in V$_3$–V$_6$ for **R**BBB

Other Common ECG Abnormalities

- **Hyperkalemia:** In order of appearance, peaked T waves, widening of PR interval, widening of QRS, and sinusoidal wave pattern → ventricular fibrillation.
- **Pulmonary embolus:** Sinus tachycardia, S1Q3T3 (S wave in lead I, Q wave in lead III, and inverted T wave in lead III).
- **Wolff-Parkinson-White syndrome:** An electrical impulse bypasses the AV node through an **accessory pathway,** excites the ventricle prematurely, and makes a **delta wave** before QRS. Can → fatal AVRT.
- **Ventricular hypertrophy:** Diagnosed as **LVH** by the Cornell criteria if the amplitude of the R wave in aVL + the amplitude of the S wave in V$_3$ ≥ 24 mm in males or > 20 mm in females. **RVH** is diagnosed with right-axis deviation and R wave in V$_1$ > 7 mm.
- **Atrial hypertrophy: Right atrial** enlargement is diagnosed if the P-wave amplitude in **lead II** > 2.5 mm; **left atrial** enlargement is diagnosed if there is a biphasic P wave in **lead V$_1$.**

> ***Management of atrial fibrillation—***
>
> **ABCD**
>
> **A**nticoagulate
> β-blockers to control rate
> **C**ardiovert/**C**alcium channel blockers
> **D**igoxin

CARDIOMYOPATHY

Intrinsic disease of the myocardium; categorized as dilated, hypertrophic, or restrictive (see Table 2.1-4). Excludes myocardial dysfunction attributable to ischemic, valvular, or hypertensive disease.

Dilated Cardiomyopathy

The most common cardiomyopathy. **Left ventricular dilatation** and **systolic dysfunction** (low ejection fraction [EF]) must be present for diagnosis. Most

A. Ventricular tachycardia

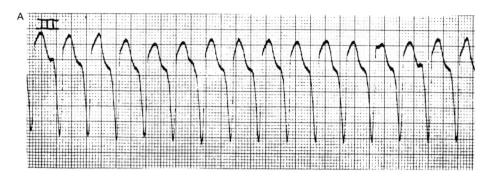

B. Ventricular fibrillation

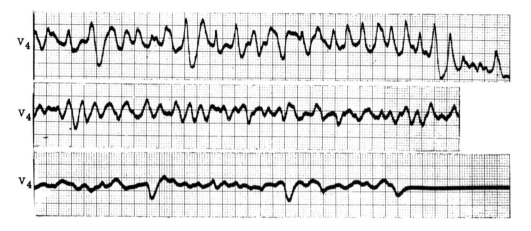

FIGURE 2.1-3. **Ventricular tachycardia and ventricular fibrillation.**

(A) Ventricular tachycardia. Note the regular, wide-complex rhythm with no discernible P waves. (B) Ventricular fibrillation. Note the erratic nature of the tracing. (Reproduced, with permission, from Saunders CE. *Current Emergency Diagnosis & Treatment*, 4th ed. Stamford, CT: Appleton & Lange, 1992:515, 517.)

TABLE 2.1-4. **Differential Diagnosis of Cardiomyopathies**

	DILATED	**HYPERTROPHIC**	**RESTRICTIVE**
Major abnormality	Impaired contractility.	Impaired relaxation.	Impaired elasticity.
Left ventricular cavity size (end diastole)	↑↑	↓	↑
Left ventricular cavity size (end systole)	↑↑	↓↓	↑
Ejection fraction	↓↓	↑ or ↔	↓ or ↔
Wall thickness	↓	↑↑	↑

cases are idiopathic, but known causes include alcohol, wet beriberi, coxsackievirus, Chagas' disease, parasites, cocaine, myocarditis, doxorubicin, HIV, and AZT use. The two most common causes of 2° dilated cardiomyopathy are ischemia and long-standing hypertension.

HISTORY/PE

- Gradual development of CHF symptoms.
- Examination may reveal cardiomegaly and an S3 as well as tricuspid and mitral regurgitation.

DIAGNOSIS

- Echocardiography is diagnostic.
- ECG may show nonspecific ST-T changes, low-voltage QRS, sinus tachycardia, and ectopy. LBBB is common.
- CXR shows an enlarged, balloon-like heart and pulmonary congestion.

TREATMENT

- Stop all alcohol usage.
- Treat symptoms of CHF and prevent disease progression (diuretics, ACEIs, β-blockers). Consider anticoagulation to ↓ thrombus risk.
- Consider an implantable cardiac defibrillator (ICD) if EF < 35%.

S3—end of rapid ventricular filling; associated with dilated cardiomyopathy.

Hypertrophic Cardiomyopathy

LVH → impaired left ventricular relaxation and filling (**diastolic dysfunction**). Left ventricular outflow tract obstruction from thickened interventricular septum → impaired left ventricular ejection of blood. The congenital form, known as idiopathic hypertrophic subaortic stenosis (IHSS), is inherited as an autosomal-dominant trait in 50% of patients and is the most common cause of sudden death in young, healthy athletes. Other causes include hypertension and aortic stenosis.

HISTORY/PE

- Syncope after exertion; dyspnea, palpitations, chest pain.
- Poor prognostic signs include arrhythmias and ↑ left atrial pressure.
- Examination may reveal mitral regurgitation, a sustained apical impulse, an S4, and a systolic ejection murmur.
- Obstruction is worsened by ↑ myocardial contractility or ↓ left ventricular filling (e.g., exercise, Valsalva maneuvers, vasodilators, dehydration).

S4—high atrial pressure/stiff ventricle; "atrial kick" associated with a hypertrophic ventricle.

DIAGNOSIS

- Echocardiography is diagnostic and shows thickened left ventricular walls and dynamic obstruction of blood flow.
- ECG shows signs of LVH.
- CXR may show a boot-shaped heart.

TREATMENT

- β-blockers are initial therapy; calcium channel blockers are second-line agents.
- Surgical options for IHSS include dual-chamber pacing, partial excision of the myocardial septum, or an ICD.
- Patients should avoid intense athletic competition and training.

Hypertrophic cardiomyopathy is the most common cause of sudden death in young, healthy athletes.

Restrictive Cardiomyopathy

- ↓ elasticity of myocardium → impaired diastolic filling without significant systolic dysfunction (normal or slightly ↓ ejection fraction).
- **Caused by infiltrative disease (e.g., sarcoidosis, hemochromatosis, amyloidosis) or by scarring and fibrosis (due to radiation or doxorubicin).**
- **Hx/PE:** Signs and symptoms of left and right heart failure occur, but symptoms of right heart failure (JVD, peripheral edema) often predominate.
- **Dx:** Cardiac biopsy.
- **Rx:** Correct the underlying cause and improve heart failure symptoms (e.g., sodium restriction, diuretics for fluid overload).

Restrictive cardiomyopathy →
myocardium that has
impaired elasticity.
Hypertrophic cardiomyopathy
*→ myocardium that is **slow***
to relax.

CONGESTIVE HEART FAILURE (CHF)

Defined as the clinical manifestation of cardiomyopathy. Occurs when the heart is unable to pump enough blood to meet the O_2 requirements of the heart and other body tissues. Risk factors include CAD, hypertension, valvular heart disease, pericardial disease, cardiomyopathy, and pulmonary hypertension. The American Heart Association/American College of Cardiology (AHA/ACC) guidelines classify heart failure according to clinical syndromes, but other common classification systems include functional severity, left versus right, and systolic versus diastolic (see Tables 2.1-5–2.1-8).

> **Causes of recurrent CHF—**
>
> **FAILURE**
>
> **F**orgot medication
> **A**rrhythmia/**A**nemia
> **I**schemia/**I**nfarct/
>   **I**nfection
> **L**ifestyle (most common
>   cause; e.g., ↑ Na⁺
>   intake, ↓ exercise)
> **U**pregulation (↑ cardiac
>   output; e.g.,
>   pregnancy,
>   hyperthyroidism)
> **R**enal failure (fluid
>   overload)
> **E**mbolus (pulmonary)

> **Caution when using**
> **β-blockers—**
>
> **ABCD**
>
> **A**sthma
> **B**lock (heart block)
> **C**OPD
> **D**iabetes

TABLE 2.1-5. **AHA/ACC classification and treatment of CHF**

STAGE	DESCRIPTION	TREATMENT
A	Patients who are at high risk of developing CHF because of the presence of risk factors, but who have no identified structural or functional abnormalities and no signs or symptoms of CHF.	Manage treatable risk factors (hypertension, smoking, hyperlipidemia, obesity, exercise, alcohol abuse). ACEIs can be used in patients with atherosclerotic vascular disease, DM, or hypertension.
B	Patients with structural heart disease (e.g., a history of MI, left ventricular systolic dysfunction, valvular disease) who have never had symptoms of CHF.	ACEIs, β-blockers.
C	Patients with structural heart disease who have prior or current symptoms of CHF (shortness of breath, fatigue, ↓ exercise tolerance).	Treatment includes diuretics, ACEIs, β-blockers, digitalis, and dietary salt restriction.
D	Patients with marked symptoms of CHF at rest despite maximal medical therapy.	Treatment options include mechanical assist devices, heart transplant, continuous IV inotropic drugs, and hospice care.

TABLE 2.1-6. New York Heart Association (NYHA) Functional Classification of CHF

CLASS	DESCRIPTION
I	No limitation of activity; no symptoms with normal activity.
II	Slight limitation of activity; comfortable at rest or with mild exertion.
III	Marked limitation of activity; comfortable only at rest.
IV	Confined to complete rest in bed or chair, as any physical activity brings on discomfort; symptoms present at rest.

Systolic Dysfunction

Defined by an EF < 50%; results from ↓ left ventricular contractile function. ↓ EF → ↑ preload (↑ left ventricular end-diastolic pressure) and, ultimately, ↑ systolic contractility according to the Frank-Starling law. Compensatory mechanisms are temporarily effective but ultimately → hypertrophy, ventricular dilatation, and ↑ myocardial work.

HISTORY/PE

- Presents with dyspnea on exertion or at rest if severe.
- Chronic cough, fatigue, lower extremity edema, orthopnea, paroxysmal nocturnal dyspnea, and/or abdominal fullness may be seen.
- Look for signs to distinguish between left- and right-sided heart failure (see Table 2.1-7).

DIAGNOSIS

- Based on clinical signs and symptoms.
- **CXR:** Look for cardiomegaly, cephalization of pulmonary vessels, pleural effusions, vascular indistinctness, and prominent hila.
- **Echocardiogram:** Shows impaired cardiac function (hypertrophic or dilated cardiomyopathy may be present).
- **ECG:** Atrial fibrillation is a common comorbid condition.
- Rule out MI in acute exacerbations. If amyloid or viral myocarditis is suspected (e.g., previous viral prodrome, young age), consider myocardial biopsy.

TREATMENT

- **Acute:**
  - Correct underlying causes (e.g., arrhythmia, alcohol-induced failure, thyroid and valvular disease).

Side effects of ACEIs—

CAPTOPRIL

Cough
Angioedema
Potassium excess
Taste changes
Orthostatic hypotension
Pregnancy
 contraindication
Rash
Indomethacin inhibition
Liver toxicity

The most common cause of right heart failure is left heart failure.

TABLE 2.1-7. Left- vs. Right-Sided Heart Failure

LEFT-SIDED CHF SYMPTOMS	RIGHT-SIDED CHF SYMPTOMS
Bilateral basilar rales	JVD
S3 gallop	Hepatomegaly
Pleural effusions	Hepatojugular reflux
Pulmonary edema	Bipedal edema

TABLE 2.1-8. **Comparison of Systolic and Diastolic Dysfunction**

	SYSTOLIC DYSFUNCTION	DIASTOLIC DYSFUNCTION
Patient age	Often < 65 years of age.	Often > 65 years of age.
Comorbidities	Dilated cardiomyopathy, valvular heart disease.	Restrictive or hypertrophic cardiomyopathy, renal disease, or hypertension.
Physical findings	Displaced PMI, S3 gallop.	Sustained PMI, S4 gallop.
CXR	Pulmonary congestion, cardiomegaly.	Pulmonary congestion, normal heart size.
ECG/echocardiography	Q waves, ↓ EF (< 40%).	LVH, normal EF (> 50%).

- Diurese aggressively with a **loop diuretic** and a non–loop diuretic (monitor K$^+$ with potassium-sparing agents).
- Use **ACEIs** in all patients who can tolerate them. β-blockers should **not** be used during **decompensated CHF**.
- **Chronic:**
  - Long-term β-blockers and ACEIs/angiotensin receptor blockers (**ARBs**) together help prevent neurohormonal remodeling of the heart.
  - Daily **aspirin** and a **statin** are recommended for ischemic heart disease to prevent further ischemic events.
  - Chronic **diuretic** therapy can prevent volume overload.
  - Low-dose **spironolactone** has been shown to ↓ mortality risk when given with **ACEIs and loop diuretics** in patients with **left ventricular systolic dysfunction** and **NYHA class III–IV heart failure.**
  - Treat arrhythmias as they arise, and limit dietary sodium and fluid intake.
  - Consider **warfarin** for severe dilated cardiomyopathy (EF < 25%), atrial fibrillation, or previous embolic episodes. Consider an ICD in patients with EF < 35%.
  - CHF that is unresponsive to maximal medical therapy may require a mechanical left ventricular assist device or cardiac transplantation.

> *Acute CHF management—*
>
> **LMNOP**
>
> **L**asix
> **M**orphine
> **N**itrates
> **O**xygen
> **P**ulmonary ventilation

Diastolic Dysfunction

- Characterized by ↓ **ventricular compliance with normal contractile function.** The ventricle is unable either to actively relax or to passively fill properly (↑ stiffness, ↓ recoil, and concentric hypertrophy). Left ventricular end-diastolic pressure ↑, cardiac output remains essentially normal, and EF is normal or ↑.
- The differences between diastolic and systolic dysfunction are summarized in Table 2.1-8.
- **History/PE:** Stable and unstable angina, shortness of breath, dyspnea on exertion, arrhythmias, MI, heart failure, sudden death.
- **Rx:** β-blockers, ACEIs, diuretics, rate control, BP management. **Digoxin is not useful in these patients.**

Major risk factors for CAD include age, gender (males > females), hypercholesterolemia, DM, hypertension, obesity, smoking, and a ⊕ family history.

CORONARY ARTERY DISEASE (CAD)

Clinical manifestations include stable and unstable angina, shortness of breath, dyspnea on exertion, arrhythmias, MI, heart failure, and sudden death.

Hypercholesterolemia is usually asymptomatic.

Side effects/ contraindications of HMG-CoA reductase inhibitors—

HMG-CoA

Hepatotoxicity
Myositis
Girl in pregnancy/**G**rowing children
Coumadin/**C**yclosporine interactions

Hypercholesterolemia

↑ blood cholesterol (defined as a total cholesterol level > 200 mg/dL), ↑ LDL, ↑ triglycerides, and ↓ HDL are risk factors for CAD. Etiologic factors include obesity, DM, alcoholism, hypothyroidism, nephrotic syndrome, hepatic disease, Cushing's disease, OCP use, diuretic use, and familial hypercholesterolemia.

HISTORY/PE

- Most patients have **no specific signs or symptoms.**
- Patients with extremely ↑ triglycerides or LDL may have **xanthomas** (eruptive nodules in skin over tendons), **xanthelasmas** (yellow fatty deposits in skin around eyes), and **lipemia retinalis** (creamy appearance of retinal vessels).

DIAGNOSIS

- Conduct a fasting lipid profile for patients > 20 years of age and repeat every five years.
- Total serum cholesterol > 200 mg/dL on two different occasions, LDL > 130 mg/dL, or HDL < 35 mg/dL is diagnostic.

TREATMENT

- Based on risk stratification (see Table 2.1-9). Risk factors include **diabetes (considered a CAD risk equivalent)**, smoking, hypertension, HDL < 40 mg/dL, age > 45 (males), age > 55 (females), and early CAD in first-degree relatives (males < 55 and females < 65).
- The first intervention should be a 12-week trial of **diet and exercise.** Commonly used lipid-lowering agents are listed in Table 2.1-10.

Angina Pectoris

Substernal chest pain due to myocardial ischemia (↑ O_2 demand or ↓ O_2 supply). **Prinzmetal's (variant) angina** mimics angina pectoris but is caused by **vasospasm** of coronary vessels. Often affects young women and classically occurs at rest in the early morning; associated with ST-segment elevations but not with cardiac enzyme elevation.

HISTORY/PE

- The classic triad consists of **substernal chest pain** or pressure **precipitated by exertion** and **relieved by rest or nitrates.**
- Pain can radiate to the arms, jaw, and neck and may be associated with shortness of breath, nausea/vomiting, or light-headedness.

TABLE 2.1-9. Risk Stratification and Target LDL

RISK CATEGORY	TARGET LDL (MG/DL)
0–1 risk factor	< 160
≥ 2 risk factors	< 130
CAD or risk equivalent	< 70

TABLE 2.1-10. Lipid-Lowering Agents

CLASS	EXAMPLES	MECHANISM OF ACTION	EFFECT ON LIPID PROFILE	SIDE EFFECTS
HMG-CoA reductase inhibitors ("statins")	Atorvastatin, simvastatin, lovastatin, pravastatin.	Inhibit the rate-limiting step in cholesterol synthesis.	↓ LDL, ↓ triglycerides.	↑ LFTs, myositis, warfarin (Coumadin) potentiation.
Lipoprotein lipase stimulators/ fibrates	Gemfibrozil.	↑ lipoprotein lipase → ↑ VLDL and triglyceride catabolism.	↓ triglycerides, ↑ HDL.	GI upset, cholelithiasis, myositis, LFT abnormalities.
Cholesterol absorption inhibitors	Ezetimibe (Zetia).	↓ absorption of cholesterol at the small intestine brush border.	↓ LDL.	Diarrhea, abdominal pain. Can → angioedema.
Niacin		↓ fatty acid release from adipose tissue; ↓ hepatic synthesis of LDL.	↓ LDL, ↑ HDL.	**Skin flushing** (can prevent by taking aspirin before); paresthesias/pruritus, GI upset, ↑ LFTs.
Bile acid resins	Cholestyramine, colestipol, colesevelam.	Bind intestinal bile acids → ↓ bile acid stores and ↑ catabolism of LDL from plasma.	↓ LDL.	Constipation, GI upset, LFT abnormalities, myalgias. Can ↓ **absorption** of other drugs from the intestine.

- Examination may reveal diaphoresis, hypertension, tachycardia, and apical systolic murmur or gallop.

DIAGNOSIS

ECG may show **ST-segment depression** or **T-wave flattening.** Check cardiac enzymes to rule out MI.

TREATMENT

- Treat acute symptoms with **morphine, O$_2$,** sublingual **nitroglycerin, ASA,** and **IV β-blockers.**
- Patients with a suspected MI must be admitted and monitored until acute MI is ruled out by serial cardiac enzymes.
- Treat chronic symptoms with nitrates, β-blockers, and calcium channel blockers. ASA ↓ the risk of MI.
- **Risk factor reduction** (e.g., smoking, cholesterol, hypertension); ACEIs for hypertension. Check lipid panel and consider starting a statin.

Unstable Angina

Angina is considered unstable if it is new, is accelerating (i.e., occurs with less exertion, lasts longer, or is less responsive to medications), or occurs at rest. It often signifies a transient vessel occlusion (i.e., disruption of an atheroscle-

The classic triad of angina is chest pain, worsened by exertion and relieved by rest or nitrates.

ST-segment depression indicates ischemia, while ST-segment elevation indicates dying myocardium.

HIGH-YIELD FACTS

CARDIOVASCULAR

rotic plaque and/or vasospasm in the area of a plaque) and an area of myocardial ischemia that can acutely progress to complete occlusion and MI.

TREATMENT

- Acute treatment is as described for stable angina; glycoprotein IIB–IIIA inhibitors (eptifibatide, tirofiban, abciximab) can also be considered.
- In addition, one should proceed to **heparinization, angiography,** and possible **revascularization** (PTCA vs. CABG).

Myocardial Infarction (MI)

Time is myocardium.

Usually caused by an occlusive thrombus or prolonged vasospasm in a coronary artery. The most common cause is an **acute thrombus on a ruptured atherosclerotic plaque.**

HISTORY/PE

- Presents with **acute-onset substernal chest pain,** often described as a **pressure or tightness,** that can **radiate to the left arm,** neck, or jaw.
- Diaphoresis, shortness of breath, light-headedness, anxiety, nausea/vomiting, and syncope may be seen.
- On examination, look for tachycardia, bradycardia, arrhythmias, **new mitral regurgitation** (ruptured papillary muscle), hypotension (cardiogenic shock), rales (pulmonary edema), and ventricular fibrillation.
- Some 20% of MI patients present with sudden death from a **lethal arrhythmia** (often ventricular fibrillation). The best predictor of survival is **left ventricular EF.**
- Be alert to atypical presentations; elderly, diabetic, postmenopausal, and postorthotopic heart transplant patients are particularly likely to have atypical, clinically silent MIs.

Elderly, diabetic, postmenopausal, and postorthotopic heart transplant patients are particularly likely to have atypical, clinically silent MIs.

DIAGNOSIS

- ECG: Look for ST-segment elevations or new LBBB.
- **Sequence of ECG changes:** Peaked T waves, ST-segment elevation, Q waves, T-wave inversion, ST-segment normalization, T-wave normalization.
- ST-segment elevations in leads II, III, and aVF are consistent with an **inferior** MI. ST-segment elevations in anterior leads (V_1–V_4) usually indicate an anterior MI. ST-segment elevations in leads I, aVL, and V_5–V_6 indicate a **lateral** MI (see Figures 2.1-4 and 2.1-5).
- **Serial cardiac enzymes:** Check troponin and CK with CK-MB fraction. Troponin I appears first and is most sensitive and specific; CK-MB appears next.

TREATMENT

- As above for unstable angina, but emergent angiography and revascularization must also be considered. If these are unavailable, consider **thrombolysis** with tPA, urokinase, or streptokinase.
- If there is single- or double-vessel disease with discrete lesions, the patient is a candidate for PTCA.
- If there is three-vessel disease, left main disease, discrete lesions not amenable to PTCA, or diffuse disease with good targets, the patient is a candidate for CABG.

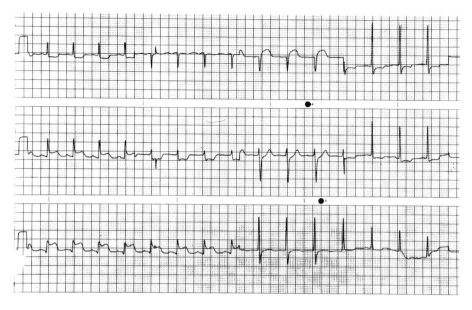

FIGURE 2.1-4. Inferior wall MI.

In this patient with acute chest pain, the ECG demonstrated acute ST-segment elevation in leads II, III, and aVF with reciprocal ST-segment depression and T-wave flattening in leads I, aVL, and V$_4$–V$_6$. (Reproduced, with permission, from Stobo J et al. *The Principles and Practice of Medicine*, 23rd ed. Stamford, CT: Appleton & Lange, 1996:20.)

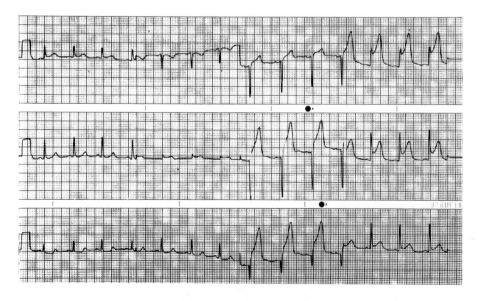

FIGURE 2.1-5. Anterior wall MI.

This patient presented with acute chest pain. ECG showed ST-segment elevation in leads aVL and V$_1$–V$_6$ and hyperacute T waves. (Reproduced, with permission, from Stobo JD et al. *The Principles and Practice of Medicine*, 23rd ed. Stamford, CT: Appleton & Lange, 1996:19.)

- Long-term treatment includes ASA, β-blockers, ACEIs, and statins. Modify risk factors with dietary changes and exercise.

COMPLICATIONS

- Reinfarction, left ventricular wall rupture, pericarditis, papillary muscle rupture (with mitral regurgitation), aneurysmal left ventricular dilatation, mural thrombi.
- **Dressler's syndrome:** An autoimmune process with fever, pericarditis, pleural effusion, leukocytosis, and ↑ ESR 2–4 weeks post-MI.
- **Lethal arrhythmia** is the most common cause of death following acute MI.

Defined as a **systolic BP > 140** and/or a **diastolic BP > 90** based on three measurements, each separated by two weeks' time (see Table 2.1-11). Classified as 1° or 2°.

1° (Essential) Hypertension

Represents 95% of cases of hypertension. Risk factors include a **family history** of hypertension or heart disease, a **high-sodium diet, smoking, obesity, race** (African-Americans > Caucasians), and **advanced age.**

HISTORY/PE

- BP elevation is **asymptomatic** until complications develop. Retinal changes, an S4 gallop, a systolic click, and/or a loud S2 may be present.
- Untreated hypertension → damage to the heart (hypertrophy, MI, CHF), brain (stroke, TIA), kidney (chronic kidney disease), vasculature (peripheral vascular disease), and eye (retinopathy).

1° hypertension is the most common cause of high blood pressure.

The BP goal in uncomplicated hypertension is < 140/< 90. For diabetics or patients with renal disease, the goal is < 130/< 80.

TABLE 2.1-11. JNC-7 Classification and Management of Hypertension[a]

BP CLASSIFICATION	SYSTOLIC BP	DIASTOLIC BP	MANAGEMENT
Normal	< 120	< 80	None.
Prehypertension	120–139	80–89	Lifestyle modification.
Stage I hypertension	140–159	90–99	Thiazide diuretic; may consider ACEIs, ARBs, β-blockers, calcium channel blockers, or a combination.
Stage 2 hypertension	≥ 160	≥ 100	Two-drug combination (usually a thiazide diuretic + an ACEI, an ARB, a β-blocker, or a calcium channel blocker).

[a] From the seventh report of the Joint National Committee on Prevention, Detection, Evaluation, and Treatment of High Blood Pressure, *Hypertension* 42(6):1206–1252, December 2003.

TREATMENT

- Rule out 2° causes of hypertension.
- Begin with lifestyle management (e.g., diet, exercise). The BP goal in otherwise healthy patients is < 140/< 90. The goal in diabetics or patients with renal disease with proteinuria is < 130/< 80.
- Diuretics (inexpensive and particularly effective in African-Americans) and β-blockers (beneficial for patients with CAD) have been shown to reduce mortality in uncomplicated hypertension. They are first-line agents unless a comorbid condition requires another medication (see Tables 2.1-12–2.1-14).
- Conduct periodic tests for end-organ complications, including renal (BUN, creatinine, microalbumin-to-creatinine ratio) and cardiac (ECG evidence of hypertrophy) complications.

2° Hypertension

Hypertension due to an **identifiable** organic cause. See Table 2.1-15 for the diagnosis and treatment of common causes.

Hypertensive Urgency and Emergency

- **Hypertensive urgency:** Defined as **BP > 180/> 130** that is asymptomatic or moderately symptomatic (headache, chest pain, syncope).
- **Hypertensive emergency:** May occur at any BP, but defined as **signs or symptoms** of impending **end-organ damage** such as acute renal failure or

> **Treatment of hypertension—**
>
> **ABCD**
>
> **A**CEIs/**A**RBs
> β-blockers
> **C**alcium channel blockers
> **D**iuretics

*ACID*azolamide → *ACID*osis.

Loops Lose calcium, while thiazides save it.

TABLE 2.1-12. Classes of Diuretics

CLASS	EXAMPLES	SITE OF ACTION	MECHANISM OF ACTION	SIDE EFFECTS
Osmotic	Mannitol.	Proximal tubule.	Creates ↑ tubular fluid osmolarity → ↑ urine flow.	Pulmonary edema, dehydration. Contraindicated in anuria and CHF.
Carbonic anhydrase inhibitors	Acetazolamide.	Proximal convoluted tubule.	$NaHCO_3$ diuresis, ↓ total body $NaHCO_3$.	Hyperchloremic metabolic acidosis, neuropathy, NH_3 toxicity, sulfa allergy.
Loop diuretics	Furosemide, ethacrynic acid, bumetanide, torsemide.	Loop of Henle.	↓ $Na^+/K^+/2Cl^-$ cotransporter; ↓ urine concentration; ↑ Ca^{2+} excretion.	Ototoxicity, hypokalemia, hypocalcemia, dehydration, gout.
Thiazide diuretics	HCTZ, chlorothiazide, chlorthalidone.	Early distal tubule.	↓ NaCl reabsorption → ↓ diluting capacity of nephron; ↓ Ca^{2+} excretion.	Hypokalemic metabolic alkalosis, hyponatremia. Hyperglycemia, hyperlipidemia, hyperuricemia, hypercalcemia.
K^+-sparing agents	Spironolactone, triamterene, amiloride.	Cortical collecting tubule.	Spironolactone is an aldosterone receptor antagonist; triamterene and amiloride block Na^+ channels.	Hyperkalemia, gynecomastia, hirsutism, sexual dysfunction.

TABLE 2.1-13.   **Major Classes of Antihypertensive Agents**

CLASS	AGENTS	MECHANISM OF ACTION	SIDE EFFECTS
Diuretics	Thiazide, loop, K^+-sparing, other (e.g., spironolactone).	Reduce extracellular fluid volume and thereby reduce vascular resistance.	Hypokalemia, hyperglycemia, hyperlipidemia, hyperuricemia (problematic in gout), azotemia.
β-adrenergic blockers	Propranolol, metoprolol, nadolol, atenolol, timolol, carvedilol, labetalol.	Reduce cardiac contractility and renin release.	Bronchospasm (in severe asthma), bradycardia, CHF exacerbation, impotence, fatigue, depression.
Centrally acting adrenergic agonists	Methyldopa, clonidine, guanabenz.	Inhibit sympathetic nervous system via central α_2-adrenergic receptors.	Somnolence, orthostasis, impotence, rebound hypertension.
α_1-adrenergic blockers	Prazosin, terazosin, phenoxybenzamine.	Cause vasodilation by blocking actions of norepinephrine on vascular smooth muscle.	Orthostasis.
Ca^{2+} channel blockers	Dihydropyridines (nifedipine, felodipine, amlodipine), diltiazem, verapamil.	Reduce smooth muscle tone and cause vasodilation; may also reduce cardiac output.	Dihydropyridines: headache, flushing, peripheral edema. Verapamil/diltiazem: reduced contractility.
Vasodilators	Hydralazine, minoxidil.	Decrease peripheral resistance by dilating arteries/arterioles.	Hydralazine: headache, lupus-like syndrome. Minoxidil: orthostasis, facial hirsutism.
ACEIs	Captopril, enalapril, fosinopril, benazepril, lisinopril.	Block aldosterone formation, reducing peripheral resistance and salt/water retention.	Cough, rashes, leukopenia, hyperkalemia.
Angiotensin II receptor antagonists	Losartan, valsartan, irbesartan.	Block aldosterone effects, reducing peripheral resistance and salt/water retention.	Rashes, leukopenia, and hyperkalemia but no cough.

hematuria; **altered mental status** or evidence of neurologic disease; intracranial hemorrhage; ophthalmologic findings (**papilledema**, vascular changes); unstable angina/MI; or pulmonary edema.

- **Malignant hypertension:** Defined as progressive **renal failure** and/or **encephalopathy** with papilledema.

DIAGNOSIS

- Cardiovascular, neurologic, ophthalmologic, and abdominal exams.
- Obtain a head and/or abdominal CT, UA, BUN/creatinine, CBC, and electrolytes to assess the extent of end-organ damage.

POPULATION	TREATMENT
Diabetes with proteinuria	ACEIs.
CHF	β-blockers, ACEIs, diuretics (including spironolactone).
Isolated systolic hypertension	Diuretics preferred; long-acting dihydropyridine calcium channel blockers.
MI	β-blockers without intrinsic sympathomimetic activity, ACEIs.
Osteoporosis	Thiazide diuretics.
BPH	α-antagonists.

Side effects of thiazides—

hyper-GLUC

hyper**G**lycemia
hyper**L**ipidemia
hyper**U**ricemia
hyper**C**alcemia

*In K⁺-sparing diuretics (**S**pironolactone, **T**riamterene, **A**miloride), the K⁺ **STA**ys.*

TREATMENT

- BP must be ↓ slowly (↓ in mean arterial pressure of only 25% over the first two hours) to prevent cerebral hypoperfusion or coronary insufficiency.
- First use **oral agents** such as β-blockers, clonidine, and ACEIs. Avoid short-acting calcium channel blockers. If insufficient, use IV agents.
- Use **IV agents** such as **nitroprusside**, nitroglycerin, labetalol, nicardipine, or hydralazine. Add a **diuretic** if there are signs of fluid overload.

PERICARDIAL DISEASE

Results from acute or chronic pericardial insult; can → pericardial effusion.

Pericarditis

Inflammation of the pericardial sac, often with an effusion. Can compromise cardiac output via tamponade or constrictive pericarditis. Causes include viral infection, TB, SLE, uremia, drugs, and neoplasms. Most commonly idiopathic. May also occur after MI (Dressler's syndrome), open heart surgery, or radiation therapy.

HISTORY/PE

- May present with pleuritic chest pain, dyspnea, cough, and fever.
- **Chest pain** is often **positional** (worsens in the supine position and with inspiration; improves with shallow breathing or leaning forward).
- Examination may reveal a pericardial **friction rub, elevated JVP**, and **pulsus paradoxus** (a fall in systolic BP > 10 mmHg on inspiration).

DIAGNOSIS

- CXR, ECG, and echocardiogram to rule out MI and pneumonia.
- ECG changes include **PR-segment depression** in precordial leads, **low voltage**, and **diffuse ST-segment elevation** (see Figure 2.1-6).
- **Pericardial thickening or effusion** on echocardiography.

Causes of 2° hypertension—

CHAPS

Cushing's syndrome
Hyperaldosteronism
Aortic coarctation
Pheochromocytoma
Stenosis of renal arteries

Look for signs of **PERIC**arditis:

Pulsus paradoxus
ECG changes
Rub
Increased JVP
Chest pain

TABLE 2.1-15. **Common Causes of 2° Hypertension**

	DESCRIPTION	MANAGEMENT
1° renal disease	Often unilateral renal parenchymal disease.	Treat with **ACEIs,** which slow the progression of renal disease.
Renal artery stenosis	Especially common in patients < 25 and > 50 years of age with recent-onset hypertension. Etiologies include **fibromuscular dysplasia** (usually in **younger** patients) and **atherosclerosis** (usually in older patients).	Diagnose with MRA or renal artery Doppler ultrasound. Treat with **angioplasty** and **stenting** if possible. Consider ACEIs as adjunctive or temporary therapy in unilateral disease. **(In bilateral disease, ACEIs can accelerate kidney failure by preferential vasodilation of the efferent arteriole.)** Open surgery is a 2° option if angioplasty is not effective or feasible.
OCP use	Common in women > 35 years of age, obese women, and those with long-standing use.	Discontinue OCPs (it can take time to see an effect).
Pheochromocytoma	An adrenal gland tumor that secretes epinephrine and norepinephrine → episodic headache, sweating, and tachycardia.	Diagnose with urinary metanephrines and catecholamine levels or plasma metanephrines. Surgical removal of tumor.
Conn's syndrome (hyperaldosteronism)	Most often due to an aldosterone-producing adrenal adenoma. Causes the triad of hypertension, unexplained hypokalemia, and metabolic alkalosis.	Surgical removal of tumor.
Cushing's syndrome	Due to an ACTH-producing pituitary tumor, an ectopic ACTH-secreting tumor, or cortisol secretion by an adrenal adenoma or carcinoma.	Surgical removal of tumor.
Coarctation of the aorta	See the Pediatrics section.	Surgical repair.

Causes of pericarditis—

CARDIAC RIND

Collagen vascular disease
Aortic dissection
Radiation
Drugs
Infections
Acute renal failure (uremia)
Cardiac (MI)
Rheumatic fever
Injury
Neoplasms
Dressler's syndrome

TREATMENT

- Treat the underlying cause (e.g., steroids/immunosuppressants for SLE, ASA/NSAIDs for viral pericarditis, dialysis for uremia).
- Small effusions can be followed, but tamponade or large effusions require **pericardiocentesis** with continuous drainage if necessary.

Cardiac Tamponade

Excess fluid in the pericardial sac → compromised ventricular filling and ↓ cardiac output. More closely related to the **rate of fluid formation** than to the size of the effusion. Risk factors include pericarditis, malignancy, SLE, TB, and trauma (commonly stab wounds medial to the left nipple).

HIGH-YIELD FACTS

CARDIOVASCULAR

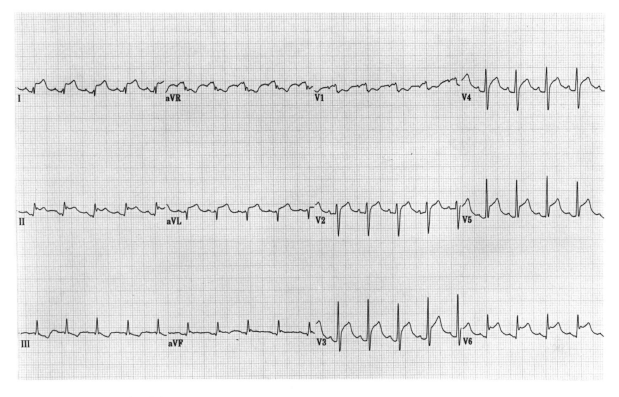

FIGURE 2.1-6. Pericarditis.

There is characteristic ST-segment elevation in all leads and PR-segment depression in the precordial leads. (Reproduced, with permission, from Stobo JD et al. *The Principles and Practice of Medicine*, 23rd ed. Stamford, CT: Appleton & Lange, 1996:85.)

HISTORY/PE

- Presents with **fatigue, dyspnea, tachycardia,** and **tachypnea** that can rapidly → shock and death.
- Examination may reveal **Beck's triad (hypotension, distant heart sounds, and distended neck veins), a narrow pulse pressure, pulsus paradoxus,** and **Kussmaul's sign** (JVD on inspiration).

DIAGNOSIS

- **Echocardiogram** shows right atrial and right ventricular diastolic collapse.
- CXR shows an enlarged, globular heart.
- ECG may show ↓ amplitude and/or **electrical alternans** (electrical axis changes with each beat).

TREATMENT

- **Aggressive volume expansion** with IV fluids.
- Urgent **pericardiocentesis** (aspirate will be **nonclotting** blood); balloon pericardotomy and pericardial window may be required.

Tamponade should be suspected in any hemodynamically unstable patient who does not respond to initial resuscitative measures.

VALVULAR HEART DISEASE

Aortic and Mitral Valve Disease

Lesions can be divided into stenotic and regurgitant (see Tables 2.1-16 and 2.1-17). Valvular disease generally presents after age 70 with the exception of

TABLE 2.1-16. Aortic Valve Disease

	RISK FACTORS	SYMPTOMS	MURMUR	PHYSICAL EXAM	TREATMENT
Aortic stenosis	Rheumatic heart disease, congenital aortic stenosis, bicuspid valve.	Classic triad of **exertional dyspnea, angina, and syncope.** Can → CHF and death.	Midsystolic crescendo-decrescendo murmur heard best at the second intercostal space, radiating to the neck.	**Pulsus parvus et tardus** (weak, delayed carotid upstroke); sustained apical beat. Paradoxically split S2.	Avoid afterload reducers. Valve replacement is curative.
Aortic regurgitation	Rheumatic heart disease, VSD, infective endocarditis, congenital bicuspid valve, Marfan's syndrome, syphilis.	Symptoms of LVH, angina, CHF due to volume overload.	Three murmurs: (1) high-pitched, blowing diastolic murmur at the left sternal border; (2) Austin Flint—low-pitched, mid-diastolic rumble; (3) midsystolic murmur at the base.	Widened pulse pressure; laterally displaced PMI.	Aortic valve replacement is curative. If not possible, treat with afterload reducers (ACEIs, vasodilators), diuretics, and digoxin.

> **Beck's triad for cardiac tamponade— the 3 D's:**
>
> **D**istant heart sounds
> **D**istended jugular veins
> **D**ecreased arterial pressure

mitral stenosis, which often presents in the fourth and fifth decades. Until recently, **rheumatic fever** (which affects the mitral valve more than the aortic valve) was the most common cause in adults; the leading cause is now mechanical degeneration.

VASCULAR DISEASE

Aortic Aneurysm

Atherosclerosis is most commonly associated with aortic aneurysms. Most are abdominal, and > 90% originate below the renal arteries.

HISTORY/PE

- Usually **asymptomatic** and discovered incidentally on exam or radiologic study.
- Risk factors include hypertension, high cholesterol, other vascular disease, family history, smoking, gender (males > females), and age.
- Examination demonstrates **pulsatile abdominal mass** or abdominal bruits.
- Ruptured aneurysm → **hypotension** and severe, **tearing abdominal pain** radiating to the back.

DIAGNOSIS

- Abdominal ultrasound for diagnosis or to follow an aneurysm over time.
- CT may be a useful adjunct to determine the precise anatomy.

TABLE 2.1-17. **Mitral Valve Disease**

	RISK FACTORS	SYMPTOMS	MURMUR	PHYSICAL EXAM	TREATMENT
Mitral stenosis	Rheumatic heart disease.	Symptoms of CHF (both left and right).	Mid-diastolic rumble with opening snap at the apex.	Atrial fibrillation, pulmonary rales, ↑ intensity of S1 and P2, right ventricular heave.	Avoid inotropic agents; use β-blockers and diuretics. Digoxin, anticoagulants for atrial fibrillation. Balloon valvuloplasty.
Mitral regurgitation	Rheumatic heart disease, MI, infective endocarditis, severe mitral valve prolapse.	Left-sided heart failure that can progress to right-sided heart failure.	High-pitched, holosystolic murmur at the apex that radiates to the axilla.	Laterally displaced PMI with left ventricular heave, atrial fibrillation, fatigue, and signs of left and right heart failure.	ACEIs, vasodilators, diuretics, digoxin; anticoagulation if atrial fibrillation; valve repair or replacement.
Mitral valve prolapse	Found in 7% of the population, especially young women.	Usually benign and asymptomatic.	Late systolic murmur with midsystolic click.	Can progress to mitral regurgitation.	Endocarditis prophylaxis with amoxicillin before dental procedures if there is associated regurgitation. Treatment of prolapse unnecessary unless symptomatic.

TREATMENT

- In asymptomatic patients, monitoring is appropriate for lesions < 5 cm.
- Surgical repair is indicated if the lesion is > 5.5 cm (abdominal) or > 6 cm (thoracic) or is enlarging rapidly.
- Emergent surgery for symptomatic or ruptured aneurysms.

Aortic Dissection

A transverse tear in the intima of a vessel → blood entering the media, creating a false lumen → a hematoma that propagates longitudinally. Most commonly due to **hypertension.** The most common sites of origin are **above the aortic valve** and **distal to the left subclavian** artery. Occurs most often in people 40–60 years of age, with a greater frequency in men than in women.

HISTORY/PE

- **Sudden tearing/stabbing** pain in the anterior chest in ascending dissection; interscapular back pain in descending dissection.

Aortic aneurysm is most commonly associated with atherosclerosis, while aortic dissection is most commonly associated with hypertension.

Hypercoagulability due to malignancy (usually adenocarcinoma) is known as Trousseau's syndrome.

- The patient is typically **hypertensive.** If a patient is hypotensive, consider pericardial tamponade or acute MI from involvement of coronary arteries.
- Signs of pericarditis or pericardial tamponade may be seen; a murmur of aortic regurgitation may be heard if the aortic valve is involved. Neurologic deficits may be seen if the aortic arch or spinal arteries are involved.

DIAGNOSIS

- ECG, CXR (widening of the mediastinum, cardiomegaly, or new left pleural effusion), CT/MRI.
- **TEE** can provide detail of the thoracic aorta, proximal coronary arteries, origins of arch vessels, presence of a pericardial effusion, and aortic valve integrity.
- There are two systems of classification for aortic dissection:
  - **DeBakey system:** Classifies dissections as involving both the ascending and descending aorta (type I), confined to the ascending aorta (type II), or confined to the descending aorta (type III).
  - **Stanford system:** Classifies dissections of the ascending aorta as type A and all others as type B.

TREATMENT

- ↓ BP and heart rate if the patient is hypertensive. Do **not** use thrombolytics.
- If the dissection involves the ascending aorta, it is a **surgical emergency**; medical therapy for dissection of the descending aorta.

Deep Venous Thrombosis (DVT)

Clot formation in the large veins of the extremities or pelvis. Predisposing factors include venous stasis due to immobilization (e.g., plane flights, bed rest), incompetent venous valves in the lower extremities, CHF, traumatic injury to the lower extremities, hypercoagulable states (e.g., malignancy, OCP use), obesity, and indwelling venous catheters.

HISTORY/PE

- Generally presents with unilateral lower extremity pain, erythema, and swelling.
- **Homans' sign:** Calf tenderness with passive foot dorsiflexion.

DIAGNOSIS

Doppler ultrasound.

TREATMENT

- **Initial anticoagulation with** IV heparin or low-molecular-weight heparin, followed by PO warfarin for a total of 3–6 months.
- Consider an **IVC filter** in patients with contraindications to anticoagulation.
- Hospitalized patients should receive DVT prophylaxis consisting of rapid mobilization, antithromboembolic stockings, leg exercises, and SQ heparin.

Peripheral Vascular Disease

Occlusion of the blood supply to the extremities by atherosclerotic plaques. The lower extremities are most commonly affected. Clinical manifestations depend on the vessels involved, the extent and rapidity of obstruction, and the presence of collateral blood flow.

HISTORY/PE

- Initially presents with **intermittent claudication** (reproducible leg pain that occurs with walking and is always relieved with rest).
- As the disease worsens, there is progression to rest pain and ischemia that affects the distal aspects of the extremities. Dorsal foot ulcerations may develop.
- A painful, cold, numb foot is characteristic of severe ischemia.
- Disease-specific presentations are as follows:
    - **Aortoiliac disease:** Buttock claudication is present and femoral pulses are absent; **impotence** is common in males.
    - **Femoropopliteal disease:** Calf claudication is present; pulses below the femoral artery are absent.
    - **Small vessel disease:** Foot pulses are absent.
    - **Acute ischemia:** Most often caused by **embolization** from the heart; acute occlusions commonly occur at bifurcations distal to the last palpable pulse.
    - **Severe chronic ischemia:** Lack of blood perfusion → muscle atrophy, pallor, cyanosis, hair loss, and gangrene/necrosis.

DIAGNOSIS

- Careful **palpation of pulses** and **auscultation for bruits** are necessary measures.
- Measurement of ankle and brachial systolic BP (**ankle-brachial index, or ABI**) can provide objective evidence of atherosclerosis (rest pain occurs with ABI < 0.4).
- Doppler ultrasound helps identify stenosis and occlusion. Doppler ankle systolic pressure readings that are > 90% of brachial readings are normal.
- Arteriography and digital subtraction angiography are necessary for surgical evaluation.

TREATMENT

- Control of underlying causes (e.g., DM) is crucial. Eliminate tobacco and institute careful hygiene and foot care. **Exercise** helps develop collateral circulation.
- Aspirin, cilostazol, and thromboxane inhibitors may improve symptoms.
- Angioplasty and stenting have a variable success rate that is dependent on the area of occlusion.
- Surgery (arterial bypass) or amputation can be employed when conservative treatment fails.

Claudication is reproducible leg pain that occurs with walking and is relieved with rest.

The 6 P's of acute ischemia:

Pain
Pallor
Pulselessness
Paralysis
Paresthesia
Poikilothermia (cold)

Peripheral vascular insufficiency inspection criteria—

SICVD

Symmetry of leg musculature
Integrity of skin
Color of toenails
Varicose veins
Distribution of hair

HIGH-YIELD FACTS

CARDIOVASCULAR

Dermatology

COMMON TERMINOLOGY FOR SKIN LESIONS

- The skin has three layers: **epidermis, dermis,** and **subcutaneous tissue.** Epidermis protects (ectodermal origin), while dermis supports (mesodermal origin).
- Epidermis is stratified squamous epithelium and has four layers: the stratum basalis (columnar basal cells), stratum spinosum (basal cells divide to become keratinocytes), stratum granulosum (keratinocytes with intracellular granules), and stratum corneum (cells die and become non-nucleated → fused cell remnants).
- See Table 2.2-1 for terms commonly used to describe the spectrum of dermatologic manifestations.

DERMATOLOGIC MANIFESTATIONS OF DIABETES

Acanthosis Nigricans

- **Velvety hyperpigmentation** of the skin associated with **insulin resistance,** endocrine disorders (diabetes, Cushing's syndrome, HAIR-AN syndrome), obesity, drugs, and malignancy (usually GI or lung cancer). May predict the development of **type 2 diabetes** later in life. Its etiology is unclear but may be related to the action of **growth factors** on skin.
- **Hx/PE:** Dark, thickened, **dirty-appearing,** velvety plaques found predominantly in the flexural areas (axillae, neck, and under the breasts and groin), often with **prominent skin lines** (see Figure 2.2-1).
- **Dx:** Histology shows **hyperkeratosis** and proliferation of **melanocytes.** Evaluation should include a fasting glucose to rule out DM.
- **Rx:** Aimed at the underlying disorder—e.g., weight reduction for obesity and insulin resistance or search for occult malignancy.

Erythrasma

- Caused by *Corynebacterium minutissimum* and other *Corynebacterium* spp; prevalent among **diabetics** and in warm climates.
- **Hx/PE:** A slowly enlarging area of pink or brown macular patches is seen, predominantly affecting the **flexor surfaces** (axilla, groin, intertriginous areas; see Figure 2.2-2). Typically not symptomatic.
- **Dx:** **Wood's light** causes lesions to **fluoresce coral pink or red** owing to porphyrins released by the bacteria. KOH prep is ⊖.
- **Rx:** Topical or oral erythromycin.

IMMUNE-MEDIATED LESIONS

Table 2.2-2 outlines the types and mechanisms of hypersensitivity reactions. Descriptions of common immune-mediated lesions follow.

Atopic Dermatitis/Eczema

A relapsing inflammatory skin disorder characterized by **pruritus.** Persistent scratching → **lichenification.**

HISTORY/PE

- Dry, scaly, itchy patches and plaques with excoriations in the **flexural areas (elbows, knees, antecubital fossae, buttocks) and neck.**

> **HAIR-AN syndrome:**
>
> **H**yperAndrogenism
> **I**nsulin **R**esistance
> **A**canthosis **N**igricans

> **Causes of generalized hyperpigmentation—**
>
> **"None of the skin is SPARED"**
>
> **S**unlight
> **P**regnancy
> **A**ddison's disease
> **R**enal failure
> **E**xcess iron (hemochromatosis)
> **D**rugs (e.g., busulfan)

Common drugs causing hyperpigmentation include minocycline, amiodarone, chloroquine, gold, chlorpromazine, bleomycin, 5-FU, and daunorubicin.

> **Gell and Coombs classification of hypersensitivity reactions—**
>
> **ACID**
>
> **A**naphylactic–type I
> **C**ytotoxic–type II
> **I**mmune complex– type III
> **D**elayed hypersensitivity– type IV

HIGH-YIELD FACTS

DERMATOLOGY

TABLE 2.2-1. **Common Terms Used to Describe Skin Lesions**

TERM	DEFINITION
Macule	Flat area of skin discoloration < 1 cm in diameter.
Papule	Elevated area of skin < 1 cm in diameter.
Plaque	Elevated area of skin > 1 cm in diameter.
Nodule	Elevated and deep (continues beneath skin) area of skin > 0.5 cm in diameter.
Cyst	Nodule containing fluid.
Vesicle	Fluid-containing skin elevation < 0.5 cm in diameter.
Wheal	Transient, pruritic, edematous papule or plaque.
Bulla	Fluid collection in elevated skin > 0.5 cm in diameter.
Pustule	Papule containing purulent fluid.
Petechiae	Nonblanching, flat, red/purple lesions caused by thrombocytopenia-associated microhemorrhages.
Purpura	Visible collection of extravasated RBCs.
Telangiectasia	Visible dilated capillaries on the surface of the skin.
Hyperkeratosis	Thickening of the stratum corneum.
Keloid	Scar tissue hypertrophy.
Scale	Thick, detached areas of stratum corneum.
Crust	Dried exudate.
Excoriation	Shallow abrasion caused by scratching.
Erosion	Loss of epidermis above the basal layer.
Ulcer	Loss of epidermis and part or all of the dermis.
Nevus	Benign growth, such as a mole, that is a cluster of melanocytes.

The allergic triad consists of atopic dermatitis, asthma, and hay fever.

- Most patients first develop symptoms in infancy.
- Triggers include skin irritants (**dry skin,** wool clothing, perfume), stress (emotional, infection), airborne allergens (dust mites, pollens), and, rarely, foods (eggs, milk, peanuts, seafood, wheat, soybeans).
- Associated with **asthma** and **allergic rhinitis.** A personal or family history of the "allergic or atopic triad" is common.

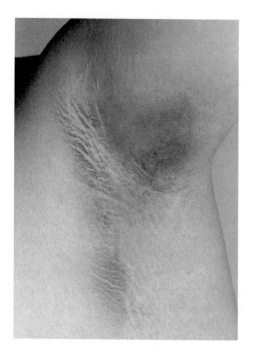

FIGURE 2.2-1. Acanthosis nigricans.

Velvety, dark brown epidermal thickening of the armpit with prominent skin fold and feathered edges. (Reproduced, with permission, from Wolff K, Johnson RA, Suurmond D. *Fitzpatrick's Color Atlas & Synopsis of Clinical Dermatology*, 5th ed. New York: McGraw-Hill, 2005:87.)

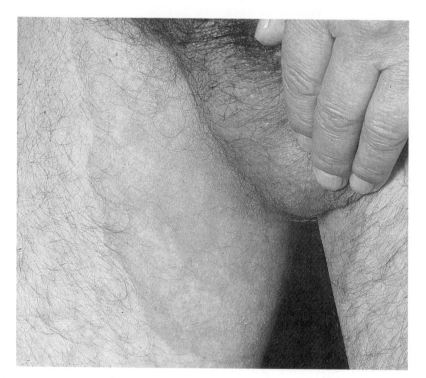

FIGURE 2.2-2. Erythrasma of the groin.

Sharply marginated, brownish-red, slightly scaling macular patches on the inguinal area (infectious intertrigo) appear bright coral-red when examined with a Wood's lamp. (Reproduced, with permission, from Wolff K, Johnson RA, Suurmond D. *Fitzpatrick's Color Atlas & Synopsis of Clinical Dermatology*, 5th ed. New York: McGraw-Hill, 2005:581.)

TABLE 2.2-2. Types and Mechanisms of Hypersensitivity Reactions

TYPE	MECHANISM	OTHER/COMMENTS
Type I	**Anaphylactic and atopic**—Antigen cross-links IgE on presensitized mast cells and basophils, triggering release of vasoactive amines (i.e., histamine). Reaction develops rapidly after antigen exposure due to preformed antibody. Examples include anaphylaxis, asthma, and local wheal and flare.	**First** and **Fast** (anaphylaxis). I, II, and III are all antibody mediated.
Type II	**Cytotoxic**—IgM, IgG bind to antigen on "enemy" cell, leading to lysis (by complement) or phagocytosis. Examples include autoimmune hemolytic anemia, Rh disease (erythroblastosis fetalis), Goodpasture's syndrome, and rheumatic fever.	Cy-**2**-toxic. Antibody and complement lead to membrane attack complex (MAC).
Type III	**Immune complex**—Antigen-antibody complexes activate complement, which attracts neutrophils; neutrophils release lysosomal enzymes. Examples include PAN, immune complex glomerulonephritis, SLE, and rheumatoid arthritis. **Serum sickness**—an immune complex disease (type III) in which antibodies to the foreign proteins are produced (takes five days). Immune complexes form and are deposited in membranes, where they fix complement (leads to tissue damage). More common than Arthus reaction. **Arthus reaction**—A local subacute antibody-mediated hypersensitivity (type III) reaction. Intradermal injection of antigen induces antibodies, which form antigen-antibody complexes in the skin. Characterized by edema, necrosis, and activation of complement. Examples include hypersensitivity pneumonitis, and thermophilic actinomycetes.	Imagine an immune complex as three things stuck together: antigen-antibody complement. Most serum sickness is now caused by drugs (not serum). Fever, urticaria, arthralgias, proteinuria, lymphadenopathy 5–10 days after antigen exposure. Antigen-antibody complexes cause the Arthus reaction.
Type IV	**Delayed (cell-mediated) type**—Sensitized T lymphocytes encounter antigen and then release lymphokines (leads to macrophage activation). Examples include TB skin test, transplant rejection, and contact dermatitis (e.g., poison ivy, poison oak).	**4th** and last—delayed. Cell mediated; therefore, it is not transferable by serum.

- Also associated with an ↑ **risk of impetigo and cellulitis**, severe **HSV-1** skin infection (**eczema herpeticum**), viral warts, and *Molluscum contagiosum*.

Eczema is an "itch that rashes."

DIAGNOSIS

Clinical impression. **IgE** levels may be ↑. Skin prick tests are not recommended.

TREATMENT

Treat with mild soaps and emollients, topical steroids, topical tacrolimus, PUVA phototherapy, and methotrexate.

Bullous Pemphigoid

Chronic blistering eruptions on an inflamed base. More common in those > 60 years of age. Due to autoantibodies to **BP1 and BP2** found in the basement membrane of the skin.

■ Prodromal erythematous, papular lesions → **large, tense, pruritic bullae** filled with serous to bloody fluid → **deep** erosions and crusts from collapsed bullae.
■ **Rarely involves the mucous membranes;** usually seen on the upper arms and thighs (see Figure 2.2-3).
■ **Pruritic,** but not usually painful.
■ ⊖ Nikolsky's sign.

DIAGNOSIS

Immunostaining shows fluorescence at the **dermal-epidermal** junction.

TREATMENT

Topical steroids for mild cases; oral steroids if severe.

Pemphigus

Shallow, painful erosions and blisters on **epidermal and mucosal** surfaces due to autoantibodies against **desmocollins and desmogleins** (transmembrane desmosomal glycoproteins) in the epidermis. **Pemphigus vulgaris** is the most common form.

HISTORY/PE

■ Slowly developing, shallow erosions on mucous membranes → skin involvement. Blisters are easily ruptured by friction or pressure → shallow ulcerations.

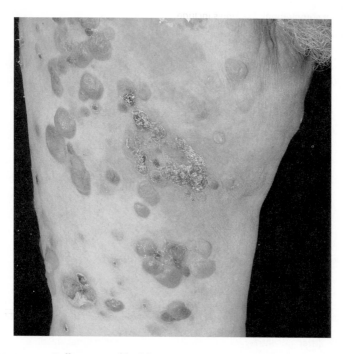

FIGURE 2.2-3. **Bullous pemphigoid.**

Multiple tense serous and partially hemorrhagic bullae can be seen. (Reproduced, with permission, from Fitzpatrick TB. *Color Atlas & Synopsis of Clinical Dermatology*, 4th ed. New York: McGraw-Hill, 2001:100.)

HIGH-YIELD FACTS

DERMATOLOGY

- Onset is between 40 and 60 years of age.
- ⊕ **Nikolsky's sign** (pressing **normal-appearing** skin with a sliding motion separates the epidermis from the basal layer and rubs skin off).
- Associated with epistaxis, hoarseness, weakness, malaise, and weight loss.
- Table 2.2-3 contrasts pemphigus with bullous pemphigoid.

DIAGNOSIS

- **Immunologic staining** of skin biopsy shows autoantibodies against epidermal **intercellular** material.
- **Acantholysis** (in which individual keratinocytes detach from their neighbors and float free) may be seen on biopsy.
- ↑ serum levels of antibodies to desmoglein 1 and 3 correlate with disease activity.

TREATMENT

- Oral steroids. Patients must continue steroids to prevent recurrence. Immunosuppressants such as azathioprine can be used to ↓ steroid dose.
- Severe cases may require plasmapheresis.
- Lesions should be cared for as burns.

Contact Dermatitis

A skin rash that develops from contact with a substance to which the patient has previously been sensitized. A delayed type IV hypersensitivity reaction. Common offending agents include poison ivy, poison oak, nickel, perfumes, soaps and detergents, and cosmetics.

HISTORY/PE

- Commonly presents with pruritus and rash, but may also present with edema, fever, lymphadenopathy, and generalized malaise.
- Erythematous, weepy, and crusted patches, plaques, or papulovesicles are grouped in linear arrays or geometric shapes with sharp angles and straight borders (see Figure 2.2-4).

TABLE 2.2-3. Pemphigus vs. Bullous Pemphigoid

	PEMPHIGUS	BULLOUS PEMPHIGOID
Location	Mucous membranes, skin.	Only the skin; usually the arms and thighs.
Autoantibody target	Desmocollins, desmogleins.	BP1 and BP2.
Location of autoantibodies	Intercellular.	Epidermal-dermal junction.
Location of blister	Intraepidermal, shallow.	Subepidermal, deep.
Nikolsky's sign	⊕	⊖
Symptoms	Painful.	Itchy.

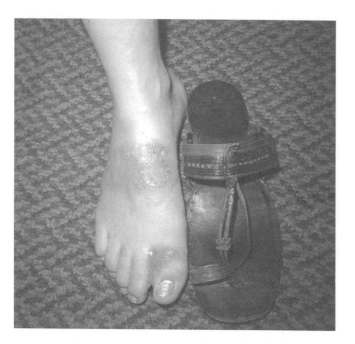

FIGURE 2.2-4. Contact dermatitis.

Shown above are erythematous papules and vesicles with serous weeping localized to areas of contact with the offending agent. (Reproduced, with permission, from Hurwitz RM. *Pathology of the Skin: Atlas of Clinical-Pathological Correlation*, 2nd ed. Stamford, CT: Appleton & Lange, 1998:3.)

- Characteristic distribution includes locations where makeup, clothing, perfume, **nickel** jewelry, and plants contact the skin.

DIAGNOSIS

Clinical impression and, if necessary, **skin patch** testing.

TREATMENT

- **Mild cases:** Cool compresses or oatmeal preparation; topical steroids 3–4 times a day to reduce pruritus.
- **Severe cases:** An extended course of systemic corticosteroids may be required; antihistamines to reduce pruritus.

Erythema Multiforme

An immune-mediated **cutaneous** disorder that is due to **drugs** (e.g., penicillin, sulfonamides, phenytoin), **infection** (especially HSV and *Mycoplasma*), **vaccinations,** or **malignancy.** Exists in a continuum with Stevens-Johnson syndrome (SJS) and toxic epidermal necrolysis (TEN) (see the discussion of SJS/TEN and Table 2.2-4).

HISTORY/PE

- Mild prodrome of malaise and myalgias.
- Lesions are most commonly seen on the extremities. Involves < 10% of body surface area (BSA).
- Raised erythematous plaques expand laterally to form target lesions (see Figure 2.2-5).

Think HSV infection with recurrent erythema multiforme.

TABLE 2.2-4. Erythema Multiforme vs. SJS and TEN

	ERYTHEMA MULTIFORME	SJS	TEN
% BSA involvement	< 10%	< 10%	> 30%
Cutaneous vs. mucosal involvement	Usually involves only skin.	Involves skin and mucosa.	Involves skin and mucosa.
Histology	Perivascular T lymphocytes; necrotic keratinocytes.	Perivascular mononuclear cells with eosinophils in the papillary dermis; degeneration of the basal layer; subepidermal blister formation.	Full-thickness, eosinophilic epidermal necrosis; cell-poor infiltrate with predominance of macrophages and dendrocytes; strong immunoreactivity for TNF-α.

- Less commonly involves the mucosa; severe mucosal involvement is defined as SJS.

DIAGNOSIS

- Look for a history of exposure to causative agents.
- Eosinophilia or ⊕ serologic tests for hepatitis, infectious mononucleosis, histoplasmosis, or *Mycoplasma*.
- Skin biopsy shows **perivascular lymphocytes** (mostly **T cells**) and **necrotic keratinocytes.**

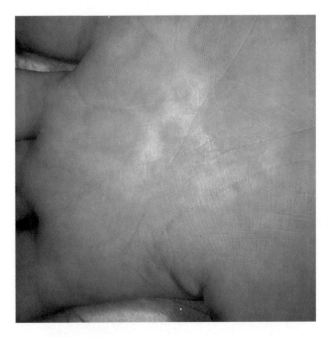

FIGURE 2.2-5. Erythema multiforme.

Evolving erythematous plaques and papules are seen with a target appearance consisting of a dull red center, a pale zone, and a darker outer ring. (Reproduced, with permission, from Hurwitz RM. *Pathology of the Skin: Atlas of Clinical-Pathological Correlation*, 2nd ed. Stamford, CT: Appleton & Lange, 1998:24.)

HIGH-YIELD FACTS

DERMATOLOGY

- Mild cases resolve spontaneously.
- If drug induced, discontinue the inciting agent.
- If due to HSV, give acyclovir.

Erythema Nodosum

Inflammation of the subcutaneous fat that produces tender **erythematous nodules,** usually on the **anterior tibial** areas (see Figure 2.2-6). Lesions result from **hypersensitivity reactions** to drugs (OCPs, NSAIDs) or from infections (α-hemolytic streptococci, coccidioidomycosis, histoplasmosis, TB, syphilis), **sarcoid, rheumatic fever,** or **IBD.** Most commonly found in young women.

HISTORY/PE

- Painful, erythematous bilateral pretibial nodules without ulceration. Rarely occurs on the face, arms, and trunk.
- Malaise, arthralgias, and fever may precede rash.

DIAGNOSIS

- Incisional wedge biopsy provides a definitive diagnosis.
- ↑ ESR, mild leukocytosis, ↑ ASO titer, or a false-⊕ VDRL may be seen.
- CXR, cultures, and Gram stain of lesion. Gram stain should be ⊖, since erythema nodosum is a reactive lesion.

NSAIDs are both a precipitating factor and a treatment for erythema nodosum.

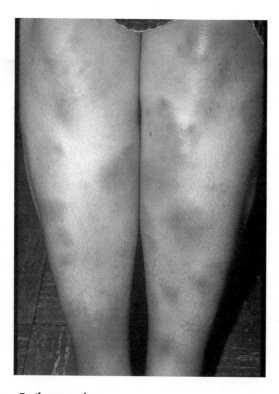

FIGURE 2.2-6. Erythema nodosum.

Erythematous plaques and nodules are commonly located on pretibial areas. Lesions are painful and indurated but heal spontaneously without ulceration. (Reproduced, with permission, from Hurwitz RM. *Pathology of the Skin: Atlas of Clinical-Pathological Correlation,* 2nd ed. Stamford, CT: Appleton & Lange, 1998:132.)

TREATMENT

- Supportive. Elevate leg, bed rest, potassium iodide, NSAIDs.
- Systemic corticosteroids may be necessary for persistent cases.

Lichen Planus

An inflammatory dermatosis involving skin and mucous membranes. Often induced by **drugs** and strongly associated with **HCV**.

HISTORY/PE

- Acute or chronic, flat-topped, purple, polygonal pruritic papules with an overlying network of white lines (**Wickham's striae**) are seen on the inner wrists and lower legs (see Figure 2.2-7).
- Reticulate white hyperkeratosis on the mucosal surfaces is also common.

DIAGNOSIS

Biopsy shows inflammation with hyperkeratosis, an ↑ granular layer, and bandlike mononuclear infiltrate in the superficial dermis.

TREATMENT

Topical steroids and oral antihistamines to reduce itch; severe cases require cyclosporine, oral prednisone, oral retinoids, and PUVA.

> **The 4 P's of lichen planus:**
>
> **P**olygonal
> **P**urple
> **P**ruritic
> **P**apules

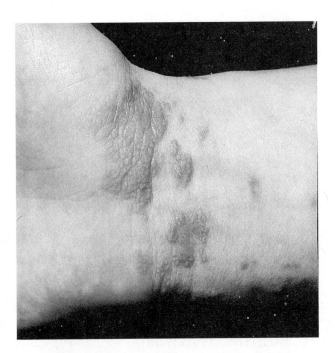

FIGURE 2.2-7. Lichen planus.

Flat-topped, polygonal, sharply defined papules of violaceous color are grouped and confluent. The surface is shiny and reveals fine white lines (Wickham's striae). (Reproduced, with permission, from Wolff K, Johnson RA, Suurmond D. *Fitzpatrick's Color Atlas & Synopsis of Clinical Dermatology*, 5th ed. New York: McGraw-Hill, 2005:125.)

Psoriasis

A **T-cell-mediated** inflammatory disorder → epidermal **hyperproliferation**.

HISTORY/PE

- Presents with dark red plaques with silvery-white scales and sharp margins classically found over the extensor surfaces (see Figure 2.2-8).
- Typically **not** pruritic.
- Characteristic nail findings include nail pitting, "oil spots," and onycholysis (lifting of the nail plate).
- Pain, tenderness, and joint stiffness occur with psoriatic arthritis (classically in the **DIP joints**).
- Fever and malaise occur with the generalized pustular form.

DIAGNOSIS

- Skin biopsy shows a **thickened epidermis** with absent granular cell layer and preservation of nuclei within a **hyperkeratotic** stratum corneum.
- **Munro microabscesses** (neutrophils in stratum corneum) are classic.
- ↑ uric acid levels, ↑ ESR, and mild anemia.

TREATMENT

- Topical steroids and topical calcipotriol for mild to moderate disease.
- Phototherapy and immunosuppressants such as methotrexate for severe or generalized disease.
- Biologic agents (e.g., infliximab, etanercept).

Seborrheic Dermatitis

A chronic superficial inflammatory disorder thought to be a reaction to *Pityrosporum* yeast.

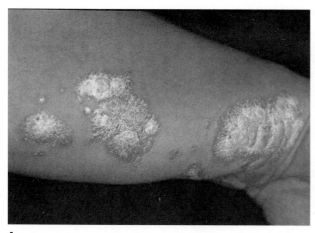

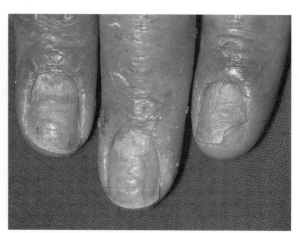

A

B

FIGURE 2.2-8. Psoriasis.

(A) Skin changes. The classic sharply demarcated plaques with silvery scales are commonly located on the extensor surfaces (e.g., elbows, knees). (B) Nail changes. Note the pitting, onycholysis, and "oil spots." (Reproduced, with permission, from Hurwitz RM. *Pathology of the Skin: Atlas of Clinical-Pathological Correlation*, 2nd ed. Stamford, CT: Appleton & Lange, 1998:15, 18.)

HISTORY/PE

- Presents with pruritus during the neonatal and postpubertal periods.
- Yellowish, greasy, and erythematous scaling patches and plaques are seen on the scalp ("**cradle cap**"), ears, and face.

TREATMENT

- Give 1% hydrocortisone and topical antifungals for the face, body, and intertriginous areas.
- Treat the scalp with medicated shampoos containing selenium sulfide or zinc pyrithione.

Stevens-Johnson Syndrome/Toxic Epidermal Necrolysis (SJS/TEN)

A life-threatening exfoliative **mucocutaneous** disease often caused by a drug-induced immunologic reaction (see Figure 2.2-9). SJS involves < 10% BSA of epidermal separation; TEN involves ≥ 30% BSA. Involvement of 10–30% is termed **overlap SJS-TEN**. The most commonly implicated agents are sulfa drugs, carbamazepine, phenytoin, valproic acid, phenobarbital, quinolones, cephalosporins, allopurinol, corticosteroids, and aminopenicillins.

HISTORY/PE

- Presents with a flulike prodrome, skin tenderness, painful mouth lesions, and a history of new-drug exposure, often within 1–3 weeks of initial exposure.
- Morbilliform rash evolves into coalescing red macules and flaccid blisters with full-thickness epidermal loss.
- ⊕ Nikolsky's sign.
- The leading cause of mortality is **sepsis** from superimposed bacterial skin infections (**S. aureus** in the early stages; gram-⊖ rods such as **Pseudomonas** in later stages).

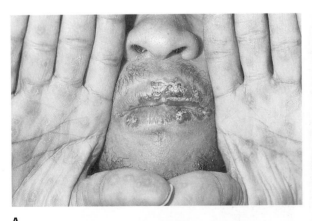
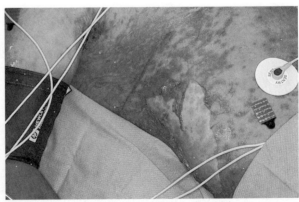

A   B

FIGURE 2.2-9. **Stevens-Johnson syndrome and toxic epidermal necrolysis.**

(A) Stevens-Johnson syndrome. Note the target lesions on the hands as well as the mucosal involvement on the lips. (B) Toxic epidermal necrolysis. The initial bullae have coalesced → extensive exfoliation of the epidermis. (Figure B courtesy of Keith Batts, MD. Reproduced, with permission, from Knoop KJ et al. *Atlas of Emergency Medicine*, 2nd ed. New York: McGraw-Hill, 2002:379, 380.)

DIAGNOSIS

- **SJS skin biopsy: Perivascular mononuclear infiltrate** with some eosinophils in the papillary dermis; degeneration of the **basal layer;** and, in severe cases, subepidermal blister formation.
- **TEN skin biopsy: Full-thickness,** eosinophilic epidermal necrosis is seen along with a cell-poor infiltrate with a predominance of **macrophages and dendrocytes** and a strong immunoreactivity for **TNF-α.**

TREATMENT

- Early diagnosis and elimination of offending agents.
- Analgesia and IVIG. The use of systemic corticosteroids is controversial.
- Hospitalize in the **burn ICU** to manage skin and fluid losses.

Vitiligo

Areas of acquired cutaneous depigmentation due to loss of **melanocytes.** Has a significant association with **autoimmune diseases.**

HISTORY/PE

- Irregular white patches due to slowly progressive loss of melanin pigment (see Figure 2.2-10).
- More common in dark-skinned people and those with a ⊕ family history.
- Associated with thyroid disease in 30% of patients.

DIAGNOSIS

- Antimelanocyte antibodies are found in some patients.
- Absence of epidermal melanocytes on skin biopsy.

With vitiligo, consider other autoimmune diseases, such as pernicious anemia, thyroid disease, Addison's disease, and type I DM.

TREATMENT

Topical artificial tanning creams, steroid/tretinoin creams, or phototherapy can be used. Lesions can be refractory.

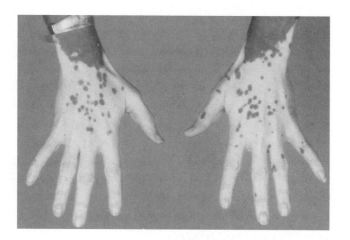

FIGURE 2.2-10.   Vitiligo.

Shown above is vitiligo in a typical acral distribution demonstrating striking cutaneous depigmentation as a result of melanocyte loss. (Reproduced, with permission, from Kasper DL et al [eds]. *Harrison's Principles of Internal Medicine*, 16th ed. New York: McGraw-Hill, 2005:288.)

Acne Vulgaris

Blockage of hair follicles by sebum and keratinous material → formation of cysts (**comedones**). Lipophilic bacteria (***Propionibacterium acnes***) within comedones break down sebum into free fatty acids → rupture of cysts and inflammatory foreign-body reaction.

HISTORY/PE

- Associated with changes in **androgen** levels.
- Found primarily during puberty; more common in males than in females.
- Open comedones (blackheads) and closed comedones (whiteheads) are found on the face, neck, arms, back, and buttocks.
- Drug-related acne is associated with lithium, steroids, OCPs, and androgens.

TREATMENT

- **Mild acne:** Topical clindamycin or erythromycin; benzoyl peroxide; topical retinoids.
- **Moderate acne:** The above regimen plus **oral antibiotics** such as tetracycline.
- **Severe nodulocystic acne:** Oral **isotretinoin** (Accutane).

*Isotretinoin is **teratogenic,** so women must have pregnancy testing before and during therapy.*

Cellulitis/Folliculitis

Skin infections typically caused by streptococci or staphylococci (most commonly *S. aureus*).

HISTORY/PE

- Folliculitis is infection of hair follicles, commonly in the distribution of facial hair.
- **Cellulitis** is infection of subcutaneous tissue. Presents with red, hot, swollen skin lesions. Fever and chills may also be present. Risk factors include diabetes, IV drug use, venous stasis, and immunocompromised states.

Pseudomonas aeruginosa causes "hot tub folliculitis."

DIAGNOSIS

Clinical impression. Wound culture may aid diagnosis. Blood cultures should be obtained if bacteremia is suspected.

TREATMENT

- For mild to moderate cases, give oral antibiotics (cephalexin or dicloxacillin) × 7–10 days.
- Hospitalize and give IV antibiotics in the presence of any signs of systemic toxicity, comorbid conditions, DM, extremes of age, or hand or orbital involvement.

Fungal Infections

Fungi can lead to a variety of skin changes.

PITYRIASIS VERSICOLOR

A common superficial fungal infection caused by *Malassezia furfur*. Also called tinea versicolor.

- **Hx/PE:** Small, scaling, hyper- or hypopigmented macules that tend to enlarge and sometimes coalesce. Lesions are usually asymptomatic but may cause mild itching. The usual sites are the chest and back.
- **Dx:** KOH prep reveals short, blunt hyphae and small spores ("spaghetti and meatballs"). Wood's light examination helps evaluate the extent of disease.
- **Rx:** Topical antifungal agents and selenium sulfide shampoo.

TINEA CORPORIS/CAPITIS

- Fungal infection of the body/scalp.
- **Hx/PE:** Pruritic, ring-shaped (also known as "ringworm"), erythematous, and scaling plaques, often with central clearing and elevated borders (see Figure 2.2-11).
- **Dx:** Hyphae are seen on KOH prep.
- **Rx:** Topical antifungal cream for tinea corporis; oral antifungals for tinea capitis and tinea unguium (nail infection).

Tinea capitis often affects children and can cause an inflammatory, granulomatous reaction of the scalp called a kerion.

Herpes Simplex

A painful, recurrent vesicular eruption of mucocutaneous surfaces due to HSV infection.

HISTORY/PE

- 1° outbreaks are longer and more severe than recurrent eruptions.
- Onset is preceded by prodromal tingling, burning, or frank pain. Also pre-

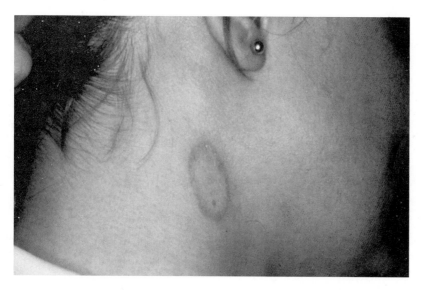

FIGURE 2.2-11. Tinea corporis.

A superficial fungal infection, seen here as an erythematous, annular, scaly plaque with central clearing. (Reproduced, with permission, from Kasper DL et al [eds.]. *Harrison's Principles of Internal Medicine*, 16th ed. New York: McGraw-Hill, 2005:1191.)

sents with lymphadenopathy, fever, discomfort, malaise, and edema of involved tissue.

- Grouped vesicles are seen on an erythematous base (see Figure 2.2-12A).
- Recurrent infections are limited to mucocutaneous areas innervated by the **involved nerve.**

DIAGNOSIS

- Multinucleated giant cells are seen on Tzanck smear (see Figure 2.2-12B).
- Because VZV has the same appearance, definitive diagnosis requires culture or DFA testing.
- The oral-labial form is due primarily to HSV-1; the genital form is due primarily to HSV-2.

TREATMENT

- Acyclovir ointment reduces the duration of viral shedding but does not prevent recurrence.
- Oral or IV acyclovir reduces both the frequency and severity of recurrences.
- Daily acyclovir suppressive therapy is used in patients with > 6 outbreaks per year.

Impetigo

A contagious and autoinoculable skin infection caused by staphylococci or streptococci. Affects children more often than adults.

HISTORY/PE

- Presents with pruritic facial lesions with **honey-colored crusts;** commonly found on the face, neck, and extremities (see Figure 2.2-13).

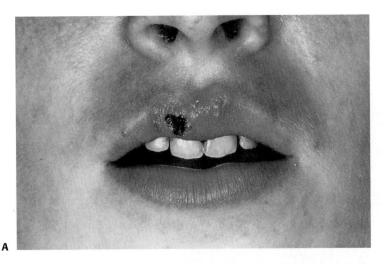 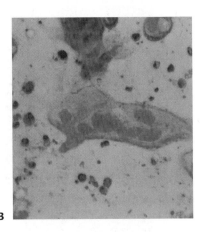

A   B

FIGURE 2.2-12. **Herpes simplex.**

(A) 1° infection. Grouped vesicles on an erythematous base on the patient's lips and oral mucosa may progress to pustules before resolving. (B) Tzanck smear. The multinucleated giant cells from vesicular fluid provide a presumptive diagnosis of HSV infection. The Tzanck smear cannot distinguish between HSV and VZV infection. (Reproduced, with permission, from Hurwitz RM. *Pathology of the Skin: Atlas of Clinical-Pathological Correlation,* 2nd ed. Stamford, CT: Appleton & Lange, 1998:145.)

- **Nonbullous impetigo:** Characterized by superficial pustules with surrounding erythema.
- **Bullous impetigo:** Begins as small, erythematous macules → thin-walled vesicles or bullae on an erythematous base. Caused by coagulase-⊕ **staphylococci** that produce **exfoliatin,** a toxin.

DIAGNOSIS

Diagnosed by clinical impression; bacterial cultures for sensitivities.

TREATMENT

- Wash lesions with mild soap.
- Topical mupirocin is effective only against coagulase-⊕ *S. aureus.*
- Systemic antibiotics have activity against both staphylococci and streptococci.
- Because of the contagion risk, patients' towels and washcloths should be segregated.

Infectious Rashes

Table 2.2-5 describes classic rashes seen with common infectious diseases.

Lice

- A parasitic infection of the scalp (*Pediculus capitis*), body (*Pediculus corporis*), or pubic area (*Phthirus pubis*).
- **History/PE:** Pruritus.
- **Dx:** Microscopic exam of hair shaft; nits fluoresce blue under Wood's lamp.
- **Rx:** Permethrin shampoo or cream; decontaminate sources of reinfection such as combs, bed sheets, and clothing.

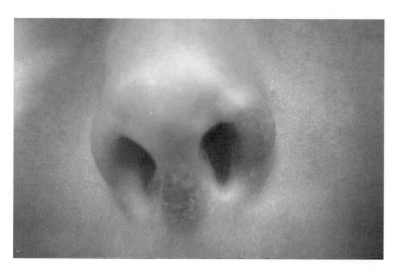

FIGURE 2.2-13. Impetigo.

Dried pustules with a superficial golden-brown crust are most commonly found around the nose and mouth. (Reproduced, with permission, from Hurwitz RM. *Pathology of the Skin: Atlas of Clinical-Pathological Correlation,* 2nd ed. Stamford, CT: Appleton & Lange, 1998:165.)

TABLE 2.2-5. **Rashes Associated with Common Infectious Diseases**

INFECTIOUS DISEASE	RASH	OTHER SYMPTOMS
Measles (rubeola)	Koplik's spots (white spots on buccal mucosa), usually occurring three days after a high fever. Also has a maculopapular rash that spreads from the head downward.	Cough, coryza (inflammation of nasal mucosa), conjunctivitis.
Rubella	Maculopapular rash spreads from the head downward.	Swelling of suboccipital and postauricular nodes; low-grade fever; malaise; arthralgias.
Erythema infectiosum (fifth disease)	"Slapped-cheek" rash of confluent erythema over the cheeks, followed by a maculopapular rash on the trunk and extremities 1–2 days later.	Low-grade fever, malaise. Caused by parvovirus B19.
Chickenpox (varicella)	Macules (usually trunk) → papules → vesicles → rupture and crusting. Crops of lesions in different stages are usually seen. The classic description is of a "dewdrop on a rose petal": a clear vesicle on an erythematous base.	Fever. Patients are at risk for bacterial superinfection of lesions.
Scarlet fever	Sandpaper-like rash on the trunk; "strawberry" tongue; circumoral pallor. The rash desquamates after a few days.	Occurs in patients with untreated streptococcal pharyngitis. Treat with penicillin to prevent rheumatic fever.
Rocky Mountain spotted fever	The rash first appears on the palms and soles and then spreads to the trunk and face.	History of tick bite; high fever, chills, headache.
Lyme disease	Erythema chronicum migrans presents with a circular lesion with central clearing, described as a "bull's eye." May also be uniformly red. Found in moist, warm areas of the body where the tick initially bites, such as the axillae, behind the knees, or in the inguinal area.	History of tick bite; fatigue, malaise, headache, arthralgias, lymphadenopathy, neurologic deficits.

Molluscum Contagiosum

A poxvirus infection most commonly found in young **children** and **AIDS** patients.

HISTORY/PE

If you see large molluscum contagiosum lesions, think HIV.

- Presents with 2- to 5-mm discrete, dome-shaped, shiny papules, frequently with central umbilication (see Figure 2.2-14).
- In children, lesions are commonly found on the trunk, extremities, and face. In adults, they are more frequently found in perianal and perigenital areas.
- If lesions are found in other areas, suspect immunocompromise.
- Lesions are asymptomatic unless they are inflamed or irritated.

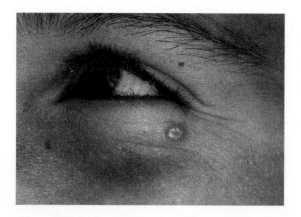

FIGURE 2.2-14. Molluscum contagiosum.

The dome-shaped, fleshy, umbilicated papule on the child's eyelid is characteristic. (Reproduced, with permission, from Hurwitz RM. *Pathology of the Skin: Atlas of Clinical-Pathological Correlation*, 2nd ed. Stamford, CT: Appleton & Lange, 1998:149.)

DIAGNOSIS

Express the contents of the papule and apply Giemsa or Wright's stain; look for large inclusion or molluscum bodies.

TREATMENT

- Lesions resolve spontaneously over months to years and are often left untreated in children.
- Curettage, liquid nitrogen cryotherapy, or application of trichloroacetic acid.

Necrotizing Fasciitis

A rapidly developing infection of skin and fascia that has high mortality without emergent treatment. Caused by group A streptococci, mixed aerobic-anaerobic bacteria, or *Clostridium perfringens*.

HISTORY/PE

- Predisposing factors include peripheral vascular disease, DM, surgery, and breaches in the skin or mucosa.
- Pain and unexplained fever may be the only presenting manifestations.
- Swelling, tenderness, induration, or bullae → friable skin with discoloration.
- Infection extends to fascia and spreads rapidly → shock and multiorgan failure if not treated (see Figure 2.2-15).
- **Fournier's gangrene** is necrotizing fasciitis of the perineal region.

DIAGNOSIS

Diagnosed by clinical impression.

TREATMENT

- Surgery to explore deep fascia and muscle and to remove necrotic tissue.
- Gram stain and culture of tissue to determine appropriate antibiotic therapy.

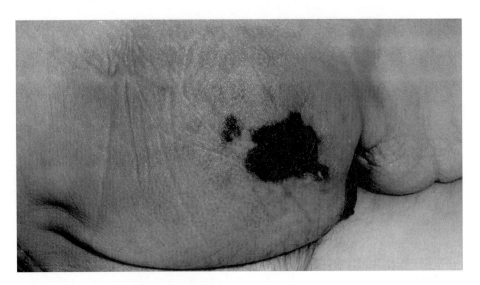

FIGURE 2.2-15. **Necrotizing fasciitis.**

Shown above is an erythematous, edematous plaque involving the entire buttock with a rapidly progressive area of necrosis. (Reproduced, with permission, from Wolff K, Johnson RA, Suurmond D. *Fitzpatrick's Color Atlas & Synopsis of Clinical Dermatology*, 5th ed. New York: McGraw-Hill, 2005:616.)

Pityriasis Rosea

A mild, self-limited cutaneous eruption associated with HHV-6.

HISTORY/PE

- Usually seen in children who present with pruritus.
- Characterized by a diffuse eruption of round to oval erythematous papules and plaques covered with a fine, "cigarette paper" white scale.
- A **Christmas-tree pattern** is seen on the trunk (see Figure 2.2-16) with a classic **herald patch** (a solitary patch that precedes the rest of the rash).

DIAGNOSIS

Consider 2° syphilis in the differential diagnosis.

TREATMENT

Lesions are self-limited, but pruritus may require treatment.

Scabies

Caused by parasitic infection with *Sarcoptes scabiei*, which burrows into the skin to lay eggs.

HISTORY/PE

- Associated with crowded and dirty living conditions. Mites are passed from person to person.
- Presents with pruritus that worsens at night and after hot showers. Symptoms result from a hypersensitivity reaction to mite feces.
- Excoriations, papules, and vesicles are seen, as are mite burrows on the wrists and between the fingers, elbows, and intertriginous areas.

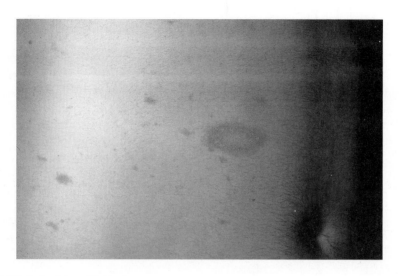

FIGURE 2.2-16. Pityriasis rosea.

The round to oval erythematous plaques are often covered with a fine white scale ("cigarette paper") and are often found on the trunk and proximal extremities. Plaques are often preceded by a larger herald patch (arrow). (Reproduced, with permission, from Hurwitz RM. *Pathology of the Skin: Atlas of Clinical-Pathological Correlation*, 2nd ed. Stamford, CT: Appleton & Lange, 1998:13.)

DIAGNOSIS

Deep scrapings of skin lesions with oil or KOH preparation reveal mites, eggs, or feces.

TREATMENT

- Treat with 5% permethrin cream; give antihistamines for pruritus.
- Treat close contacts; wash bedding and clothing to prevent reinfestation.

Varicella Zoster

1° infection with VZV causes chickenpox (see Table 2.2-5). Latent infection in the sensory **dorsal root ganglia** may reactivate → herpes zoster or "shingles."

HISTORY/PE

- Herpes zoster commonly occurs in the elderly or immunocompromised.
- A prodrome of fever, dysesthesias, malaise, and headache precedes vesicular eruption by days.
- Painful, unilateral vesicular eruptions occur in a dermatomal distribution (see Figure 2.2-17).

DIAGNOSIS

Usually clinical, but a Tzanck smear can be done to look for multinucleated giant cells if the diagnosis is uncertain.

TREATMENT

Antivirals (acyclovir, valacyclovir) within 72 hours of appearance of lesions. Give IV antivirals if patients are immunocompromised; otherwise, oral antivirals are sufficient.

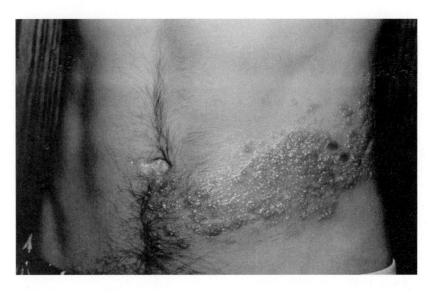

FIGURE 2.2-17. Varicella zoster.

The unilateral dermatomal distribution of the grouped vesicles on an erythematous base is characteristic. (Reproduced courtesy of the Yale University Department of Dermatology.)

HPV (most commonly HPV 16, 18, 31 and 33) also causes cervical cancer.

Verrucae (Warts)

- Caused by HPV.
- **Hx/PE:** Usually occurs in older children; commonly found on the hands.
- **Rx:** Salicylic acid, liquid nitrogen, curettage.

LICHEN SCLEROSUS

A chronic, benign disorder that is characterized by inflammation and epithelial thinning. Commonly affects the skin in the anogenital area.

HISTORY/PE

- Occurs primarily in **postmenopausal** women. May be pruritic and painful.
- White, sharply demarcated, confluent macules, papules, and plaques are seen.
- Nongenital involvement is characterized by dilated sweat ducts with keratin plugs (dells). Lesions may also be found on the trunk, neck, and oral mucosa.
- There is a risk of developing **squamous cell carcinoma** in rare cases.

DIAGNOSIS

Biopsy shows **hyperkeratotic** epidermis with follicular plugging, progressing to atrophy.

TREATMENT

Short-term, high-potency topical glucocorticoids or oral hydrochloroquine.

NEUROCUTANEOUS SYNDROMES

Neurocutaneous diseases (phakomatoses) commonly affect the skin, nervous system, and eyes (see Table 2.2-6).

TABLE 2.2-6.　Neurocutaneous Syndromes

DISEASE	CUTANEOUS MANIFESTATIONS	NONDERMATOLOGIC SYMPTOMS
Tuberous sclerosis	Shagreen patches (thickened areas of skin), ash leaf spots (hypopigmentation), angiofibromas (red papules around the nose).	Periventricular tubers, seizures, mental retardation, kidney or heart tumors.
Neurofibromatosis	Café-au-lait spots, neurofibromas, axillary freckling.	Meningiomas, acoustic neuromas, Lisch nodules (iris lesions), optic nerve gliomas, renovascular hypertension, scoliosis, seizures.
Sturge-Weber syndrome	Port-wine stain on the face (hemangioma) over the distribution of CN V_1.	Seizures, mental retardation, visual impairment.
von Hippel–Lindau syndrome	Hemangiomas.	Retinal vascular hamartomas, renal cell cancer, pheochromocytomas, polycythemia.

PRECANCEROUS AND CANCEROUS LESIONS

Abnormal skin lesions must be identified and biopsied to prevent skin cancer. The prognosis and treatment vary depending on the type of lesion.

Seborrheic Keratosis

- A benign epithelial tumor with a "stuck-on" appearance. Usually brown in color (see Figure 2.2-18); often found on the face, trunk, and upper extremities.
- **Hx/PE:** Melanoma may look like seborrheic keratosis but has different surface characteristics. Melanomas have a smooth surface that varies in elevation, color, density, and shade. Seborrheic keratoses have a uniform appearance over the entire surface.
- **Rx:** Requires no further treatment after diagnosis but **can be removed with cryosurgery or curettage for cosmetic purposes.**

When numerous seborrheic keratoses acutely erupt, it is known as the "sign of Leser-Trélat" and can be a sign of underlying malignancy (e.g., gastric cancer).

Basal Cell Carcinoma

The most common skin cancer; commonly found on the head and neck. Associated with sun exposure.

HISTORY/PE

- Presents as a bleeding or scabbing sore that heals and recurs.
- Pearly-colored papules of variable sizes are seen with translucent external surfaces covered with fine telangiectasias (see Figure 2.2-19).

DIAGNOSIS

- Arises from basal keratinocytes and grows by direct extension.
- Does not usually metastasize, but destroys normal tissue.
- Skin biopsy shows characteristic basophilic cells palisading with retraction.
- Has five histologic patterns: nodular, micronodular, infiltrative, superficial, and morpheaform.

HIGH-YIELD FACTS

DERMATOLOGY

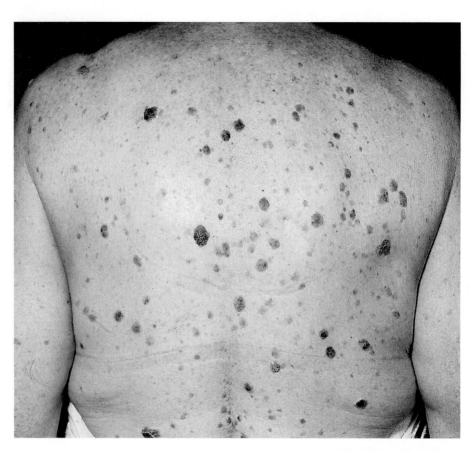

FIGURE 2.2-18. **Seborrheic keratoses.**

Multiple brown, warty papules and nodules are seen on the back, characterized by a "stuck-on" appearance. (Reproduced, with permission, from Fitzpatrick TB. *Color Atlas & Synopsis of Clinical Dermatology*, 4th ed. New York: McGraw-Hill, 2001:195.)

TREATMENT

- Therapy depends on the size and location of the tumor, histologic type, and clinical presentation.
- Options include curettage, surgical excision, Mohs' micrographic surgery (serial excisions with fresh-tissue microscopic examination to maximize cosmesis), cryosurgery, and radiation.
- Prevent with UVA/UVB sunscreens and avoidance of prolonged sun exposure.

Actinic Keratosis

- A premalignant lesion that results from sun exposure and is confined to the epidermis.
- Hx/PE:
  - Presents as asymptomatic, rough papules with poorly demarcated erythematous bases and areas of white, superficial scaling (see Figure 2.2-20).
  - Can progress to squamous cell carcinoma.
- **Dx:** Skin biopsy shows areas of dysplastic squamous epithelium (hyperkeratosis, with cells of the lower epidermis showing loss of polarity, pleomorphism, and hyperchromatic nuclei) without invasion into the dermis.

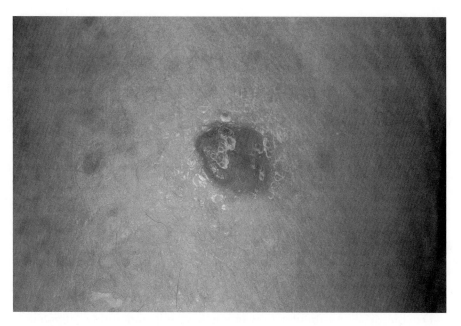

FIGURE 2.2-19. Basal cell carcinoma.

Seen above is an erythematous, fleshy, telangiectatic nodule with a translucent surface. (Reproduced, with permission, from Hurwitz RM. *Pathology of the Skin: Atlas of Clinical-Pathological Correlation*, 2nd ed. Stamford, CT: Appleton & Lange, 1998:362.)

- Rx:
  - Cryosurgery, topical 5-FU, curettage, or chemical peel.
  - Prevent with UVA/UVB sunscreens and avoidance of prolonged sun exposure.

Squamous Cell Carcinoma

- Risk factors include exposure to sun, ionizing radiation, actinic keratosis, immunosuppression, arsenic, and industrial carcinogens.

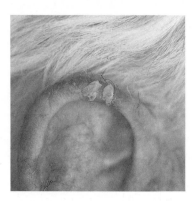

FIGURE 2.2-20. Actinic keratosis.

The discrete patch above has an erythematous base and a rough white scale. (Reproduced, with permission, from Hurwitz RM. *Pathology of the Skin: Atlas of Clinical-Pathological Correlation*, 2nd ed. Stamford, CT: Appleton & Lange, 1998:359.)

- **Hx/PE:**
  - Presents as slowly evolving and asymptomatic small, red, exophytic nodules with varying degrees of scaling or crusting (see Figure 2.2-21).
  - Commonly found on the scalp, the backs of the hands, and the superior surface of the pinna.
  - Occasionally bleed or become painful.
- **Dx:** Biopsy shows irregular masses of anaplastic epidermal cells proliferating down to the dermis.
- **Rx:**
  - Surgical excision, Mohs' micrographic surgery, or radiation.
  - Prevent with UVA/UVB sunscreens and avoidance of prolonged sun exposure.

Kaposi's Sarcoma

- Caused by HHV-8; almost always seen in patients with AIDS.
- **Hx/PE:** Reddish-purple, thin, oval plaques are seen on the skin and mucosa (see Figure 2.2-22).
- **Dx:** Biopsy shows proliferation of small vessels and slitlike intercellular spaces with extravasated RBCs.
- **Rx:** Antiretrovirals for HIV; chemotherapy for lesions (radiation, intralesional vinblastine, liquid nitrogen cryotherapy).

Melanoma

An aggressive malignancy of melanocytic origin (see Figure 2.2-23). Risk factors include sun exposure, fair skin, family history, xeroderma pigmentosum, a large number of nevi, and the presence of dysplastic nevi.

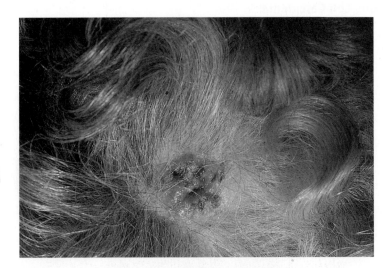

FIGURE 2.2-21.   Squamous cell carcinoma.

Note the crusting and ulceration of this erythematous plaque. Most lesions are exophytic nodules with erosion or ulceration. (Reproduced, with permission, from Hurwitz RM. *Pathology of the Skin: Atlas of Clinical-Pathological Correlation*, 2nd ed. Stamford, CT: Appleton & Lange, 1998:360.)

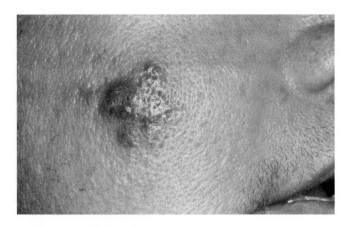

FIGURE 2.2-22. Kaposi's sarcoma.

A single violaceous patch is seen on the face of an HIV-⊕ patient. (Courtesy of George Turiansky, MD. Reproduced, with permission, from Knoop KJ et al. *Atlas of Emergency Medicine*, 2nd ed. New York: McGraw-Hill, 2002:655.)

HISTORY/PE

- A pigmented skin lesion that has recently changed in size or appearance should raise concern.
- Generally asymptomatic until late in the disease process, but may present with pruritus and mild discomfort.
- Lesions are found on sun-exposed areas as well as on the plantar aspect of the feet.
- Characterized by the **ABCDs of melanoma** (see mnemonic).

> **The ABCDs of melanoma:**
>
> **A**symmetric shape
> **B**orders irregular
> **C**olor variegated
> **D**iameter > 6 mm

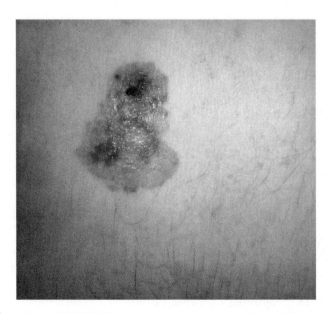

FIGURE 2.2-23. Melanoma.

Note the asymmetry, border irregularity, color variation, and large diameter of this plaque. (Reproduced, with permission, from Hurwitz RM. *Pathology of the Skin: Atlas of Clinical-Pathological Correlation*, 2nd ed. Stamford, CT: Appleton & Lange, 1998:432.)

TABLE 2.2-7.   **Types of Malignant Melanoma**

	SUPERFICIAL SPREADING	NODULAR	ACRAL-LENTIGINOUS	LENTIGO MALIGNA
Appearance	Dark brown, variegated, irregular borders; asymmetric shape.	Uniform, dark, "blueberry-like" nodule.	Marked variegation of brown/black macule or papule.	Flat, **"geographic" shape;** brown/black with "stain-like" appearance.
Distribution	Back, legs.	Any area; **arises rapidly.**	**Palms, soles, mucous membranes, nails.**	Head, neck, hands, **sun-exposed areas.**
Epidemiology	30s–50s, M = F, fair-skinned, **70% of all melanomas.**	50s, M = F.	60s, **M > F, more common in Asians and African-Americans.**	60s, M = F, fair-skinned.

- Melanomas are classified according to type (see Table 2.2-7).

DIAGNOSIS

Skin biopsy shows melanocytes with marked cellular atypia (vacuolated cytoplasm, hyperchromatic nuclei with prominent nucleoli, and pleomorphism) and melanocytic invasion into dermis.

TREATMENT

- Surgical excision is the treatment of choice.
- Depth of invasion (Breslow stage) and histologic evidence of ulceration are the most important factors involved in the staging of nonmetastatic lesions.
- Depending on depth, lymph node dissection may be necessary.
- Systemic chemotherapy is used for metastatic disease.

Mycosis Fungoides

A cutaneous T-cell lymphoma of unknown etiology.

HISTORY/PE

- Begins as thin, scaling patches, often in sun-protected areas, that → plaques → nodules → tumors and lymphadenopathy (see Figure 2.2-24).
- Extensive infiltration is associated with a lion-like facies.
- Causes intractable pruritus.

DIAGNOSIS

- Biopsy shows infiltrate of atypical lymphocytes with convoluted cerebriform nuclei in the upper dermis and microabscesses in the epidermis (Pautrier's microabscesses).

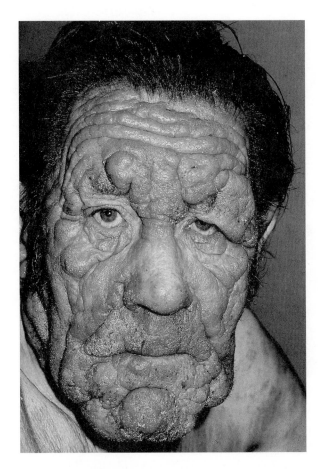

FIGURE 2.2-24. Mycosis fungoides.

Massive nodular infiltration of the face → a leonine facies. (Reproduced, with permission, from Fitzpatrick TB. *Color Atlas & Synopsis of Clinical Dermatology*, 4th ed. New York: McGraw-Hill, 2001:541.)

- Immunostaining shows T cells (CD3+, CD4+), not B cells.
- Eosinophilia, ↑ LDH.

TREATMENT

PUVA photochemotherapy, topical nitrogen mustard, total-body electron beam irradiation, ultra-high-potency topical steroids, systemic and topical retinoids.

COMPLICATIONS

Sézary's syndrome (peripheral blood involvement), sepsis 2° to skin infection, transformation to high-grade lymphoma.

ROSACEA

A chronic disorder of pilosebaceous units involving ↑ reactivity of capillaries to heat. Has a female predominance and is more common among those with fair skin.

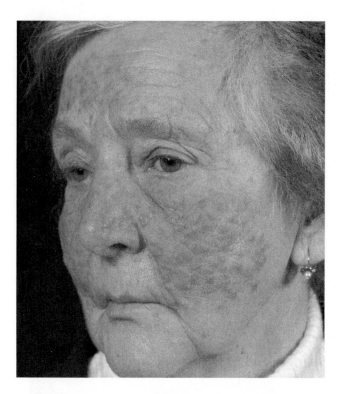

FIGURE 2.2-25. Rosacea.

Note the prominent facial erythema, telangiectasias, scattered papules, and small pustules. (Reproduced, with permission, from Wolff K, Johnson RA, Suurmond D. *Fitzpatrick's Color Atlas & Synopsis of Clinical Dermatology*, 5th ed. New York: McGraw-Hill, 2005:11.)

HISTORY/PE

- Small papules/pustules, erythema, and telangiectasias are distributed symmetrically, predominantly on the cheeks, chin, and forehead (see Figure 2.2-25). Facial flushing is worsened by hot liquids, spicy foods, alcohol, heat, caffeine, and sun exposure.
- Men can develop **rhinophyma** (large, porous, lobulated nose).

TREATMENT

- Avoid precipitating factors.
- Topical metronidazole, sulfur lotions, and oral tetracycline or isotretinoin are options.

Endocrinology

Type 1 Diabetes Mellitus (Type 1 DM)

Due to autoimmune pancreatic β-cell destruction → insulin deficiency and abnormal fuel metabolism.

HISTORY/PE

- **Classic symptoms: Polyuria** (especially nocturia), **polydipsia, polyphagia,** rapid weight loss. Patients may also present with **ketoacidosis.**
- Usually occurs in nonobese children or young adults.
- Associated with HLA-DR3 and -DR4.

DIAGNOSIS

At least one of the following is required to make the diagnosis:

- Fasting plasma glucose ≥ 126 mg/dL on two separate occasions.
- Random plasma glucose ≥ 200 mg/dL plus symptoms.
- Two-hour postprandial glucose ≥ 200 mg/dL after a glucose tolerance test on two separate occasions.

TREATMENT

- Insulin (see Table 2.3-1) and self-monitoring of blood glucose.
- Routine HbA_{1c} (goal $HbA_{1c} < 7$), frequent BP checks, foot checks, annual dilated-eye exams, annual microalbuminuria screening, lipid profile every 2–5 years.

COMPLICATIONS

Table 2.3-2 outlines the acute, chronic, and treatment-related complications of DM.

Type 2 Diabetes Mellitus (Type 2 DM)

Dysfunction in glucose metabolism similar to that of type 1 DM. Best characterized as varying degrees of insulin deficiency and resistance.

> *Symptoms of diabetic ketoacidosis—*
>
> **DKA**
>
> **D**ehydrated
> **K**etones/**K**ussmaul breathing/**K** drops
> **A**cidosis/**A**cetone breath

TABLE 2.3-1. Types of Insulin

INSULIN	ONSET	PEAK EFFECT	DURATION
Regular	30–60 minutes	2–4 hours	5–8 hours
Humalog (lispro)	5–10 minutes	0.5–1.5 hours	6–8 hours
NovoLog (aspart)	10–20 minutes	1–3 hours	3–5 hours
NPH or Lente	2–4 hours	6–10 hours	18–28 hours
Ultralente	3–5 hours	10–16 hours	12–20 hours
Lantus	1–4 hours	No discernible peak	20–24 hours

TABLE 2.3-2.   Complications of DM

COMPLICATION	DESCRIPTION
Complications of treatment	
Dawn phenomenon	Early-morning hyperglycemia caused by ↓ effectiveness of insulin at that time. **Move P.M. insulin closer to bedtime to treat.**
Acute complications	
Diabetic ketoacidosis (DKA)	Hyperglycemia-induced crisis that occurs most commonly in **type 1 DM.** Often precipitated by stress (including infections, MI, trauma, or alcohol) or by noncompliance with insulin therapy. May present with **abdominal pain, vomiting, Kussmaul respirations,** and a **fruity, acetone breath odor.** Patients are severely dehydrated with many electrolyte abnormalities and may also develop mental status changes. Treatment includes fluids, potassium, **insulin,** and treatment of the initiating event or underlying disease process.
Nonketotic hyperglycemia (NKH)	Presents as **profound dehydration,** mental status changes, hyperosmolarity, and extremely high plasma glucose (> 600 mg/dL) without acidosis. Occurs in **type 2 DM;** precipitated by acute stress (dehydration, infections) and often fatal. Treatment includes **aggressive fluid and electrolyte replacement** and insulin. Treat the initiating event.
Chronic complications	
Retinopathy (nonproliferative, proliferative)	Appears when diabetes has been present for at least **3–5 years.** Preventive measures include control of hyperglycemia and hypertension, annual eye exams, and **laser photocoagulation therapy for retinal neovascularization.**
Diabetic nephropathy	Characterized by glomerular hyperfiltration followed by **microalbuminuria.** Preventive measures include **ACEIs** and BP and glucose control.
Neuropathy	Peripheral, symmetric, sensorimotor neuropathy → burning pain, foot trauma, infections, and diabetic ulcers. Treat with preventive **foot care** and **analgesics.** Late complications due to autonomic dysfunction include delayed gastric emptying, esophageal dysmotility, impotence, and orthostatic hypotension.
Macrovascular complications	Cardiovascular, cerebrovascular, and peripheral vascular disease. Cardiovascular disease is the most common cause of death in diabetic patients. Goal BP is < 130/< 75; ↓ LDL to < 100 mg/dL; ↓ triglycerides to < 150 mg/dL. Patients should also be started on low-dose ASA.

HISTORY/PE

- Patients typically present with symptoms of hyperglycemia.
- Onset is more **insidious.** Patients often present with complications.
- **Nonketotic hyperglycemia** is possible with very poor glycemic control.
- Usually occurs in older adults with obesity (often truncal); associated with a strong genetic predisposition.

DIAGNOSIS

- Diagnostic criteria: Same as type 1 DM.
- Follow-up testing:
    - Patients without risk factors: Test at 45 years of age; retest every three years.
    - Patients with impaired fasting glucose (> 110 mg/dL but < 126 mg/dL): Frequent retesting.

TREATMENT

- Diet, weight loss, exercise.
- **Oral agents** (monotherapy or combination if uncontrolled):
  - **Sulfonylurea (glipizide and glyburide):** Insulin secretagogues. Hypoglycemia and weight gain are side effects.
  - **Meglitinides (repaglinide and nateglinide):** Action is similar to that of sulfonylureas. Short acting.
  - **Metformin:** Inhibits hepatic gluconeogenesis; ↑ peripheral sensitivity to insulin. Side effects include weight loss, GI upset, and, rarely, lactic acidosis. Contraindicated in the elderly (> 80 years of age) and in those with renal disease.
  - **Thiazolidinediones (the "glitazones"):** ↑ insulin sensitivity. Side effects include weight gain, edema, and potential hepatotoxicity.
  - **α-glucosidase inhibitors:** ↓ intestinal absorption of carbohydrates. Rarely used owing to the side effect of flatulence.
- Insulin (alone or in conjunction with oral agents).
- Statins for hypercholesterolemia; glucose control and fibric acid derivatives for hypertriglyceridemia.
- **Strict BP control.** ACEIs are usually first-line agents.

COMPLICATIONS

See Table 2.3-2 for an outline of the complications of DM.

Metabolic Syndrome

- Also known as insulin resistance syndrome or Syndrome X. Associated with an ↑ risk of CAD and mortality from a cardiovascular event.
- **Hx/PE: Abdominal obesity, high BP, impaired glycemic control, dyslipidemia.**
- **Dx:** Must meet three out of five of the following criteria:
  - Abdominal obesity (↑ waist girth).
  - Triglycerides ≥ 150 mg/dL.
  - HDL cholesterol < 40 mg/dL in men and < 50 mg/dL in women.
  - BP ≥ 130/85 mmHg or administration of antihypertensive drugs.
  - Fasting glucose ≥ 110 mg/dL.
- **Rx:** Intensive weight loss, aggressive cholesterol lowering, BP control.

THYROID DISORDERS

Testing of Thyroid Function

TFTs include the following (see also Table 2.3-3):

- **Radioactive iodine uptake (RAIU) and scan:** Determines the level of iodine uptake by the thyroid. Useful in differentiating thyrotoxic states.
- **Total T_4 measurement:** Not an adequate screening test. Ninety-nine percent of circulating T_4 is bound to thyroxine-binding globulin (TBG). Total T_4 levels can be altered by disorders of the binding proteins.
- **T_3 resin uptake (T3RU):** Used with total T_4 or T_3 to correct for changes in TBG levels (e.g., the free thyroxine index = total $T_4 \times$ T3RU).
- **Free T_4 measurement:** The preferred screening test for thyroid hormone levels.
- **TSH measurement:** The single best test for assessing thyroid function. High TSH levels → 1° hypothyroidism. Low TSH levels → 1° hyperthyroidism.

Free T_4 is a better measure of thyroid hormone than total T_4 because it is not affected by changes in TBG.

TABLE 2.3-3.   **Common Thyroid Function Abnormalities**

Diagnosis	TSH	T$_4$	T$_3$	Causes
1° hyperthyroidism	↓	↑	↑	Graves' disease, toxic multinodular goiter (TMNG), toxic adenoma, amiodarone, molar pregnancy, postpartum thyrotoxicosis, postviral thyroiditis.
1° hypothyroidism	↑	↓	↓	Hashimoto's thyroiditis, hypothyroid phase of thyroiditis, iatrogenic factors (radioactive thyroid ablation or excision with inadequate supplementation, external radiation), lithium, amiodarone, iodide, infiltrative disease.

Hyperthyroidism

Causes of thyrotoxicosis (↑ levels of T$_3$/T$_4$ due to any cause) in which the thyroid overproduces thyroid hormone, including **Graves' disease**, TMNG, and toxic adenomas.

- **Hx/PE:** Weight loss, ↑ appetite, **heat intolerance, nervousness, palpitations,** ↑ **bowel frequency,** insomnia, menstrual abnormalities. Exam reveals warm, moist skin; goiter; sinus **tachycardia** or **atrial fibrillation;** thyroid bruit; fine **tremor; lid lag;** and hyperactive reflexes. Exophthalmos and pretibial myxedema are seen only in Graves' disease (see Figure 2.3-1).

- **Dx:** See Table 2.2-3.
- **Rx:**
  - **Three main treatments: Radioactive** ^{131}I **thyroid ablation, thyroidectomy,** and **antithyroid drugs** (methimazole or propylthiouracil).
  - Give **propranolol** for β-adrenergic symptoms while awaiting the resolution of hyperthyroidism.
  - Give levothyroxine to prevent hypothyroidism for patients who have undergone ablation or surgery.

TSH receptor antibodies are seen in patients with Graves' disease.

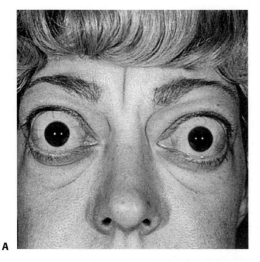

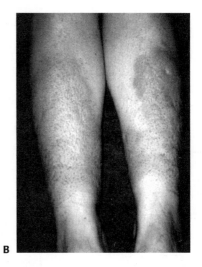

FIGURE 2.3-1.   Physical signs of Graves' disease.

(A) Graves' ophthalmopathy. (B) Pretibial myxedema. (Reproduced, with permission, from Greenspan FS, Strewler GJ [eds]. *Basic and Clinical Endocrinology,* 5th ed. Stamford, CT: Appleton & Lange, 1997, Figs. 7-41 and 7-42.)

HIGH-YIELD FACTS

ENDOCRINOLOGY

Hypothyroidism

- **Hashimoto's thyroiditis** is the most common cause (see Table 2.3-3). Anti-TPO antibodies are ⊕.
- Myxedema coma refers to severe hypothyroidism with ↓ mental status, hypothermia, and other symptoms.
- Hx/PE: Weakness, fatigue, **cold intolerance, constipation,** weight gain, **depression,** menstrual irregularities, **hoarseness.** Exam may reveal **dry, cold, puffy skin;** edema; **bradycardia;** and delayed relaxation of DTRs.
- Dx: See Table 2.2-3.
- Rx:
  - **Uncomplicated hypothyroidism (e.g., Hashimoto's disease):** Administer levothyroxine.
  - **Subacute thyroiditis:** Usually self-limited; treat with NSAIDs or with oral steroids for severe cases.
  - **Myxedema coma:** IV levothyroxine and IV hydrocortisone (unless adrenal insufficiency has been excluded).

Thyroiditis

- Inflammation of the thyroid gland. Common types are subacute granulomatous, radiation, lymphocytic, postpartum, and drug-induced (e.g., amiodarone) thyroiditis.
- **Hx/PE: In subacute and radiation,** presents with **tender thyroid,** malaise, and URI symptoms.
- Dx: Thyroid dysfunction (typically hyperthyroidism followed by hypothyroidism), all with ↓ uptake on RAIU.
- Rx:
  - β-blockers for hyperthyroidism; levothyroxine for hypothyroidism.
  - **Subacute thyroiditis: Anti-inflammatory medication.**

Thyroid Neoplasms

Thyroid nodules are very common and show an ↑ incidence with age. Most are benign.

HISTORY/PE

- Usually **asymptomatic** on initial presentation.
- **If hyperfunctioning:** Hyperthyroidism, local symptoms (dysphagia, dyspnea, cough, choking sensation), ⊕ family history (especially **medullary thyroid cancer**).
- An ↑ risk of malignancy is associated with a **history of neck irradiation,** "cold" nodules (on radionuclide scan), firm and fixed solitary nodules, and **rapidly growing nodules** with **hoarseness.**
- Check for anterior cervical lymphadenopathy. Carcinoma will likely be palpable, **firm, fixed,** and **nontender.**
- Medullary thyroid carcinoma is associated with multiple endocrine neoplasia (MEN) types II and III.

DIAGNOSIS

- TSH and **TFTs** (TSH to exclude hyperfunction).
- **Ultrasound** determines if the nodule is solid or cystic; a radioactive scan determines whether it is hot or cold (cancers are usually cold and solid). Hot nodules are never cancerous and should not be biopsied.

- The best method of assessing a nodule for malignancy is **fine-needle aspiration** (FNA); has high sensitivity and moderate specificity.

TREATMENT

- **Benign FNA:** Follow with physical exam/ultrasound.
- **Malignant FNA:** Surgical resection; if papillary or follicular, radioactive iodine ablation.
- **Indeterminate FNA:** Perform a lobectomy and wait for final pathology.
- Medullary thyroid cancer has a poorer prognosis than papillary and follicular types. Anaplastic thyroid cancer has an extremely poor prognosis.

Multiple Endocrine Neoplasia (MEN)

Associated with an autosomal-dominant inheritance. Subtypes are as follows:

- **MEN type I (Wermer's syndrome):** Pancreatic (e.g., Zollinger-Ellison syndrome, insulinomas, VIPomas), parathyroid, and pituitary tumors.
- **MEN type II (Sipple's syndrome):** Medullary carcinoma of the thyroid, pheochromocytoma, parathyroid gland hyperplasia.
- **MEN type III (formerly MEN IIB):** Medullary carcinoma of the thyroid, pheochromocytoma, oral and intestinal ganglioneuromatosis (mucosal neuromas), marfanoid habitus.

BONE AND MINERAL DISORDERS

Osteoporosis

A common metabolic bone disease characterized by low bone mass and microarchitectural disruption.

HISTORY/PE

Commonly asymptomatic. Patients may present with **hip fractures, vertebral compression fractures** (→ loss of height and progressive thoracic kyphosis), and/or distal radius fractures after minimal trauma (see Figure 2.3-2). Most often affects thin, postmenopausal women, especially Caucasians and Asians. **Smoking,** excessive caffeine intake, a history of amenorrhea, and **steroid use** are associated with an ↑ risk.

DIAGNOSIS

- **Lab tests:** ↑ markers of bone turnover (urinary N-telopeptides and deoxypyridinoline)
- **X-rays:** Global demineralization after > 30% of bone density is lost.
- **DEXA:** Significant osteopenia (bone mineral density < 2.5 SDs from normal), most commonly in the vertebral bodies, proximal femur, and distal radius.

TREATMENT

Prevention with **calcium supplementation** and vitamin D. Smoking cessation and weight-bearing exercises help maintain bone density. Bisphosphonates (e.g., alendronate, risedronate), selective estrogen receptor modulators (e.g., raloxifene), and intranasal calcitonin may be used to ↑ bone density.

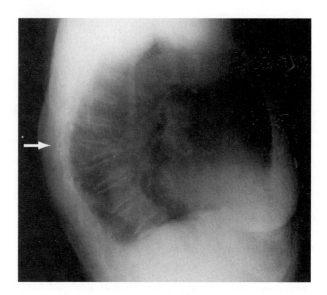

FIGURE 2.3-2. **Radiographic findings in osteoporosis.**

Lateral spine x-ray shows severe osteopenia and a severe wedge-type deformity (severe anterior compression). (Reproduced, with permission, from Kasper DL et al [eds]. *Harrison's Principles of Internal Medicine*, 16th ed. New York: McGraw-Hill, 2005:2269.)

Paget's Disease

- Characterized by an ↑ rate of bone turnover. Causes both excessive resorption and excessive formation of bone → a "mosaic" lamellar bone pattern. Suspected to be due to viral infection and/or genetic factors. Found in roughly 4% of men and women > 40 years of age.
- **Hx/PE:** Usually asymptomatic, but may present with **aching bone or joint pain,** headaches, skull deformities, fractures, or nerve entrapment → loss of hearing.
- **Dx:** Based on clinical history, characteristic radiographic changes (see Figure 2.3-3), and lab findings. Radionuclide bone scan is the most sensitive test. Lab abnormalities include ↑ serum alkaline phosphatase with normal calcium and phosphate.
- **Rx: The majority of patients are asymptomatic and require no treatment.** There is no cure for Paget's disease. Bisphosphonates and calcitonin are used to slow osteoclastic bone resorption.

Hyperparathyroidism

- Eighty percent of cases are due to a single **adenoma** and 15% to parathyroid hyperplasia.
- **Hx/PE:** Most cases are **asymptomatic,** but signs and symptoms may include **stones** (nephrolithiasis), **bones** (bone pain, myalgias, arthralgias, fractures), abdominal **groans** (abdominal pain, nausea, vomiting, PUD, pancreatitis), and **psychiatric overtones** (fatigue, depression, anxiety, sleep disturbances).
- **Dx: Hypercalcemia, hypophosphatemia,** hypercalciuria. PTH is inappropriately ↑ relative to ionized calcium (see Table 2.3-4).
- **Rx: Parathyroidectomy** if symptomatic or if certain criteria are met. For acute hypercalcemia, give **IV fluids** (with a loop diuretic if renal or heart failure), **IV bisphosphonate, and calcitonin.**

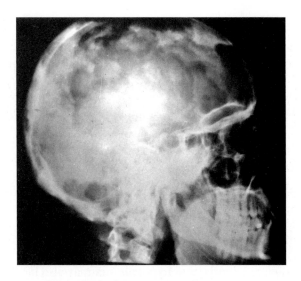

FIGURE 2.3-3. **Radiographic findings in Paget's disease.**

Skull of a 58-year-old woman with Paget's disease of bone. (Reproduced, with permission, from Kasper DL et al [eds]. *Harrison's Principles of Internal Medicine*, 16th ed. New York: McGraw-Hill, 2005:2280.)

PITUITARY AND HYPOTHALAMIC DISORDERS

Cushing's Syndrome

Most commonly due to hypersecretion of ACTH from a pituitary adenoma (known as Cushing's disease, or **central** hypercortisolism). Other causes include ectopic ACTH secretion from neoplasia (e.g., carcinoid tumor, small cell lung cancer), excess adrenal secretion of cortisol (e.g., bilateral adrenal hyperplasia, adrenal cancer), and iatrogenic factors (exogenous corticosteroids).

TABLE 2.3-4. **Functions and Mechanisms of PTH**

SOURCE	FUNCTIONS	MECHANISMS	REGULATION
Chief cells of parathyroid.	↑ bone resorption of calcium and phosphate. ↑ kidney reabsorption of calcium in the distal convoluted tubule. ↓ kidney reabsorption of phosphate. ↑ 1,25-(OH)$_2$ vitamin D (cholecalciferol) production by stimulating kidney 1α-hydroxylase.	PTH ↑ serum Ca^{2+}, ↓ serum (PO$_4$)$^{3-}$, and ↑ urine (PO$_4$)$^{3-}$. PTH stimulates both osteoclasts and osteoblasts.	↓ in free serum Ca^{2+} ↑ PTH secretion.

HISTORY/PE

- **Hypertension, central obesity,** muscle wasting, thin skin with purple striae, psychological disturbances, **hirsutism, moon facies, "buffalo hump."**
- **Depression,** oligomenorrhea, growth retardation, proximal weakness, acne, **excessive hair growth,** symptoms of **diabetes** (2° to glucose intolerance).

DIAGNOSIS

Diagnosis is as follows (see also Table 2.3-5):

- **Screen: 24-hour free urine cortisol or low-dose dexamethasone suppression test**—abnormal if A.M. cortisol is persistently ↑ after overnight suppression.
- **Differentiate: High-dose dexamethasone suppression test**—cortisol is suppressed only in patients with Cushing's disease.
- Hyperglycemia, glycosuria, and **hypokalemia** may also be present.

TREATMENT

- **Surgical resection** of the hypersecretory source (pituitary, adrenal).
- Pituitary radiotherapy may also be considered.
- Blockers of adrenal steroidogenesis (**ketoconazole, metyrapone**).

Acromegaly

An adult condition due to a benign pituitary growth hormone (GH) adenoma. Children with excess GH production present with **gigantism.**

HISTORY/PE

- **Enlargement of the jaw, hands, and feet; coarsening of facial features.** May → carpal tunnel syndrome, diastolic dysfunction, hypertension, and arthritis.
- **Bitemporal hemianopsia** due to compression of the optic chiasm by a pituitary adenoma.
- Excess GH may also → **glucose intolerance** or **diabetes.**

DIAGNOSIS

- MRI of the pituitary shows a sellar lesion.
- Serum GH levels may be ↑, but this finding is unreliable.
- Screen by measuring insulin-like growth factor I (IGF-I) levels (↑); confirm the diagnosis with an oral glucose tolerance test (GH levels will remain ↑ despite glucose stimulation).

TABLE 2.3-5. Laboratory Findings in Cushing's Syndrome

	CUSHING'S DISEASE (PITUITARY HYPERSECRETION)	EXOGENOUS STEROID USE	ECTOPIC ACTH SECRETION	ADRENAL CORTISOL HYPERSECRETION
ACTH	↑	↓	↑	↓
Urinary free cortisol	↑	↑	↑	↑

TREATMENT

- Transsphenoidal surgical resection or irradiative ablation of the tumor.
- Octreotide, pergolide, and pegvisomant can be used for symptomatic management of refractory cases.

Prolactinoma

- **Hx/PE:** Hypogonadism manifested by infertility, oligomenorrhea, or amenorrhea. Galactorrhea or bitemporal hemianopsia may be prominent.
- **Dx:** Serum prolactin level is typically > 200 mg/mL.
- **Rx:**
  - **Dopamine agonists:** Cabergoline, bromocriptine, or pergolide.
  - **Surgery:** Should be considered when medical treatment has failed or in the presence of visual field defects.

ADRENAL GLAND DISORDERS

Adrenal Insufficiency

- **1°:** Most commonly caused by autoimmune adrenal cortical destruction (**Addison's disease**) → deficiencies of mineralocorticoids and glucocorticoids. **Autoimmune destruction** may occur as part of a polyglandular autoimmune syndrome (hypothyroidism, type 1 DM, vitiligo, premature ovarian failure, testicular failure, pernicious anemia). Other causes of 1° adrenal insufficiency include congenital enzyme deficiencies, adrenal hemorrhage, TB, and other infections.
- **2°:** Caused by ↓ ACTH production by the pituitary; most often due to **abrupt cessation of chronic glucocorticoid treatment.**

HISTORY/PE

- Most symptoms are nonspecific.
- **Weakness, fatigue,** and **anorexia with weight loss** are common. GI manifestations, hypotension, and salt craving are also seen.
- **Hyperpigmentation** (due to ↑ ACTH secretion) is seen in Addison's disease.

DIAGNOSIS

- **Hyponatremia** and **eosinophilia** (1° or 2°).
- **Hyperkalemia** (specific to 1°).
- Diagnosis is confirmed with plasma **cortisol levels:**
  - Low plasma cortisol levels (< 20 < g/dL) during a period of high physiologic stress is confirmatory.
  - A random plasma cortisol level > 20 µg/dL excludes the diagnosis.
  - **Confirmatory test with synthetic ACTH stimulation test:** A plasma cortisol level > 20 µg/dL excludes the diagnosis.

TREATMENT

- **Glucocorticoid replacement, with mineralocorticoid** replacement if 1°.
- ↑ steroids during periods of stress (e.g., major surgery, trauma, infection). Avoid 2° adrenal insufficiency by tapering off steroids slowly.

> **The 4 S's of adrenal crisis management:**
>
> **S**alt: 0.9% saline
> **S**teroids: IV hydrocortisone 100 mg every 8 hours
> **S**upport
> **S**earch for the underlying illness

Pheochromocytoma

- Tumors of chromaffin tissue of either the adrenal medulla or extra-adrenal sites that secrete catecholamines, mimicking activation of the sympathetic nervous system. May be associated with von Hippel-Lindau syndrome, neurofibromatosis, or MEN II/III syndromes.
- Hx/PE: Intermittent tachycardia, palpitations, chest pain, diaphoresis, hypertension, headache, tremor, anxiety.
- Dx: CT or MRI often demonstrates a suprarenal mass. Screen with plasma free metanephrines (metanephrine and normetanephrine) or 24-hour urinary metanephrines. MIBG scan is sometimes helpful.
- Rx: **Surgical resection.** Preoperatively, use α-adrenergic blockade to ↓ the incidence of intraoperative hypertension. Use β-blockade second to control tachycardia. Never give β-blockade first; otherwise, unopposed α-adrenergic stimulation → ↑ BP.

Hyperaldosteronism

- Results from excessive secretion of aldosterone from the zona glomerulosa of the adrenal cortex. Usually due to unilateral adrenal adenoma (**Conn's syndrome**). Can be due to adrenocortical hyperplasia.
- Hx/PE: **Hypertension, headache, polyuria,** and **muscle weakness**; tetany and/or paresthesias; peripheral edema in severe cases.
- Dx: **Hypokalemia, mild hypernatremia,** metabolic alkalosis, hypomagnesemia, **low plasma renin,** ↑ 24-hour urine aldosterone; CT or MRI may reveal an adrenal mass.
- Rx: Laparoscopic or open **adrenalectomy** for adrenal tumors (after correcting BP and potassium). Treat with **spironolactone** (an aldosterone receptor antagonist) for bilateral hyperplasia.

Congenital Adrenal Hyperplasia

- A family of inherited disorders → cortisol deficiency.
- Most cases are due to **21-hydroxylase deficiency (autosomal recessive)** → ↓ cortisol production. In severe cases, mineralocorticoid deficiency with salt wasting may develop.
- Other causes include 11- and 17-hydroxylase deficiencies. Cortisol deficiency stimulates ACTH synthesis and → overproduction of adrenal androgens.
- Hx/PE: **Ambiguous genitalia** in female infants; **virilization** (if manifested later in life). **Macrogenitosomia** in male infants; precocious puberty (if manifested later in life), hypertension (with 11- and 17-hydroxylase deficiencies).
- Dx: High levels of cortisol precursors and androgens in blood and urine.
- Rx:
  - **Medical:** Cortisol administration to ↓ ACTH and adrenal androgens. Fludrocortisone for severe 21-hydroxylase deficiency.
  - **Surgical:** May be required in the case of ambiguous genitalia in female infants.

Epidemiology and Preventive Medicine

Defined as any error in the design, implementation, or analysis of a study → conclusions differing from the truth.

Selection Bias

Produces a sample that is not representative of the study **population** of interest; → **overestimation or underestimation** of the association between an exposure and outcome. Subtypes are as follows:

- **Self-selection bias:** Patients who choose or do not choose to participate (**nonrespondent bias**) may yield results that are not representative of the population. As an example, patients with refractory disease may be more likely than others to enroll in an experimental study.
- **Enrollment bias:** Subjects are assigned to a study group in a nonrandom fashion. An example would be **assignment of healthier patients to the intervention group.**

Information Bias

Yields misclassification of subjects on the basis of exposure and/or outcome; → differing quality of data between study groups. Subtypes are as follows:

- **Lead-time bias: A disease is diagnosed earlier without actually prolonging true survival** (the natural course of the disease is not altered).
- **Measurement bias:** Information gathering distorts data; → distorted results and conclusions. An example would be an assay that inaccurately estimates a biological parameter.
- **Responder bias:** Participants' responses to subjective questions are affected by their awareness of their study arm.
- **Observer bias:** An observer's evaluation of a participant's response to treatment may be affected by awareness of the hypothesis. Eliminated with **double-blind** study design.
- **Recall bias: Errors of memory** that occur in retrospective cohort or case-control studies. People who develop a disease or who have a ⊖ outcome may be more likely to remember risk factors or to exaggerate their history of exposures.

Confounding

Variables associated with an exposure that also cause the outcome and → overestimation or underestimation of the relationship between exposure and outcome.

- **Example:** If vitamin consumption is associated with a healthy diet, it may appear that individuals who take vitamins are protected from a particular disease when it is actually diet that is the protective factor.
- **Reduced by study design** (randomization or matching for case control) or by statistical adjustment (e.g., multivariate analysis).

EVALUATION OF SCREENING AND DIAGNOSTIC TEST PERFORMANCE

Sensitivity

The probability that a diseased patient will have a ⊕ test result.

- Calculated as true positives ÷ the total number of people **with** the disease (see Figure 2.4-1).

	Disease Present	No Disease	
Positive test	a	b	$PPV = a / (a + b)$
Negative test	c	d	$NPV = d / (c + d)$
	Sensitivity = $a / (a + c)$ Specificity = $d / (b + d)$		

FIGURE 2.4-1.   Sensitivity, specificity, PPV, and NPV.

- A sensitive test is good for **ruling out (SnOUT)** a disease.
- High sensitivity = good **screening test** (↓ **false negatives**).

SnOUT: **Sen**sitive tests rule **OUT** disease.
SpIN: **Sp**ecific tests rule **IN** disease.

Specificity

The probability that a nondiseased person will have a ⊖ test result.

- Calculated as true negatives ÷ the total number of people **without** the disease (see Figure 2.4-1).
- High specificity = good for **ruling in (SpIN)** a disease (good **confirmatory test**).
- For quantitative tests, there is often a **trade-off between sensitivity and specificity**. The ideal test is both sensitive and specific (see Figure 2.4-2).

Positive Predictive Value (PPV)

The probability that a patient with a ⊕ test result has the disease.

- Calculated as true positives ÷ the total number of people who tested ⊕.
- A test will have a higher PPV for diseases with a **high prevalence** (fewer false positives).

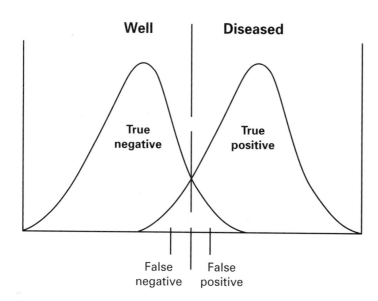

FIGURE 2.4-2.   Graphical representation of the balance between sensitivity and specificity.

Negative Predictive Value (NPV)

The probability that a patient with a ⊖ test result is disease free.

- Calculated as true negatives ÷ the total number of people who tested ⊖.
- A test will have a higher NPV for diseases with a **low prevalence** (the relative number of false negatives to true negatives will be lower).

Both PPV and NPV are affected by the prevalence of the disease.

Incidence and Prevalence

- **Incidence:** The number of **new cases** in a given at-risk population over a specified period of time.
- **Prevalence:** The number of existing cases at a moment in time. Prevalence reflects incidence and disease duration.

Reliability and Validity

- **Reliability,** or precision, is the reproducibility of results.
- **Inter-rater reliability** measures the similarity of results when tests are interpreted by different people.
- **Test-retest probability (intraobserver variability)** assesses the similarity of results when a single person interprets a test repeatedly.
- **Validity,** or accuracy, measures how well a test measures what it intends to measure. New diagnostic tests are compared to a **gold standard test,** which is considered the most valid and reliable (although typically not the most convenient or safe) test available.

STUDY DESIGNS

Case-Control Study

An observational study in which cases (with disease) and controls (without disease) are identified. Information about **past** exposure is used to calculate an **odds ratio (OR).**

- Advantages:
  - Small study groups.
  - Inexpensive.
  - Useful for **rare diseases or outcomes.**
  - Can be used to examine multiple potential etiologic factors.
- Limitations:
  - Data may be inaccurate owing to **recall bias** and **survivorship bias** (those with more aggressive disease may already have died).
  - Prevalence, incidence, and relative risk (RR) **cannot be calculated.**

Cohort Study

An observational study in which a cohort of exposed and nonexposed individuals are **followed to determine if disease develops. Usually prospective, but can also be retrospective.**

- Advantages:
  - Data are collected in real time.
  - ↓ recall bias.
  - Allows the effects of **rare exposures** and **multiple outcomes** of an exposure to be examined.
  - **RR, incidence,** and OR can be determined.

- **Limitations:**
  - Studies are time consuming, require many subjects, and are very expensive.
  - **Selection bias** and confounding variables may complicate result interpretation (exposure is not randomly distributed).
  - Rare diseases cannot be studied.
  - Losses occur to follow-up.

Cross-Sectional Study

A survey of the population at **a single point in time.**

- **Advantages:** Can be used to **estimate disease prevalence** and to form hypotheses.
- **Limitations:** Because risk factors and presence of disease are determined simultaneously, causal relationships cannot be established (vs. case-control and cohort studies).

Meta-analysis

A statistical combination of data from several studies (often via a literature search).

- **Advantages:**
  - Can ↑ the statistical power of a study to allow for the evaluation of small differences.
  - May resolve conflicting studies in the literature.
- **Limitations:**
  - Cannot overcome the limitations of individual studies.
  - One must make sure that the pooled data evaluate similar populations and interventions.
  - Analyses are complicated because errors are introduced when means and variances from different studies are combined.

Randomized Controlled Clinical Trial (RCCT)

An experimental, **prospective** study in which subjects are assigned to a treatment or control group. **Randomization** ↓ bias and confounding. May be **blinded** (the patient does not know to which group he/she is assigned) or **double blinded** (neither the patient nor the researcher knows the group assignment).

- **Advantages:**
  - **Highest-quality** study.
  - Minimizes the effect of bias and confounding.
  - Can potentially demonstrate a causal relationship.
- **Limitations:**
  - Very costly and time intensive.
  - May be difficult to blind some interventions (e.g., education, exercise, surgery).
  - For ethical reasons, one cannot compare a new treatment to a placebo if there is a standard of care.

Randomization minimizes bias and confounding; double-blinded studies prevent observation bias.

STUDY ANALYSES

Table 2.4-1 outlines basic terminology and concepts used in the course of study analysis. Table 2.4-2 summarizes the fundamental concepts underlying hypothesis testing.

TABLE 2.4-1. Description of Epidemiological Terms

TERM	DESCRIPTION
Attributable risk (AR)	Absolute difference in the incidence rate (IR) of a disease in exposed vs. unexposed populations. Used in cohort studies. Computed as the IR of disease in exposed − IR of disease in unexposed.
RR	Used in cohort studies to determine the likelihood of developing a disease when a patient is exposed to a risk factor. Computed as the IR of disease in exposed ÷ IR of disease in unexposed.
OR	Determines the likelihood of disease among individuals with an exposure compared to those without the exposure (exactly equal to the OR of exposure in those with disease vs. those without). Used in both case-control and cohort studies. OR = ad/bc (see Figure 2.4-3).
Number needed to treat (NNT)	The number of people in the general population who must be treated to prevent disease in one patient. Inverse of the absolute risk reduction associated with an intervention. NNT = 1 ÷ (rate in untreated group − rate in treated group).

PUBLIC HEALTH

Disease Prevention

- **1° prevention:** Health-promoting measures to ↓ the development (↓ the incidence) of disease.
- **2° prevention:** The detection of a disease when it is asymptomatic or mild to prevent its complications.
- **3° prevention:** The reduction of morbidity associated with the presence of disease.

Leading Causes of Mortality

Table 2.4-3 summarizes the leading causes of mortality in different age groups.

- Excluding skin cancers, prostate and breast cancer are the most common cancers in men and women, respectively.
- Lung and colorectal cancers are the second and third most common types in both genders.

TABLE 2.4-2. Hypothesis Testing

	NULL HYPOTHESIS IS TRUE	NULL HYPOTHESIS IS FALSE
Accept null hypothesis	Correct conclusion	Type II error (β)
Reject null hypothesis	Type I error (α)	Correct conclusion (power = $1 - \beta$)

	Disease Develops	No Disease
Exposure	a	b
No exposure	c	d

$$RR = \frac{a/(a+b)}{c/(c+d)}$$

$$OR = ad/bc$$

FIGURE 2.4-3. RR and OR.

- Lung cancer is the most common cause of death from cancer in all groups.
- Since the 1950s, deaths from lung cancer have ↑, while deaths from gastric, colorectal, and cervical cancer have ↓.

Health Care Screening

Table 2.4-4 summarizes recommended health care screening measures by age group.

Cancer Screening

Table 2.4-5 outlines cancer screening recommendations by modality.

Colorectal Cancer Screening

- Screening of the general population should begin at 50 years of age. Currently, screening recommendations with regard to colorectal cancer vary

Body mass index (BMI) = weight (kg) ÷ height (m²)

- Normal: 18.5–24.9
- Overweight: 25.0–29.9
- Class I obesity: 30.0–34.9
- Class II obesity: 35.0–39.9
- Class III obesity (extreme): > 40

Approximately one-third of the population is at a healthy weight, one-third is overweight, and one-third is obese.

TABLE 2.4-3. Leading Causes of Death by Age

AGE GROUP	VARIABLE
All ages	Heart disease, cancer, stroke, chronic lower respiratory disease, accidents, diabetes.
< 1 year	Congenital anomalies, disorders related to low birth weight, SIDS, maternal complications.
1–4 years	Injuries, congenital anomalies, neoplasms, homicide, heart disease.
5–14 years	Injuries, neoplasms, congenital anomalies, homicide, suicide, heart disease.
15–24 years	Injuries, homicide, suicide, neoplasms, heart disease.
25–44 years	Injuries, neoplasms, heart disease, suicide, **HIV,** homicide.
45–64 years	Neoplasms, heart disease, injuries, stroke, diabetes, chronic lower respiratory disease.
≥ 65 years	Heart disease, neoplasms, stroke, COPD, influenza and pneumonia, diabetes.

Adapted from the National Center for Health Statistics, *Health 2003.*

TABLE 2.4-4. Screening Measures by Age

Age Group	Measures
Birth–10 years	Height and weight, BP, vision screening, hemoglobinopathy screen (at birth), phenylalanine level (at birth), TSH and/or T_4 (at birth), lead level (at least one time before six years of age).
11–24 years	Height and weight, BP, Pap smear, chlamydia and gonorrhea (GC) screen (if sexually active), rubella serology or vaccination (women only); screen for risky behaviors, including substance abuse.
25–64 years	Height and weight, BP (every two years), cholesterol (every five years), Pap smear and bimanual pelvic exam, fecal occult blood test (FOBT), sigmoidoscopy or colonoscopy, mammography, rubella serology or vaccination (women only); screen for alcohol abuse and depression.
≥ 65 years	Height and weight, BP, FOBT, sigmoidoscopy or colonoscopy, Pap smear, vision and hearing screening; screen for alcohol abuse and depression.

(e.g., FOBT; sigmoidoscopy + FOBT; colonoscopy + FOBT; double-contrast barium enema + FOBT).

- All polyps identified on endoscopy should be removed entirely and reviewed by pathology.
- Patients with **large or multiple adenomas** on endoscopy should have a follow-up colonoscopy within three years.
- Patients with a **first-degree relative** with a history of colorectal cancer should begin screening at 40 years or 10 years before the earliest diagnosis of cancer.
- Patients with **IBD of eight years' duration** should consider surveillance with colonoscopy.
- Patients with a family history of **familial adenomatous polyposis (FAP)** should be screened by genetic analysis; if the mutation is present, perform frequent screening with colonoscopy starting at 10 years of age.
- Patients with **FAP** or long-standing **ulcerative colitis** (≥ 10 years) should be counseled about prophylactic colectomy, particularly if there is evidence of dysplasia.

The influenza vaccine is a killed-virus vaccine that is encouraged for pregnant women in their second or third trimester. The measles and varicella vaccines contain live attenuated virus and are contraindicated in pregnancy.

Influenza A Vaccine

A trivalent killed-virus vaccine that is administered annually.

- Recommended for the following:
  - All persons ≥ 65 years of age (especially those in **chronic care facilities**).
  - Children 6 months to 18 years of age.
  - Pregnant women (second and third trimester).
  - Health care workers.
- Patients with cardiopulmonary disease, DM, hemoglobinopathies, renal dysfunction, or an immunocompromised status.
- **Avoid** in those with egg allergies.

Pneumococcal Vaccine

- The standard vaccine (PPV23) is used in adults but is not effective in children < 2 years of age.

TABLE 2.4-5. **Screening Recommendations**

MODALITY	RECOMMENDATION[a]
Colonoscopy	Once every 10 years in patients ≥ 50 years of age; screening ≥ 40 years for high-risk patients. Preferred modality if there is a known history of dysplasia.
Flexible sigmoidoscopy	Once every five years in patients ≥ 50 years of age; screening ≥ 40 years for high-risk patients.
FOBT	Once yearly in patients ≥ 50 years of age; screening ≥ 40 years for high-risk patients.
Bimanual pelvic exam	Once every 1–3 years in patients 20–40 years of age; once yearly in patients ≥ 40 years of age.
Pap smear	Once every 1–3 years if sexually active or ≥ 21 years of age.
Mammography	Once every 1–2 years in patients ≥ 40 years of age; once yearly in patients ≥ 50 years of age (controversial).
Endometrial tissue sampling	Not recommended as a screening test; indicated for postmenopausal bleeding.
CXR	Not recommended as a screening test.
Skin exam	Insufficient evidence.
DRE	Offer to high-risk patients at 40 years and to others at 50 years of age (controversial).
PSA	Offer to high-risk patients at 40 years and to others at 50 years of age (controversial).
Clinical breast exam	Offer to patients at 40 years of age or earlier if they are high risk (controversial).

[a] Different medical societies have various recommendations regarding cancer screening. Refer to the National Cancer Institute's Web site for a recent summary of recommendations: www.nci.nih.gov/cancer_information/testing.

Adapted from the National Guideline Clearinghouse, www.guidelines.gov.

- A conjugate vaccine (PPV7) has been approved for children < 2 years of age.
- PPV23 is recommended for the following:
    - All persons ≥ 65 years of age.
    - Native Americans and Alaskans.
    - Patients with chronic cardiopulmonary disease, DM, nephrotic syndrome, cirrhosis, asplenia (e.g., sickle cell disease), or immunosuppression.
- Five-year revaccination is recommended for patients who are medically high risk or for adults > 65 years of age if their first vaccination was before age 65.

Reportable Diseases

Many diseases must be reported to the CDC, including HIV, AIDS, syphilis, gonorrhea, chlamydia, measles, mumps, rubella, diphtheria, tetanus, pertussis, viral hepatitis, TB, Lyme disease, cholera, varicella, salmonella, shigella, coccidioidomycosis, and cryptosporidiosis.

Ethics and Legal Issues

GENERAL PRINCIPLES

- **Autonomy:** Clinicians are obligated to respect patients as individuals and to honor their preferences in medical care.
- **Beneficence:** Physicians have a responsibility to act in the patient's best interest ("the physician is a fiduciary"). Patient autonomy may conflict with beneficence.
- **Nonmaleficence:** "Do no harm." If the benefits of an intervention outweigh the risks, however, a patient may make an informed decision to proceed.

DISCLOSURE

- Patients have a right to know about their medical status, prognosis, and treatment options (full disclosure). A patient's family cannot require that a doctor withhold information from the patient.
- **Physicians are obligated to inform patients of mistakes made in their medical treatment.**
- A doctor may withhold information only if the patient requests not to be told or in the rare case when a physician determines that disclosure would severely harm the patient or undermine informed decision-making capacity (**therapeutic privilege**).

CONFIDENTIALITY

- Information disclosed by a patient to his/her physician and information about a patient's medical condition are confidential and cannot be divulged without express patient consent.
- A patient may waive the right to confidentiality (e.g., with insurance companies).
- It is ethically and legally necessary to override confidentiality in the following situations:
    - **Patient intent to commit a violent crime (Tarasoff decision):** Physicians have a **duty to protect** the intended victim through reasonable means (e.g., warn the victim, notify police).
    - Suicidal patients.
    - Child and elder abuse.
    - Infectious diseases (duty to warn public officials and identifiable people at risk).
    - Gunshot and knife wounds (duty to notify the police).
    - Impaired automobile drivers (e.g., the department of motor vehicles requires that licensed drivers be seizure free for at least six months).

INFORMED CONSENT

- Defined as willing acceptance (without coercion) of a medical intervention by a patient after adequate discussion with a physician about the **nature** of the intervention, **indications, risks, benefits,** and potential **alternatives** (including no treatment).
- **Patients may change their minds at any time.** Exceptions include the following:
    - When emergency treatment is required (consent is implied).
    - When patients lack decision-making capacity (consent can be obtained from a surrogate decision maker).

- **Competence:** Refers to a person's legal capacity to make decisions and be held accountable in a court of law. Competence is assessed by the courts and may be used interchangeably with the term *decision-making capacity*.
- **Decision-making capacity:** A medical term that refers to the ability of a patient to understand relevant information, appreciate the medical situation and its consequences, communicate a choice, and deliberate rationally about one's values in relation to the decision.
    - Patients who have decision-making capacity have the right to refuse or discontinue treatment (e.g., Jehovah's Witnesses can refuse blood products).
    - Incompetent patients, as assessed by the courts, or temporarily incapacitated patients (e.g., intoxicated patients with altered mental status) cannot accept or refuse treatment.

MINORS

- **Consent for treatment** is implied in life-threatening situations when parents cannot be contacted.
- Emancipated minors do not require parental consent for medical care. Minors are emancipated if they are married or in the armed services.
- Minors are considered emancipated for the purposes of obtaining medical care for **pregnancy, sexually transmitted infections,** or **drug or alcohol abuse.**
- If a parent requests information about an emancipated minor, confidentiality can be broken only with the patient's permission or if the minor is a danger to him/herself or to others.
- **Refusal of treatment:** A parent has the right to refuse treatment for his/her child as long as those decisions do not pose a serious threat to the child's well-being (e.g., refusing immunizations is not considered a serious threat). If a decision is not in the best interest of the child, a physician may seek a court order to provide treatment against parental wishes. In emergent situations, if withholding treatment jeopardizes the child's safety, treatment can be initiated on the basis of legal precedent.

END-OF-LIFE ISSUES

Written Advance Directives

- **Living will:** Addresses a patient's wishes to withhold or withdraw life-sustaining treatment in the event of terminal disease or a persistent vegetative state. Examples include **DNR** (do not resuscitate) and **DNI** (do not intubate) orders.
- **Durable power of attorney:** Legally designates a surrogate health care decision maker if a patient lacks decision-making capacity. **More flexible** than a living will. Surrogates should make decisions consistent with the person's stated wishes.
- If no living will or DPOA exists, decisions should be made by close family members (spouse, adult children, parents, and adult siblings), friends, or personal physicians, in that order.

Withdrawal of Care

- Patients and their decision makers have the right to forgo life-sustaining treatment.

*DNR/DNI orders do **not** mean "do not treat."*

- There is **no ethical distinction between withholding and withdrawing life-sustaining interventions.** These include ventilation, fluids, nutrition, and medications (e.g., antibiotics).
- It is ethical to provide palliative treatment to relieve pain and suffering even if such treatment may hasten a patient's death.

Euthanasia and Physician-Assisted Suicide

- **Euthanasia** is the administration of a lethal agent with the intent to end life.
    - It is opposed by the AMA Code of Medical Ethics and **is illegal.**
    - Patients who request euthanasia should be evaluated for inadequate pain control and comorbid depression.
- **Physician-assisted suicide** is prescribing a lethal agent to a patient who will self-administer it to end his/her own life. This is currently legal only in the state of Oregon.

Futility

Physicians are not ethically obligated to provide treatment and may **refuse** a family's request for further intervention on the grounds of futility under the following circumstances:

- There is no pathophysiologic rationale for treatment.
- Maximal intervention is currently failing.
- A given intervention has already failed.
- Treatment will not achieve the goals of care.

It is ethical to provide palliative treatment even though it may hasten a patient's death.

CONFLICT OF INTEREST

- Occurs when physicians find themselves having two interests in a given situation.
- **Example:** A physician may own stock in a pharmaceutical company (financial interest) that produces a drug he is prescribing to his patient (patient care interest).
- Physicians should disclose existing conflicts of interest to affected parties (e.g., patients, institutions, the audience of a journal article).

MALPRACTICE

The 4 D's of malpractice:

Duty
Dereliction
Damage
Direct cause

- The essential elements of a civil suit under negligence include the **four D's:**
    - The physician has a **D**uty to the patient.
    - **D**ereliction of duty occurs.
    - There is **D**amage to the patient.
    - **D**ereliction is the **D**irect cause of damage.
- Unlike a criminal suit, in which the burden of proof is "beyond a reasonable doubt," the burden of proof in a malpractice suit is "the preponderance of the evidence."

Gastrointestinal

Cholelithiasis and Biliary Colic

Colic results from transient cystic duct blockage from impacted stones. Risk factors include the **4 F's**—**F**emale, **F**at, **F**ertile, and **F**orty—but the disorder is common and can occur in any patient. Other risk factors include OCP use, rapid weight loss, a ⊕ family history, chronic hemolysis (pigment stones), small bowel resection, and TPN.

HISTORY/PE

- Patients present with **postprandial abdominal pain** (usually in the **RUQ**) that radiates to the right subscapular area or the epigastrium.
- Pain is abrupt, followed by gradual relief, and often associated with **nausea and vomiting,** fatty food intolerance, dyspepsia, and flatulence.
- Gallstones may be asymptomatic in up to 80% of patients. Examination may reveal RUQ tenderness and a palpable gallbladder.

DIAGNOSIS

- Plain x-rays are rarely diagnostic; only 10–15% of stones are radiopaque.
- **RUQ ultrasound** may show gallstones (85–90% sensitive).
- Consider an upper GI series to rule out a hiatal hernia or ulcer.

TREATMENT

- **Cholecystectomy** is curative and can be performed electively.
- Patients may require preoperative ERCP for common bile duct stones.
- Treat nonsurgical candidates with **dietary modification** (avoid triggers such as fatty foods).

COMPLICATIONS

Recurrent biliary colic, acute cholecystitis, choledocholithiasis, acute cholangitis, gallstone ileus, gallstone pancreatitis.

Acute Cholecystitis

Prolonged blockage of the cystic duct, usually by an impacted stone → obstructive distention, inflammation, superinfection, and possibly gangrene of the gallbladder (acute gangrenous cholecystitis). **Acalculous cholecystitis** occurs in the absence of cholelithiasis in chronically debilitated patients, those on TPN, and trauma or burn victims.

HISTORY/PE

- Patients present with **RUQ pain, nausea, low-grade fever, and vomiting.** Symptoms are typically more severe and of longer duration than those of biliary colic.
- RUQ tenderness, inspiratory arrest during deep palpation of the RUQ (**Murphy's sign**), low-grade fever, leukocytosis, mild icterus, and possibly guarding or rebound tenderness may be present on examination.

DIAGNOSIS

- CBC, amylase, lipase, and an LFT panel should be obtained.
- Ultrasound may demonstrate stones, bile sludge, pericholecystic fluid, a thickened gallbladder wall, gas in the gallbladder, and an ultrasonic Murphy's sign (see Figure 2.6-1).

Pigmented gallstones result from hemolysis.

Only 10–15% of gallstones are radiopaque.

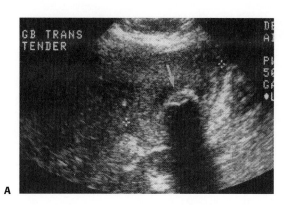
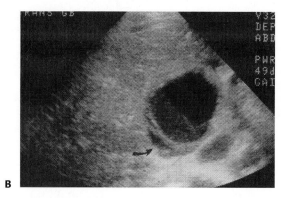

FIGURE 2.6-1. Acute cholecystitis, ultrasound.

(A) Note the sludge-filled, thick-walled gallbladder with a hyperechoic stone and acoustic shadow (arrow). (B) This patient exhibits sludge and pericholecystic fluid (arrow) but no gallstones. (Reproduced, with permission, from Grendell J. *Current Diagnosis and Treatment in Gastroenterology,* 1st ed. Stamford, CT: Appleton & Lange, 1996:212.)

In patients with significant medical problems (including DM), delay cholecystectomy until acute inflammation resolves.

- Obtain a **HIDA scan** when ultrasound is equivocal (see Figure 2.6-2); non-visualization of the gallbladder on HIDA scan suggests acute cholecystitis.

TREATMENT

- Hospitalize patients, administer **IV antibiotics** and **IV fluids,** and replete electrolytes.
- Perform **early cholecystectomy** (within 72 hours of symptom onset) along with either a preoperative ERCP or an **intraoperative cholangiogram** to rule out common bile duct stones.
- Since 50% of cases resolve spontaneously, hemodynamically stable patients with significant medical problems (e.g., DM) can initially be managed medically with a four- to six-week delay in surgical treatment.

COMPLICATIONS

Gangrene, empyema, perforation, gallstone ileus, fistulization, sepsis, abscess formation.

Choledocholithiasis

- Gallstones in the common bile duct. Symptoms vary according to the degree of obstruction, the duration of the obstruction, and the extent of bacterial infection.
- **Hx/PE:** Although sometimes asymptomatic, it often presents with biliary pain, jaundice, episodic colic, fever, and pancreatitis.
- **Dx:** The hallmark is ↑ **alkaline phosphatase** and **total bilirubin,** which may be the only abnormal lab values.
- **Rx:** Management generally consists of ERCP with sphincterotomy followed by semielective cholecystectomy.

Acute Cholangitis

An acute bacterial infection of the biliary tree that commonly occurs 2° to **obstruction,** usually from **gallstones (choledocholithiasis)** or 1° sclerosing cholangitis (progressive inflammation of the biliary tree associated with ulcerative colitis). Gram-⊖ enterics (e.g., *E. coli, Enterobacter, Pseudomonas*) are

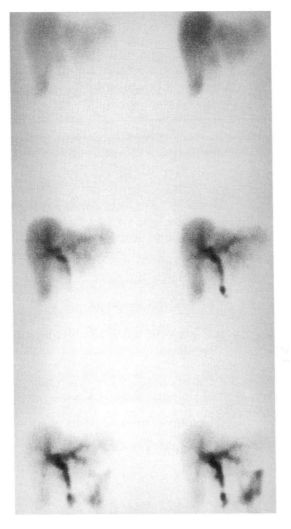

FIGURE 2.6-2. Acute cholecystitis, HIDA scan.

IV dye is taken up by hepatocytes and is conjugated and excreted into the common bile duct. The gallbladder is not visualized, although activity is present in the liver, common duct, and small bowel, suggesting cystic duct obstruction due to acute cholecystitis. (Reproduced, with permission, from Grendell J. *Current Diagnosis and Treatment in Gastroenterology*, 1st ed. Stamford, CT: Appleton & Lange, 1996:217.)

commonly identified pathogens. Risk factors include bile duct stricture, ampullary carcinoma, and pancreatic pseudocyst.

HISTORY/PE

- Charcot's triad—RUQ pain, jaundice, and fever/chills—is classic.
- Reynolds' pentad—Charcot's triad plus shock and altered mental status—may be present in acute suppurative cholangitis and suggests sepsis.

DIAGNOSIS

- Look for leukocytosis, ↑ bilirubin, and ↑ alkaline phosphatase.
- Obtain blood cultures to rule out sepsis. Ultrasound or CT may be a useful adjunct, but diagnosis is often clinical.
- ERCP is both diagnostic and therapeutic (biliary drainage).

Charcot's triad consists of RUQ pain, jaundice, and fever/chills.

Reynolds' pentad consists of RUQ pain, jaundice, fever/chills, shock, and altered mental status.

TREATMENT

- Patients often require **ICU admission** for monitoring, hydration, BP support, and broad-spectrum **IV antibiotic treatment.**
- Patients with acute suppurative cholangitis require **emergent bile duct decompression** via ERCP sphincterotomy, percutaneous transhepatic drainage, or open decompression.

DISORDERS OF THE SMALL BOWEL

Diarrhea

Defined as the production of **> 200 g of feces per day along with a change in stool consistency.** Risk factors include viral/bacterial GI infection, systemic infection, sick contacts, immunosuppression, recent antibiotic use, and recent travel.

HISTORY/PE

The presentation of common diarrheas is as follows (see also Table 2.6-1):

- **Acute diarrhea:** Acute onset with < 3 weeks of symptoms; usually infectious and self-limited. Causes include *E. coli, Salmonella, Shigella, S. aureus, Campylobacter, Vibrio cholera, Giardia,* pseudomembranous colitis (*C. difficile*), and HIV-related diseases (*Cryptosporidium, Isospora*).
- **Chronic diarrhea:** Insidious onset with > 6 weeks of symptoms; usually due to disrupted secretion (e.g., carcinoid, VIPomas), malabsorption (e.g., lactose intolerance, celiac sprue, bacterial overgrowth, IBD), or altered motility. See Figure 2.6-3 for a diagnostic algorithm.
- **Pediatric diarrhea:** Most commonly due to **rotavirus infection (winter),** but may also be due to any adult causes.

Avoid antimotility agents in patients with bloody diarrhea, high fever, or systemic toxicity.

DIAGNOSIS

- Acute diarrhea usually does not require laboratory investigation unless the patient has a high fever, bloody diarrhea, or diarrhea lasting > 4–5 days.
- Send stool for fecal leukocytes, bacterial culture, *C. difficile* toxin, and O&P.
- Consider sigmoidoscopy in patients with bloody diarrhea.

TREATMENT

- **Acute diarrhea:** When bacterial infection is not suspected, treat with antidiarrheals (e.g., loperamide, bismuth salicylate) and oral **fluids** with electrolyte replacement.
- If the patient has evidence of systemic infection (e.g., fever, chills, malaise), avoid antimotility agents and consider antibiotics after stool studies have been sent.
- **Chronic diarrhea:** Identify the underlying cause and treat symptoms with loperamide, opioids, octreotide, or cholestyramine.
- **Pediatric diarrhea:** For children who cannot take medication or PO fluids, hospitalize, give IV fluids, and treat the underlying cause.

Acute diarrhea is generally infectious and self-limited.

Irritable Bowel Syndrome (IBS)

An idiopathic **functional disorder** characterized by abdominal pain and changes in bowel habits that ↑ with stress and are **relieved by bowel move-**

TABLE 2.6-1. **Causes of Infectious Diarrhea**

Infectious Agent	History	PE	Comments	Treatment
Campylobacter	**Most common etiology of infectious diarrhea.** Ingestion of contaminated food or water. Affects young children and young adults. Generally lasts 7–10 days.	Fecal RBCs and WBCs.	Rule out appendicitis and IBD.	Erythromycin.
Clostridium difficile	Recent treatment with antibiotics (cephalosporins, **clindamycin**). Affects hospitalized adult patients. **Watch for toxic megacolon.**	Fever, abdominal pain, possible systemic toxicity. Fecal RBCs and WBCs.	Most commonly in the large bowel, but can also involve the small bowel. Identify *C. difficile* toxin in the stool.	PO metronidazole or PO vancomycin; IV metronidazole if the patient cannot tolerate oral medication.
Entamoeba histolytica	Ingestion of contaminated food or water, history of travel in developing countries. Incubation period can last up to three months.	Severe abdominal pain, fever. Fecal RBCs and WBCs.	Chronic amebic colitis mimics IBD.	Steroids can → fatal perforation. Treat with metronidazole.
E. coli O157:H7	Ingestion of contaminated food (raw meat). Affects children and the elderly. Generally lasts 5–10 days.	Severe abdominal pain, low-grade fever, vomiting. Fecal RBCs and WBCs.	It is important to rule out GI bleed and ischemic colitis. HUS is a possible complication.	Avoid antibiotic therapy.
Salmonella	Ingestion of contaminated poultry or eggs. Affects young children and elderly patients. Generally lasts 2–5 days.	Prodromal headache, fever, myalgia, abdominal pain. Fecal WBCs.	Sepsis is a concern as 5–10% of patients become bacteremic. Sickle cell patients are susceptible to invasive disease → osteomyelitis.	Treat bacteremia or at-risk patients (e.g., sickle cell) with oral quinolone or TMP-SMX.
Shigella	Extremely contagious; transmitted between people by fecal-oral route. Affects young children and institutionalized patients.	Fecal RBCs and WBCs.	May → severe dehydration. Can also → febrile seizures in the very young.	Treat with TMP-SMX to ↓ person-to-person spread.

HIGH-YIELD FACTS

GASTROINTESTINAL

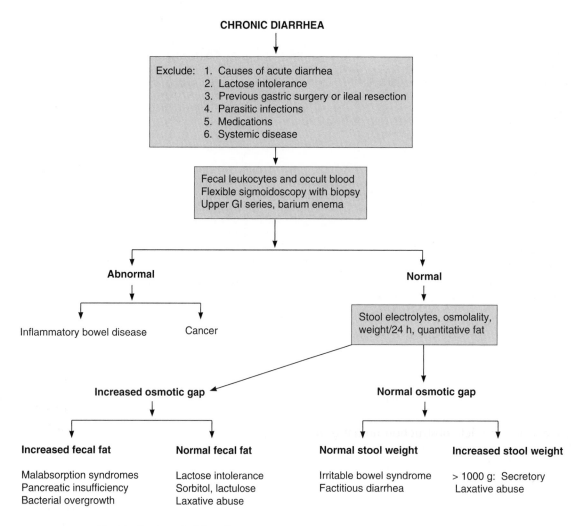

CHRONIC DIARRHEA

Exclude:
1. Causes of acute diarrhea
2. Lactose intolerance
3. Previous gastric surgery or ileal resection
4. Parasitic infections
5. Medications
6. Systemic disease

Fecal leukocytes and occult blood
Flexible sigmoidoscopy with biopsy
Upper GI series, barium enema

Abnormal

Inflammatory bowel disease   Cancer

Normal

Stool electrolytes, osmolality, weight/24 h, quantitative fat

Increased osmotic gap

Increased fecal fat

Malabsorption syndromes
Pancreatic insufficiency
Bacterial overgrowth

Normal fecal fat

Lactose intolerance
Sorbitol, lactulose
Laxative abuse

Normal osmotic gap

Normal stool weight

Irritable bowel syndrome
Factitious diarrhea

Increased stool weight

> 1000 g: Secretory
          Laxative abuse

FIGURE 2.6-3.   Chronic diarrhea decision diagram.

(Reproduced, with permission, from Tierney LM. *Current Medical Diagnosis & Treatment*, 39th ed. New York: McGraw-Hill, 2000:566.)

Half of all patients with IBS have comorbid psychiatric disturbances.

IBS is a diagnosis of exclusion.

ments. Most common in the second and third decades, but since the syndrome is chronic, patients may present at any age. Half of all IBS patients who seek medical care have **comorbid psychiatric disorders** (e.g., depression, anxiety).

HISTORY/PE

- Patients present with **abdominal pain,** a change in bowel habits (**diarrhea and/or constipation**), abdominal distention, stools with mucus, and **relief of pain with a bowel movement.**
- IBS rarely awakens patients from sleep; vomiting, significant weight loss, and constitutional symptoms are also uncommon.
- Examination is usually **unremarkable** except for mild abdominal tenderness.

DIAGNOSIS

- A **diagnosis of exclusion** based on clinical history.
- Tests to rule out other GI causes include CBC, TSH, electrolytes, stool cultures, abdominal films, and barium contrast studies.
- Manometry can assess sphincter function.

TREATMENT

- **Psychological:** Patients need **reassurance** from their physicians. They should not be told that their symptoms are "all in their head."
- **Dietary:** Fiber supplements (psyllium) may help.
- **Pharmacologic:** Treat with TCAs, **antidiarrheals** (loperamide), **antispasmodics** (dicyclomine, anticholinergics), or tegaserod for those with constipation-predominant IBS.

Small Bowel Obstruction (SBO)

Defined as blocked passage of bowel contents through the small bowel. Fluid and gas can build up proximal to the obstruction → fluid and electrolyte imbalances and significant abdominal discomfort. The obstruction can be complete or partial, and strangulation of the bowel may occur. SBO may arise from adhesions from a prior abdominal surgery (60% of cases) or from hernias (10–20%), neoplasms (10–20%), intussusception, gallstone ileus, stricture due to IBD, volvulus, or cystic fibrosis (CF).

HISTORY/PE

- Patients typically experience cramping abdominal pain with a recurrent **crescendo-decrescendo pattern** at 5- to 10-minute intervals.
- Vomiting typically follows the pain; early emesis is bilious and nonfeculent if the obstruction is proximal but **feculent** if it is distal.
- In partial obstruction there is continued passage of flatus but no stool, whereas in complete obstruction no flatus or stool is passed (**obstipation**).
- Abdominal exam often reveals distention, tenderness, prior surgical scars, or hernias.
- Bowel sounds are characterized by **high-pitched tinkles** and **peristaltic rushes.**
- Later in the disease, peristalsis may disappear. Fever, hypotension, rebound tenderness, and tachycardia suggest a surgical emergency.

DIAGNOSIS

- CBC may demonstrate leukocytosis if there is strangulation of bowel.
- Chemistries often reflect dehydration and metabolic alkalosis due to vomiting. Lactic acidosis is particularly worrisome, as it suggests necrotic bowel and the need for emergent surgical intervention.
- Abdominal films often demonstrate a **stepladder pattern of dilated small-bowel loops, air-fluid levels** (see Figure 2.6-4), and a paucity of gas in the colon. The presence of radiopaque material at the cecum is suggestive of gallstone ileus.

TREATMENT

- **Partial obstruction:** Supportive care may be sufficient and should include NPO status, NG suction, IV hydration, correction of electrolyte abnormalities, and Foley catheterization to monitor fluid status.
- Surgery is required in cases of complete SBO, vascular compromise (necrotic bowel), or symptoms lasting > 3 days without resolution.
    - Exploratory laparotomy may be performed with lysis of adhesions; resection of necrotic bowel; and evaluation for stricture, IBD, and hernias.
    - There is a 2% mortality risk for a nonstrangulated SBO; strangulated SBO is associated with up to a 25% mortality rate depending on the time between diagnosis and treatment.

The leading cause of SBO in adults is adhesions.

The leading cause of SBO in children is hernias.

Never let the sun rise or set on a complete SBO.

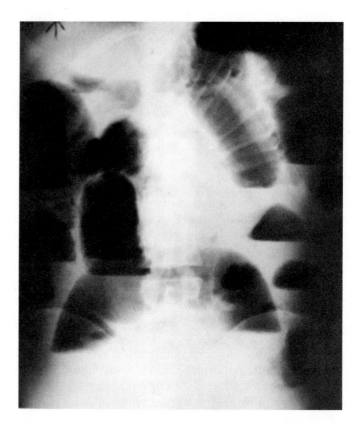

FIGURE 2.6-4. **Acute mechanical obstruction of the small intestine (upright film).**

Note the air-fluid levels, marked distention of bowel loops, and absence of colonic gas. (Reproduced, with permission, from Kasper DL et al [eds]. *Harrison's Principles of Internal Medicine*, 16th ed. New York: McGraw-Hill, 2005:1804.)

- A second-look laparotomy or laparoscopy may be performed 18–36 hours after initial surgical treatment to reevaluate bowel viability.

Ileus

Loss of peristalsis **without structural obstruction.** Risk factors include recent surgery/GI procedures, severe medical illness, immobility, **hypokalemia** or other electrolyte imbalances, **hypothyroidism,** DM, and medications that slow GI motility (e.g., **anticholinergics, opioids**).

HISTORY/PE

- Presenting symptoms include diffuse, constant, moderate abdominal discomfort; **nausea and vomiting** (especially with eating); and an **absence of flatulence or bowel movements.**
- Examination may reveal diffuse tenderness and **abdominal distention, no peritoneal signs,** and ↓ or absent bowel sounds.
- A **rectal examination is required** to rule out fecal impaction in elderly patients.

DIAGNOSIS

- Diffusely **distended loops of small and large bowel on supine AXR** with air-fluid levels on upright view.

Look for air throughout the small and large bowel on AXR.

126

- A Gastrografin study can rule out partial obstruction; CT can rule out neoplasms.

TREATMENT

- ↓ the use of narcotics and any other drugs that reduce **bowel motility.**
- Temporarily ↓ or discontinue oral feeds.
- Initiate **NG suction/parenteral feeds** as necessary.
- Replete electrolytes as needed.

Anticholinergics, opioids, and hypokalemia slow GI motility.

Malabsorption

- Inability to absorb nutrients as a result of an underlying condition such as **celiac disease, Whipple's disease, short bowel syndrome, pancreatic insufficiency, lactose intolerance,** and **infection.** The small bowel is most commonly involved.
- ↓ absorption of protein, fat, carbohydrates, and the smaller vitamins and minerals can be present.
- Hx/PE: Presents with **frequent, loose, watery stools** and/or **pale, foul-smelling, bulky stools** associated with abdominal pain, **flatus, bloating,** weight loss, **nutritional deficiencies,** and fatigue.
- Rx: Etiology dependent. Severely affected patients may receive TPN, immunosuppressants, and anti-inflammatory medications.

Carcinoid Syndrome

- Due to liver metastasis of serotonin and substance P from **carcinoid tumors** (from hormone-producing enterochromaffin cells) that most commonly arise from the ileum and appendix.
- Hx/PE: **Cutaneous flushing, diarrhea, wheezing,** and **cardiac valvular lesions** are the most common manifestations. Symptoms usually follow eating, exertion, or excitement.
- Dx: High urine levels of the serotonin metabolite 5-HIAA are diagnostic. Chest and abdominal CT scans can localize the tumor.
- Rx: Treatment includes **octreotide** (for symptoms) and reduction of tumor mass.

Cutaneous flushing, diarrhea, wheezing, and cardiac valvular lesions are the most common manifestations of carcinoid tumors.

DISORDERS OF THE LARGE BOWEL

Diverticular Disease

Outpouchings of mucosa and submucosa (false diverticula) that herniate through the colonic muscle layers in areas of high intraluminal pressure; most commonly found in the sigmoid colon. **Diverticulosis is the most common cause of acute lower GI bleeding in patients > 40 years of age.** Risk factors include a **low-fiber and high-fat diet,** advanced age (65% occur in those > 80 years of age), and connective tissue disorders (e.g., Ehlers-Danlos, Marfan's syndromes). **Diverticulitis** is due to inflammation and, potentially, perforation of a diverticulum.

HISTORY/PE

- Often **asymptomatic,** but can manifest with constipation, **LLQ abdominal pain,** and **abnormal bowel habits.**
- Bleeding is painless and sudden, generally presenting as hematochezia with symptoms of anemia (fatigue, light-headedness, dyspnea on exertion).

Diverticular disease is the most common cause of acute lower GI bleeding in patients > 40 years of age.

Diverticular disease must be distinguished from colon cancer with perforation.

Avoid flexible sigmoidoscopy and barium enemas in the initial stages of diverticulitis because of perforation risk.

- Uncomplicated diverticular disease presents with a benign exam.
- Diverticulitis presents as an acute, mild-to-severe, steady or cramping pain commonly localized to the **LLQ** with fever, nausea, and vomiting. Perforation is a serious complication.

DIAGNOSIS

- CBC may show **leukocytosis.**
- Diagnosis is based on AXR, colonoscopy, or barium enema. Invasive techniques must be avoided in those with early diverticulitis owing to perforation risk.
- In patients with severe disease or in those who show lack of improvement, CT may reveal abscess or free air.

TREATMENT

- **Uncomplicated diverticular disease:** Patients can be followed and placed on a **high-fiber diet** or fiber supplements.
- **Diverticular bleeding:** Bleeding usually stops spontaneously; transfuse and hydrate as needed. If bleeding does not stop, angiography with embolization or **surgery** is indicated.
- **Diverticulitis:** Treat with **bowel rest** (NPO), NG tube placement, and **broad-spectrum antibiotics** (metronidazole and a fluoroquinolone or a second- or third-generation cephalosporin) if the patient is stable. Avoid barium enema and flexible sigmoidoscopy if diverticulitis is suspected.
- For perforation, perform immediate surgical resection of diseased bowel with 1° anastomosis or temporary colostomy with a Hartmann's pouch and mucous fistula.

Large Bowel Obstruction (LBO)

Table 2.6-2 describes features that distinguish SBO from LBO. Figure 2.6-5 demonstrates the classic radiographic findings of LBO.

Colon and Rectal Cancer

The second leading cause of cancer mortality in the United States after lung cancer. There is an ↑ incidence with age, with a peak incidence at 70–80 years. Risk factors and screening protocols are summarized in Table 2.6-3.

HISTORY/PE

- Without screening, colon and rectal cancer typically presents with symptoms after a prolonged period of silent growth.
- Abdominal pain is the most common presenting complaint. Other features depend on location.
  - **Right-sided lesions:** Often bulky, ulcerating masses that → **anemia from chronic occult blood loss.** Patients may complain of weight loss, anorexia, diarrhea, weakness, or vague abdominal pain. Obstruction is rare.
  - **Left-sided lesions:** Typically **"apple-core" obstructing** masses (see Figure 2.6-6). Patients complain of a **change in bowel habits** (e.g., ↓ stool caliber, constipation, obstipation) and/or blood-streaked stools. Obstruction is common.

TABLE 2.6-2. Characteristics of Small and Large Bowel Obstruction

VARIABLE	SBO	LBO
History	Moderate to severe acute abdominal pain; **copious emesis.** Cramping pain with distal SBO. Fever, signs of dehydration, and hypotension may be seen.	Constipation/obstipation, deep and cramping abdominal pain, nausea/vomiting (less than SBO but more commonly **feculent**).
PE	**Abdominal distention** (distal SBO), abdominal tenderness, visible peristaltic waves, fever, hypovolemia. Look for **surgical scars/hernias;** perform a rectal exam. **High-pitched "tinkly" bowel sounds;** later, absence of bowel sounds.	Sigificant **distention,** tympany, tenderness; examine for peritoneal irritation or mass; fever or signs of shock suggest perforation/peritonitis or ischemia/strangulation. **High-pitched "tinkly" bowel sounds;** later, absence of bowel sounds.
Causes	**Adhesions** (postsurgery), hernias, neoplasm, volvulus, intussusception, gallstone ileus, foreign body, Crohn's disease, CF, stricture, hematoma.	**Colon cancer,** diverticulitis, volvulus, fecal impaction, benign tumors. **Assume colon cancer until proven otherwise.**
Differential	LBO, paralytic ileus, gastroenteritis.	SBO, paralytic ileus, appendicitis, IBD.
Diagnosis	CBC, lactic acid, electrolytes, AXR (see Figure 2.6-4); contrast studies (determine if it is partial or complete), CT scan.	CBC, electrolytes, lactic acid, AXR (see Figure 2.6-5), CT scan; water contrast enema (if perforation is suspected); sigmoidoscopy/colonoscopy if stable.
Treatment	Hospitalize. Partial SBO can be treated conservatively with **NG decompression** and NPO status. Patients with complete SBO should be managed aggressively with NPO status, NG decompression, IV fluids, and **surgical correction.**	Hospitalize. Obstruction can be treated with a Gastrografin enema, colonoscopy, or a **rectal tube;** however **surgery** is usually required. Gangrenous colon usually requires partial colectomy with a diverting colostomy. Treat the underlying cause (e.g., neoplasm).

HIGH-YIELD FACTS

GASTROINTESTINAL

- **Rectal lesions:** Usually present with bright red blood per rectum, and may have tenesmus and/or rectal pain. Can coexist with hemorrhoids, so rectal cancer must be ruled out in all patients with rectal bleeding.

DIAGNOSIS

- Order a CBC (often shows microcytic anemia) and stool occult blood.
- Perform sigmoidoscopy to evaluate rectal bleeding and all suspicious left-sided lesions.
- Rule out synchronous right-sided lesions with colonoscopy. If colonoscopy is incomplete, rule out additional lesions with an air-contrast barium enema.
- Determine the degree of invasion in **rectal cancer** with endoscopic ultrasound.
- Whole-body CT/MRI is used to stage colon cancer according to Dukes' criteria.
- Order CXR, LFTs, and an abdominal CT for metastatic workup. Metastases may arise from direct extension (to local viscera), hematogenous

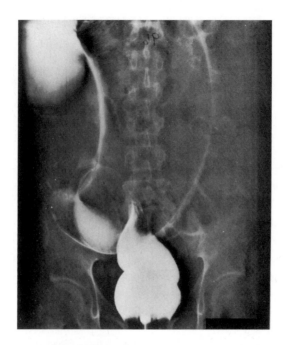

FIGURE 2.6-5. **Large bowel obstruction.**

Barium study shows the "bird-beak" sign, with juxtaposed adjacent bowel walls in the dilated loop pointing toward the site of obstruction. (Reproduced, with permission, from Way L. *Current Surgical Diagnosis & Treatment*, 10th ed. Stamford, CT: Appleton & Lange, 1994:676.)

spread (40–50% go to the liver, but spread may also occur to bone, lungs, and brain), and lymphatic spread (to pelvic lymph nodes).

TREATMENT

- **Preoperative bowel prep:** Mechanical stool evacuation (e.g., Golytely) and oral antibiotics (neomycin, erythromycin).

TABLE 2.6-3. **Risk Factors and Screening for Colorectal Cancer**

RISK FACTORS	SCREENING
Age.	A DRE should be performed yearly for patients ≥ 50 years of age. Up to 10% of all lesions are palpable with DRE.
Hereditary syndromes—familial adenomatous polyposis (100% risk), Gardner's disease, hereditary nonpolyposis colorectal cancer (HNPCC).	Stool guaiac should be performed every year for patients ≥ 50 years of age. Up to 50% of ⊕ guaiac tests are due to colorectal cancer.
Family history.	Sigmoidoscopy performed every 3–5 years for those ≥ 50 years of age can be used to identify and biopsy 50–75% of lesions.
IBD—ulcerative colitis carries a higher risk than does Crohn's disease.	Perform colonoscopy every 10 years in patients ≥ 40 years of age with a family history of colon cancer or polyps, or 10 years prior to the
Adenomatous polyps—villous polyps progress more often than tubular polyps and sessile more than pedunculated polyps. Lesions > 2 cm carry an ↑ risk.	age at diagnosis of the youngest family member with colorectal cancer.
Past history of colorectal cancer.	Colonoscopy every 10 years ≥ 50 years of age can be performed instead of sigmoidoscopy.
High-fat, low-fiber diet.	

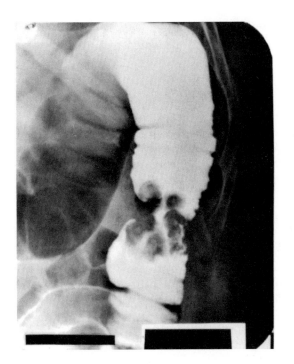

FIGURE 2.6-6. Colon carcinoma.

The encircling carcinoma appears as an "apple-core" filling defect in the descending colon on barium enema x-ray. (Reproduced, with permission, from Way L. *Current Surgical Diagnosis & Treatment*, 10th ed. Stamford, CT: Appleton & Lange, 1994:658.)

- **Colonic lesions:** Surgical resection of the lesion with 3- to 5-cm margins. The lymphatic drainage and mesentery at the origin of the arterial supply are also resected. 1° anastomosis of bowel can usually be performed.
- **Rectal lesions:** The resection technique depends on the proximity of the lesion to the anal verge (junction between the anal canal and the anal skin).
    - **Abdominoperineal resection:** For low-lying lesions < 10 cm from the anal verge, the rectum and anus are resected and a permanent colostomy is placed.
    - **Low anterior resection:** For proximal lesions > 10 cm from the anal verge, a 1° anastomosis between the colon and rectum is created.
    - **Wide local excision:** For small, low-stage, well-differentiated tumors in the lower third of the rectum.
    - **Adjuvant chemotherapy:** Used in cases of colon cancer with ⊕ nodes. Radiation is ineffective for colon cancer but is a useful adjuvant in rectal cancer.
    - Follow with serial CEA levels (diagnostically nonspecific, but useful for monitoring recurrence), colonoscopy, LFTs, CXR, and abdominal CT (for metastasis).

Iron deficiency anemia in an elderly male is colorectal cancer until proven otherwise.

ESOPHAGEAL DISEASE

Dysphagia/Odynophagia

Difficulty swallowing (dysphagia) or pain with swallowing (odynophagia) due to abnormalities of the oropharynx or esophagus. Etiologic factors include achalasia, peptic stricture, esophageal webs or rings, carcinoma, scleroderma, spastic motility disorders, Sjögren's syndrome, medications, and radiation injury.

HISTORY/PE

- Oropharyngeal dysphagia usually involves **liquids** more than solids and may be accompanied by dysarthria or dysphonia.
- Esophageal dysphagia usually involves solids more than liquids for most obstructive causes and is generally progressive; achalasia presents with **both** liquid and solid dysphagia.
- Examine for masses (e.g., goiter, tumor) and anatomical defects.

DIAGNOSIS

- **Oropharyngeal dysphagia:** Cine-esophagram.
- **Esophageal dysphagia:** Barium swallow followed by endoscopy, manometry, and/or pH monitoring. If an obstructive lesion is suspected, proceed directly to endoscopy with biopsy.
- **Odynophagia:** Upper endoscopy.

TREATMENT

Etiology dependent. For achalasia, consider botulinum toxin injection, calcium channel blockers, or balloon dilatation as temporizing measures or esophageal myotomy for long-term treatment.

Esophageal Cancer

- **Squamous cell carcinoma** and **adenocarcinoma are equally common types of esophageal cancer.** The latter is associated with Barrett's esophagus (columnar metaplasia of the distal esophagus 2° to chronic GERD).
- Risk factors include alcohol use, male gender, smoking, and age > 50 years.
- **Hx/PE:** Progressive dysphagia, initially to solids and later to liquids, is commonly seen. Weight loss, odynophagia, GERD, GI bleeding, and vomiting are also seen.
- **Dx:** Barium study shows narrowing of the esophagus with an irregular border protruding into the lumen. EGD and biopsy confirm the diagnosis. MRI or CT are used to evaluate for metastases.
- **Rx:** Chemoradiation therapy is used, but prognosis is poor. Surgical resection can be beneficial in some cases. Patients may require an endoscopically placed esophageal stent for palliation and improved quality of life.

Gastroesophageal Reflux Disease (GERD)

Symptomatic reflux of gastric contents into the esophagus, most commonly as a result of **transient LES relaxation.** Can be due to an incompetent LES, gastroparesis, or hiatal hernia. Risk factors include ↑ intra-abdominal pressure (e.g., obesity, pregnancy), scleroderma, alcohol, caffeine, nicotine, chocolate, and fatty foods.

HISTORY/PE

- Patients present with **heartburn** that commonly occurs 30–90 minutes **after a meal, worsens with reclining,** and often improves with antacids, sitting, or standing.
- Sour taste ("water brash"), laryngitis, dysphagia, and cough or wheezing.

Squamous esophageal cancer is associated with tobacco and alcohol use.

Esophageal webs are associated with iron deficiency anemia (Plummer-Vinson syndrome).

Candidal esophagitis is associated with AIDS.

BARRett's—

Becomes
Adenocarcinoma,
Results from **R**eflux.

- Examination is usually **normal** unless a systemic disease (e.g., Raynaud's syndrome, scleroderma) is present.

DIAGNOSIS

- History and clinical impression.
- Diagnosis may include an AXR, CXR, barium swallow (of limited usefulness, but can diagnose hiatal hernia), esophageal manometry, and 24-hour pH monitoring.
- **EGD** with biopsies should be performed if the patient has long-standing symptoms (to rule out Barrett's esophagus and adenocarcinoma).

TREATMENT

- **Lifestyle:** Weight loss, head-of-bed elevation, and avoidance of nocturnal meals and substances that ↓ LES tone.
- **Health maintenance:** Monitor for Barrett's esophagus and esophageal adenocarcinoma with **serial EGD and biopsy.**
- **Pharmacologic:** Start with **antacids** in patients with intermittent disease; use **H₂ receptor antagonists** (cimetidine, ranitidine) or **PPIs** (omeprazole, lansoprazole) in patients with chronic and frequent symptoms.
- **Surgical:** For refractory or severe disease, **Nissen fundoplication** may offer significant relief.

COMPLICATIONS

Esophageal ulceration, esophageal stricture, aspiration of gastric contents, upper GI bleeding, **Barrett's esophagus.**

GASTRIC DISEASE

Hiatal Hernia

- Herniation of a portion of the stomach upward into the chest through a diaphragmatic opening. There are two common types:
    - **Sliding hiatal hernias (95%):** The gastroesophageal junction and a portion of the stomach are displaced above the diaphragm.
    - **Paraesophageal hiatal hernias (5%):** The gastroesophageal junction remains below the diaphragm, while a neighboring portion of the fundus herniates into the mediastinum.
- **Hx/PE:** May be asymptomatic. Those with sliding hernias may present with GERD.
- **Dx:** Incidental finding on CXR is common, but frequently diagnosed by barium swallow or EGD.
- **Rx:**
    - **Sliding hernias:** Medical therapy and lifestyle modifications to ↓ GERD symptoms.
    - **Paraesophageal hernias:** Surgical gastropexy (attachment of the stomach to the rectus sheath and closure of the hiatus) is recommended to prevent gastric volvulus.

Gastritis

Inflammation of the stomach lining. Subtypes are as follows:

- **Acute gastritis:** Rapidly developing, superficial lesions that are often due to **NSAIDs,** alcohol, *H. pylori* infection, and stress from severe illness (e.g., burns, CNS injury).

Risk factors for GERD include hiatal hernia and ↑ intra-abdominal pressure.

GERD can mimic asthma.

Patients with GERD should avoid caffeine, alcohol, chocolate, garlic, onions, mints, and nicotine.

HIGH-YIELD FACTS

GASTROINTESTINAL

- Chronic gastritis:
  - **Type A (10%):** Occurs in the fundus and is due to **autoantibodies to parietal cells.** Associated with other autoimmune disorders, including pernicious anemia and thyroiditis, as well as with an ↑ risk of gastric adenocarcinoma.
  - **Type B (90%):** Occurs in the antrum and may be caused by NSAID use or *H. pylori* **infection.** Often asymptomatic, but associated with an ↑ risk of PUD and gastric cancer.

HISTORY/PE

Patients may be asymptomatic or may complain of indigestion, nausea, vomiting, hematemesis, or melena.

DIAGNOSIS

- Upper endoscopy can help visualize the gastric lining.
- *H. pylori* infection can be detected by urease breath test, serum IgG antibody (indicating exposure, not current infection), urine *H. pylori* stool antigen, or endoscopic biopsy.

TREATMENT

- ↓ intake of offending agents; antacids, sucralfate, H_2 blockers, and/or PPIs may help.
- Use triple therapy (amoxicillin, clarithromycin, omeprazole) to treat *H. pylori* infection.
- Give a prophylactic H_2 blocker for patients at risk for stress ulcers (e.g., ICU patients).

Gastric Cancer

- This malignant tumor is the second most common cause of cancer-related death worldwide. They are generally adenocarcinomas, which exhibit two morphologic types:
  - **Intestinal type:** Thought to arise from intestinal metaplasia of **gastric mucosal cells.** Risk factors include a diet high in nitrites and salt and low in fresh vegetables (antioxidants), *H. pylori* colonization, and chronic gastritis.
  - **Diffuse type:** Tends to be poorly differentiated and not associated with *H. pylori* infection or chronic gastritis. Risk factors are largely unknown.
- **Hx/PE:** Advanced cases generally present with abdominal pain, early satiety, and weight loss. Five-year survival is < 10%.
- **Dx:** Early gastric carcinoma is largely asymptomatic and is discovered serendipitously with endoscopic examination of high-risk individuals.
- **Rx:** Successful treatment rests entirely on early detection and surgical removal of the tumor.

Peptic Ulcer Disease (PUD)

Damage to the gastric or duodenal mucosa caused by impaired mucosal defense and/or ↑ acidic gastric contents. *H. pylori* plays a causative role in > 90% of duodenal ulcers and 70% of gastric ulcers. Other risk factors include **corticosteroid, NSAID, alcohol,** and **tobacco** use. Males are affected more often than females.

HISTORY/PE

- Classically presents with chronic or periodic **dull, burning epigastric pain** that **improves with meals** (especially duodenal ulcers), worsens 2–3 hours after eating, and can radiate to the back.
- Patients may also complain of nausea, hematemesis ("coffee-ground" emesis), or blood in the stool (melena or hematochezia).
- Examination may reveal varying degrees of **epigastric tenderness** and, if there is active bleeding, ⊕ stool guaiac.
- An acute perforation can present with a rigid abdomen, rebound tenderness, guarding, or other signs of peritoneal irritation.

DIAGNOSIS

- **AXR to rule out perforation** (free air under the diaphragm) and CBC to assess for GI bleeding (low or ↓ hematocrit).
- **Upper endoscopy** with biopsy to confirm PUD and to rule out active bleeding or gastric adenocarcinoma (10% of gastric ulcers); barium swallow is an alternative.
- *H. pylori* testing includes urease breath test, serum IgG (less expensive but less sensitive and indicates exposure, not active infection), stool *H. pylori* antigen test, or endoscopic biopsy.
- In recurrent or refractory cases, serum gastrin can be used to screen for Zollinger-Ellison syndrome (patients must discontinue PPI use prior to testing).

TREATMENT

- **Acute:**
  - Rule out active bleeding with serial hematocrits, rectal exam with stool guaiac, and NG lavage.
  - Monitor the patient's hematocrit and BP and initiate IV hydration, transfusion, IV PPIs, endoscopy, and surgery as needed.
  - If perforation is likely, **emergent surgery** is indicated.
- **Pharmacologic:**
  - Involves protecting the mucosa, ↓ acid production, and eradicating *H. pylori* infection.
  - Treat mild disease with antacids or with sucralfate, bismuth, and misoprostol (a prostaglandin analog) for mucosal protection. PPIs or H$_2$ receptor antagonists may be used to ↓ acid secretion.
  - Patients with confirmed *H. pylori* infection should receive triple therapy (amoxicillin, clarithromycin, and omeprazole).
- Discontinue use of exacerbating agents. Patients with recurrent or severe disease may require chronic symptomatic therapy.
- **Endoscopy and surgery:**
  - Patients with symptomatic gastric ulcers for **> 2 months** that are **refractory** to medical therapy should have either an endoscopy or an upper GI series with barium to rule out gastric adenocarcinoma.
- Refractory cases may require a surgical procedure such as **parietal cell vagotomy** (the most selective and preferred surgical approach).

COMPLICATIONS

Hemorrhage (posterior ulcers that erode into the gastroduodenal artery), gastric outlet obstruction, perforation (usually anterior ulcers), intractable pain.

The leading cause of lower GI bleed is upper GI bleed.

Rule out Zollinger-Ellison syndrome with serum gastrin levels in cases of GERD and PUD that are refractory to medical management.

Misoprostol can help patients with PUD who require NSAID therapy (e.g., patients with arthritis).

Complications of PUD—

HOPI

Hemorrhage
Obstruction
Perforation
Intractable pain

Zollinger-Ellison Syndrome

- A rare condition characterized by **gastrin-producing tumors** in the duodenum and/or pancreas → oversecretion of gastrin.
- ↑ gastrin → production of high levels of **gastric acid** by the gastric mucosa → recurrent/intractable **ulcers** in the stomach and duodenum.
- In 25–50% of cases, gastrinomas are associated with MEN I.
- **Hx/PE:** Patients may present with unresponsive, recurrent **gnawing, burning abdominal pain** as well as with **diarrhea,** nausea, vomiting, fatigue, weakness, weight loss, and **GI bleeding.**
- **Dx:** Measurement of serum gastrin level and endoscopic examination of the gastric mucosa.
- **Rx:**
  - Requires ↓ **acid production.** H₂ blockers are typically ineffective, but a moderate- to high-dose PPI often controls the symptoms.
  - Surgical repair of peptic ulcers and/or removal of tumor can be beneficial in refractory cases.
  - Since roughly 50% of gastrinomas are malignant, close **follow-up** is mandatory.

Zollinger-Ellison syndrome is associated with MEN I syndrome in roughly 25–50% of cases.

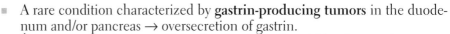
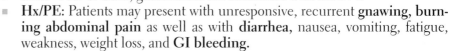

GASTROINTESTINAL BLEEDING

Bleeding from the GI tract may present as hematemesis, hematochezia, and/or melena. Table 2.6-4 presents the features of upper and lower GI bleeding.

TABLE 2.6-4.   Features of Upper and Lower GI Bleeding

VARIABLE	UPPER GI BLEEDING	LOWER GI BLEEDING
History/PE	Hematemesis, melena > hematochezia, depleted volume status (e.g., tachycardia, light-headedness, hypotension).	Hematochezia > melena, but can be either.
Diagnosis	NG tube and NG lavage; endoscopy if stable.	Rule out upper GI bleed with NG tube and NG lavage. Colonoscopy if stable.
Common causes	**Gastritis,** PUD, Mallory-Weiss tear, esophageal varices, vascular abnormalities, neoplasm, esophagitis.	**Diverticulosis** (most common), AV malformations, neoplasm, IBD, anorectal disease, mesenteric ischemia.
Initial treatment	Protect the airway (may need intubation). Stabilize the patient with IV fluids, blood (hematocrit is not an accurate measure of acute blood loss).	Similar to upper GI bleed.
Long-term management	Endoscopy followed by therapy directed at underlying cause (e.g., H₂ blockers or PPIs for PUD; sclerotherapy or banding for varices).	Rule out upper GI source; anoscopy or sigmoidoscopy; colonoscopy; manage etiology (e.g., surgical resection for tumor or diverticula, medical therapy for IBD).

Consists of **Crohn's disease and ulcerative colitis** (see Figure 2.6-7). Most common in whites and **Ashkenazi Jews,** appearing most frequently during the teens to early 30s or in the 60s. Table 2.6-5 summarizes the features of IBD.

INGUINAL HERNIAS

Abnormal **protrusions of abdominal contents** (usually the small intestine) into the inguinal region through a weakness or defect in the abdominal wall. Defined as **direct** or **indirect** on the basis of their relationship to the inguinal canal.

- **Indirect:** Herniation of abdominal contents through the internal and then **external inguinal rings** and eventually into the scrotum (in males).
  - The **most common hernia in both genders.**
  - Due to a **congenital patent processus vaginalis.**
- **Direct:** Herniation of abdominal contents through the floor of **Hesselbach's triangle** (see Figure 2.6-8).
  - Hernial sac contents do not traverse the internal **inguinal ring;** they herniate directly through the abdominal wall and are contained within the **aponeurosis** of the **external oblique muscle.**
  - Most often due to an acquired defect in the **transversalis fascia** from mechanical breakdown that ↑ with age.

Hesselbach's triangle is an area bounded by the inguinal ligament, inferior epigastric artery, and rectus abdominis.

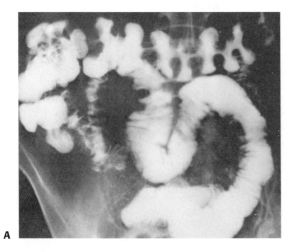

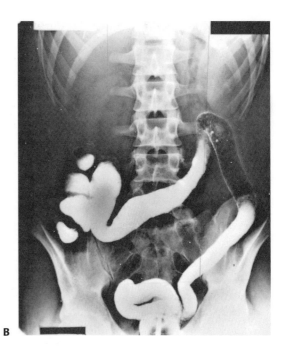

FIGURE 2.6-7. **Inflammatory bowel disease.**

(A) Crohn's disease. Barium enema x-ray reveals deep transverse fissures, ulcers, and edema of the bowel. (B) Ulcerative colitis. Barium enema x-ray demonstrates shortening of the colon, loss of haustra ("lead pipe" appearance), and fine serrations of the bowel edges from small ulcers. (Reproduced, with permission, from Stobo JD et al. *The Principles and Practice of Medicine,* 23rd ed. Stamford, CT: Appleton & Lange, 1996:135.)

TABLE 2.6-5. Features of Ulcerative Colitis and Crohn's Disease

VARIABLE	ULCERATIVE COLITIS	CROHN'S DISEASE
Site of involvement	The **rectum** is always involved. May extend proximally in a **continuous fashion.** Inflammation and ulceration are **limited to the mucosa and submucosa.**	May involve **any portion** of the GI tract, particularly the **ileocecal region,** in a **discontinuous pattern** ("skip lesions"). The rectum is often spared. **Transmural** inflammation.
History/PE	**Bloody diarrhea,** lower abdominal cramps, tenesmus, urgency. Exam may reveal orthostatic hypotension, tachycardia, abdominal tenderness, frank blood on rectal exam, and extraintestinal manifestations.	Abdominal pain, abdominal mass, low-grade fever, weight loss, watery diarrhea. Exam may reveal fever, abdominal tenderness or mass, **perianal fissures, fistulas,** and extraintestinal manifestations.
Extraintestinal manifestations	Aphthous stomatitis, episcleritis/uveitis, arthritis, **1° sclerosing cholangitis, toxic megacolon,** erythema nodosum, and pyoderma gangrenosum.	Same as ulcerative colitis, as well as nephrolithiasis and fistulas to the skin, biliary tract, or urinary tract or between bowel loops.
Diagnosis	CBC, AXR, stool cultures, O&P, stool assay for *C. difficile.* Colonoscopy can show diffuse and continuous rectal involvement, friability, edema, and **pseudopolyps.** Definitive diagnosis can be made with biopsy.	Same laboratory workup as ulcerative colitis. Colonoscopy may show aphthoid, linear, or stellate ulcers, strictures, **"cobblestoning,"** and **"skip lesions."** "Creeping fat" may also be present. Definitive diagnosis can be made with biopsy.
Treatment	**Sulfasalazine** or **5-ASA** (mesalamine); corticosteroids and immunosuppressants for refractory disease. **Total colectomy is curative** for long-standing or fulminant colitis or toxic megacolon.	**Sulfasalazine;** corticosteroids and immunosuppression indicated if no improvement. Surgical resection may be necessary for suspected perforation; **may recur** anywhere in the GI tract.
Incidence of cancer	**Markedly ↑ risk of colorectal cancer** in long-standing cases (monitor with frequent fecal occult blood screening and colonoscopy after eight years of disease).	Incidence of 2° malignancy is much lower than in ulcerative colitis.

TREATMENT

- Because of the risk of **incarceration** and **strangulation,** surgical management (open or laparoscopic) is indicated unless specific contraindications are present.
- Repair of a direct inguinal hernia involves correcting the defect in the transversalis fascia.
- Indirect inguinal hernias are repaired by isolating and ligating the hernial sac and reducing the size of the internal inguinal ring to allow only the spermatic cord structures in males to pass through.

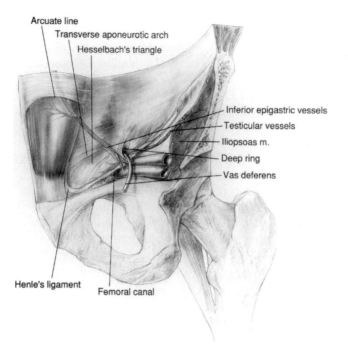

Arcuate line
Transverse aponeurotic arch
Hesselbach's triangle

Inferior epigastric vessels
Testicular vessels
Iliopsoas m.
Deep ring
Vas deferens

Henle's ligament
Femoral canal

FIGURE 2.6-8. **Hesselbach's triangle.**

(Reproduced, with permission, form Schwartz LS. *Principles of Surgery*, 7th ed. New York: McGraw-Hill, 1999:1588.)

LIVER DISEASE

Hepatitis

Inflammation of the liver. Jaundice is a major clinical feature and arises when there is excess bilirubin circulating in the blood. In adults, jaundice is pathological, indicating either overload or damage to the liver or an inability to excrete bilirubin through the biliary system. Causes of jaundice include the following:

- Obstruction of the biliary system (by infection, stone, stricture, or tumor).
- Hepatitis (viral, drug induced, autoimmune).
- Alcoholic cirrhosis, pancreatic cancer, hemolytic anemia, and congenital disorders of bilirubin metabolism (Gilbert's syndrome, Dubin-Johnson syndrome, Crigler-Najjar syndrome).

History/PE

- Acute hepatitis often starts with a viral prodrome of nonspecific symptoms (e.g., **malaise,** fever, joint pain, fatigue, URI symptoms, **nausea, vomiting,** changes in bowel habits) followed by **jaundice** and RUQ tenderness.
- Examination often reveals **jaundice,** scleral icterus, **tender hepatomegaly,** possible splenomegaly, and lymphadenopathy.
- Chronic hepatitis usually gives rise to symptoms indicative of chronic liver disease (jaundice, cirrhosis, fatigue). At least 80% of those infected with HCV and 10% of those with HBV will develop chronic hepatitis.
- Other etiologies of chronic hepatitis include HDV (with HBV), autoimmune hepatitis, alcoholic hepatitis, drug-induced disease (e.g., INH, methyldopa, acetaminophen), right-sided heart failure, Wilson's disease, hemochromatosis, α_1-antitrypsin deficiency, and neoplasms.

139

DIAGNOSIS

- **Normal WBC count (with relative leukocytosis)**, dramatically ↑ **ALT and AST**, and ↑ bilirubin/alkaline phosphatase are present in the acute form.
- In chronic hepatitis, ALT and AST are ↑ for > 6 months with concurrent alkaline phosphatase/bilirubin ↑ and hypoalbuminemia. In severe cases, PT will be prolonged, as all clotting factors except factor VIII are produced by the liver.
- The diagnosis of viral hepatitis is made by **hepatitis serology** (see Table 2.6-6 and Figure 2.6-9 for description and timing of serologic markers) and in chronic or severe cases by liver biopsy.
- ANA, anti–smooth muscle antibody, and antimitochondrial antibody indicate autoimmune hepatitis. Iron saturation (hemochromatosis) and ceruloplasmin (Wilson's disease) can identify other causes.

TREATMENT

- Treatment is etiology specific; monitor for resolution of symptoms over time.
- Steroids for severe alcoholic hepatitis.
- **Immunosuppression** with steroids and other agents (azathioprine) for autoimmune hepatitis.
- **IFN-α, lamivudine (3TC), and adefovir** for chronic HBV infection; peginterferon **and ribavirin** for chronic HCV infection.
- **Liver transplantation** is the treatment of choice for patients with end-stage liver failure.
- ICU management and emergent transplant for fulminant hepatic failure.

COMPLICATIONS

Cirrhosis, liver failure, hepatocellular carcinoma (3–5%), death within five years (50%).

An AST/ALT ratio > 2 suggests alcoholic hepatitis.

Some 80% of patients with HCV infection will develop chronic hepatitis.

The sequelae of chronic hepatitis include cirrhosis, liver failure, and hepatocellular carcinoma.

Table 2.6-6. Key Hepatitis Serologic Markers

SEROLOGIC MARKER	DESCRIPTION
IgM HAVAb	IgM antibody to HAV; best test to detect active hepatitis A.
HBsAg	Antigen found on surface of HBV; continued presence indicates carrier state.
HBsAb	Antibody to HBsAg; **provides immunity** to hepatitis B.
HBcAg	Antigen associated with core of HBV.
HBcAb	Antibody to HBcAg; positive during **window period.** IgM HBcAb is an indicator of recent disease.
HBeAg	A second, different antigenic determinant in the HBV core. Important indicator of transmissibility. (**BE**ware!)
HBeAb	Antibody to e antigen; indicates low transmissibility.

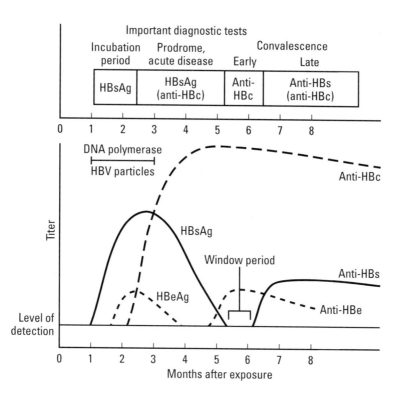

FIGURE 2.6-9. **Hepatitis B time course with serologic markers.**

Portal Hypertension

Defined as portal pressure 5 mmHg greater than the pressure in the IVC. Causes are as follows:

- **Presinusoidal:** Splenic or portal vein thrombosis, schistosomiasis, granulomatous disease.
- **Sinusoidal:** Cirrhosis, granulomatous disease.
- **Postsinusoidal:** Right heart failure, constrictive pericarditis, hepatic vein thrombosis.
- **Budd-Chiari syndrome:** Hepatic vein thrombosis 2° to hypercoagulability; treatment includes clot lysis, TIPS, or hepatic transplantation. Has a poor prognosis.

HISTORY/PE

- Presents with **jaundice, ascites, spontaneous bacterial peritonitis, hepatic encephalopathy** (e.g., asterixis, altered mental status), **gastroesophageal varices,** and renal dysfunction.
- Examination may reveal the stigmata of portal hypertension (see Figures 2.6-10 and 2.6-11).

DIAGNOSIS

- Includes LFTs, alkaline phosphatase, bilirubin, albumin, and PT/PTT to assess hepatic function.
- Serum ferritin, ceruloplasmin, α_1-antitrypsin, and ultrasound may help identify additional causes, such as hemochromatosis, Wilson's disease, α_1-antitrypsin deficiency, and Budd-Chiari syndrome, respectively.
- Indirect hepatic vein wedge pressure (a measure of portal pressure) is ↑.
- The etiology of ascites can be established by measurement of the **serum-**

Gut, butt, and caput—the 3 anastomoses commonly seen in cirrhosis.

Alcoholism, chronic hepatitis, and other chronic liver diseases → cirrhosis.

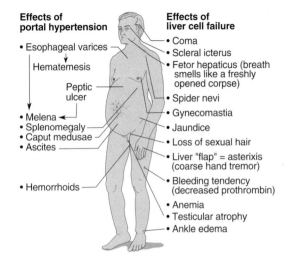

Effects of portal hypertension
- Esophageal varices
  - Hematemesis
- Peptic ulcer
- Melena
- Splenomegaly
- Caput medusae
- Ascites
- Hemorrhoids

Effects of liver cell failure
- Coma
- Scleral icterus
- Fetor hepaticus (breath smells like a freshly opened corpse)
- Spider nevi
- Gynecomastia
- Jaundice
- Loss of sexual hair
- Liver "flap" = asterixis (coarse hand tremor)
- Bleeding tendency (decreased prothrombin)
- Anemia
- Testicular atrophy
- Ankle edema

FIGURE 2.6-10. Presentation of cirrhosis/portal hypertension.

(Adapted, with permission, from Chandrasoma P, Taylor CE. *Concise Pathology*, 3rd ed. Stamford, CT: Appleton & Lange, 1998:654.)

ascites albumin gradient (**SAAG** = ascites albumin − serum albumin); see Table 2.6-7.

TREATMENT

- Aimed at ameliorating the complications of portal hypertension.
- **Ascites:**
  - Sodium restriction and diuretics (furosemide and spironolactone).

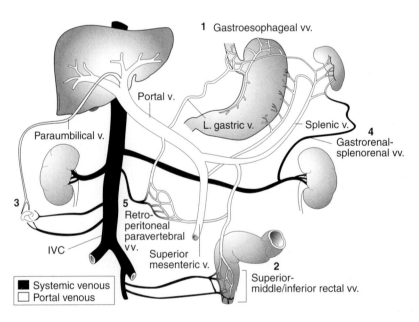

FIGURE 2.6-11. Portosystemic anastomoses.

1. Left gastric–azygos → esophageal varices. 2. Superior–middle/inferior rectal → hemorrhoids. 3. Paraumbilical–inferior epigastric → caput medusae (navel). 4. Gastrorenal-splenorenal. 5. Retroperitoneal paravertebral.

TABLE 2.6-7. **Serum-Ascites Albumin Gradient**

SAAG > 1.1	SAAG < 1.1

Ascites is due to an imbalance between hydrostatic and oncotic pressures:
   Chronic liver disease
   Massive hepatic metastases
   CHF
	Ascites is due to protein leakage:
	   Nephrotic syndrome
	   Tuberculosis
	   Malignancy (e.g., ovarian cancer)

- Rule out infectious and neoplastic causes; perform paracentesis to obtain the SAAG, CBC, and cultures.
- If possible, treat underlying liver disease.
- **Spontaneous bacterial peritonitis:**
  - Check peritoneal fluid if there is a possibility of infection. The fluid is ⊕ if there are > 250 PMNs/mL or > 500 WBCs.
  - Treat with **IV antibiotics** (e.g., third-generation cephalosporin) to cover both gram-⊕ (*Enterococcus*) and gram-⊖ (*E. coli, Klebsiella*) organisms until a causative organism is identified.
- **Hepatorenal syndrome:** A diagnosis of exclusion; difficult to treat and often requires dialysis.
- **Hepatic encephalopathy:** ↓ protein consumption; treat with **lactulose** and/or **metronidazole.**
- **Esophageal varices:** Monitor for GI bleeding; treat medically (β-blockers), endoscopically (band ligation and sclerotherapy), or surgically (portocaval shunt).

Spontaneous bacterial peritonitis is diagnosed by > 250 PMNs/mL or > 500 WBCs in the ascitic fluid.

Hepatocellular Carcinoma

One of the most common cancers worldwide despite its relatively low incidence in the United States. 1° risk factors for the development of hepatocellular carcinoma in the United States are **cirrhosis** and **chronic hepatitis** (HBV or HCV). In developing countries, **aflatoxins** (in various food sources) are also major risk factors.

HISTORY/PE

- Patients commonly present with **RUQ tenderness, abdominal distention,** and signs of chronic liver disease such as **jaundice, easy bruisability,** and **coagulopathy.**
- **Examination usually reveals a nodular cirrhotic liver.**

DIAGNOSIS

- Diagnosis is often suggested by the presence of a mass on **ultrasound** or **CT** as well as by ↑ LFTs and significantly ↑ α-fetoprotein (AFP) levels.
- Liver biopsy for definitive diagnosis.

TREATMENT

- For small tumors that are detected early, aggressive tumor resection or **orthotopic liver transplantation** may be successful.
- Chemotherapy and radiation are generally not effective, although they may be used to shrink large tumors prior to surgery (**neoadjuvant therapy**).

Complications of hepatocellular carcinoma include GI bleeding, liver failure, and metastasis.

- Monitor tumor recurrence with serial AFP levels. Prevent exposure to hepatic carcinogens and vaccinate against hepatitis in high-risk individuals.

Hemochromatosis

Caused by hyperabsorption of iron with parenchymal hemosiderin accumulation in the liver, pancreas, heart, adrenals, testes, pituitary, and kidneys. It is an **autosomal-recessive** disease that usually occurs in males of northern European descent and is rarely recognized before the fifth decade. 2° hemochromatosis may occur with iron overload and is common in patients receiving **chronic transfusion therapy** (e.g., for α-thalassemia) as well as in **alcoholics** (alcohol ↑ iron absorption).

HISTORY/PE

- Patients may present with abdominal pain or **symptoms of DM, hypogonadism, arthropathy of the MCP joints, heart failure,** or cirrhosis.
- Exam may reveal **bronze skin pigmentation**, pancreatic dysfunction, **cardiac dysfunction** (CHF), hepatomegaly, and testicular atrophy.

DIAGNOSIS

- Evaluate for ↑ **serum iron,** percent saturation of iron, and ferritin with ↓ serum transferrin.
- Fasting transferrin saturation (serum iron divided by transferrin level) > 45% is the most sensitive diagnostic test.
- **Glucose intolerance** and mildly ↑ AST and alkaline phosphatase can be present.
- Perform a **liver biopsy** (to determine hepatic iron index), hepatic MRI, or hemochromatosis mutation C282Y screen.

TREATMENT

- **Weekly phlebotomy;** when serum iron levels ↓, perform maintenance phlebotomy every 2–4 months.
- **Deferoxamine** can be used for maintenance therapy.

COMPLICATIONS

Cirrhosis, hepatocellular carcinoma, cardiomegaly → CHF and/or conduction defects, DM, impotence, arthropathy, hypopituitarism.

Wilson's Disease (Hepatolenticular Degeneration)

> **Wilson's disease—**
>
> **ABCD**
>
> **A**sterixis
> **B**asal ganglia
> deterioration
> **C**eruloplasmin ↓,
> **C**irrhosis, **C**opper ↑,
> **C**arcinoma
> (hepatocellular),
> **C**horeiform
> movements
> **D**ementia

- ↓ ceruloplasmin and **excessive deposition of copper** in the liver and brain due to a deficient copper-transporting protein. Linked to an autosomal-recessive defect on chromosome 13. Usually occurs in patients < 30 years of age; 50% of patients are symptomatic by 15 years of age.
- Hx: Patients present with hemolytic anemia, **liver abnormalities** (jaundice 2° to hepatitis/cirrhosis), and neurologic (loss of coordination, **tremor,** dysphagia) as well as **psychiatric** (psychosis, anxiety, mania, depression) **abnormalities.**
- PE: May reveal **Kayser-Fleischer rings** in the cornea (green-to-brown deposits of copper in Descemet's membrane) as well as jaundice, hepatomegaly, asterixis, choreiform movements, and rigidity.
- Dx: ↓ **serum ceruloplasmin,** ↑ urinary copper excretion, ↑ hepatic copper.
- Rx: **Dietary copper restriction** (avoid shellfish, liver, legumes), **penicillamine** (a copper chelator that ↑ urinary copper excretion; administer with pyridoxine), and possibly oral zinc (↑ fecal excretion).

Pancreatitis

Table 2.6-8 lists the important features of acute and chronic pancreatitis. Table 2.6-9 lists Ranson's criteria for predicting mortality associated with acute pancreatitis.

T A B L E   2 . 6 - 8 .   **Features of Acute and Chronic Pancreatitis**

VARIABLE	ACUTE PANCREATITIS	CHRONIC PANCREATITIS
Pathophysiology	Leakage of pancreatic enzymes into pancreatic and peripancreatic tissue, often 2° to gallstone disease or alcoholism.	Irreversible parenchymal destruction → pancreatic dysfunction.
Time course	Abrupt onset of severe pain.	Persistent, recurrent episodes of severe pain.
Risk factors	**Gallstones, alcoholism,** hypercalcemia, hypertriglyceridemia, trauma, drug side effects (thiazide diuretics), viral infections, post-ERCP, scorpion bites.	**Alcoholism** (90%), gallstones, hyperparathyroidism, congenital malformation (pancreas divisum). May also be idiopathic.
History/PE	**Severe epigastric pain (radiating to the back),** nausea, vomiting, weakness, fever, shock. Flank discoloration (**Grey Turner sign**) and periumbilical discoloration (**Cullen's sign**) may be evident on exam.	Recurrent episodes of **persistent epigastric pain,** anorexia, nausea, constipation, flatulence, **steatorrhea,** DM.
Diagnosis	↑ **amylase,** ↑ **lipase,** ↓ **calcium** if severe; **"sentinel loop"** or **"colon cutoff"** sign on AXR. Ultrasound or CT may show enlarged pancreas with stranding, abscess, hemorrhage, necrosis, or pseudocyst.	↑ or normal amylase and lipase, **glycosuria, pancreatic calcifications,** and mild ileus on AXR and CT (**"chain of lakes"**).
Treatment	Removal of offending agent if possible. Standard supportive measures: IV fluids/electrolyte replacement, analgesia, bowel rest, NG suction, nutritional support, O_2, "tincture of time." IV antibiotics, respiratory support, and surgical debridement if necrotizing pancreatitis is present.	Analgesia, exogenous lipase/trypsin and medium-chain fatty-acid diet, avoidance of causative agents (EtOH), celiac nerve block, surgery for intractable pain or structural causes.
Prognosis	85–90% mild, self-limited; 10–15% severe, requiring ICU admission; mortality may approach 50% in severe cases.	Can have chronic pain and pancreatic exocrine and endocrine dysfunction.
Complications	**Pancreatic pseudocyst, fistula formation,** hypocalcemia, renal failure, pleural effusion, chronic pancreatitis, sepsis. Mortality 2° to acute pancreatitis can be predicted with Ranson's criteria (see Table 2.6-9).	**Chronic pain,** malnutrition/weight loss, pancreatic cancer.

TABLE 2.6-9.   Ranson's Criteria for Acute Pancreatitis[a]

ON ADMISSION	AFTER 48 HOURS
"GA LAW":	**"C HOBBS":**
Glucose > 200 mg/dL	**C**a²⁺ < 8.0 mg/dL
Age > 55 years	**H**ematocrit decrease by > 10%
LDH > 350 IU/L	**O**₂ Pao₂ < 60 mmHg
AST > 250 IU/dL	**B**ase excess > 4 mEq/L
WBC > 16,000/mL	**B**UN increase > 5 mg/dL
	Sequestered fluid > 6 L

[a] The risk of mortality is 20% with 3–4 signs, 40% with 5–6 signs, and 100% with ≥ 7 signs.

Pancreatic Cancer

Roughly 90% are pancreatic head adenocarcinomas. Risk factors include smoking, chronic pancreatitis, a first-degree relative with pancreatic cancer, and a high-fat diet. Most commonly seen in men in their 60s.

HISTORY/PE

- Presents with abdominal pain radiating toward the back, as well as with jaundice, loss of appetite, nausea, vomiting, weight loss, weakness, fatigue, and indigestion.
- Examination may reveal a palpable, nontender gallbladder (**Courvoisier's sign**) or migratory thrombophlebitis (**Trousseau's sign**).

DIAGNOSIS

The classic presentation of pancreatic cancer is painless, progressive jaundice.

Use CT to detect a pancreatic mass, dilated pancreatic and bile ducts, the extent of vascular involvement, and metastases. If a mass is not visualized, use ERCP or endoscopic ultrasound for better visualization, and consider fine-needle aspiration.

TREATMENT

- Most patients present with metastatic disease, and treatment is palliative.
- Some 10–20% of pancreatic head tumors have no evidence of metastasis and may be resected using the Whipple procedure (pancreaticoduodenectomy).
- Chemotherapy with 5-FU and gemcitabine may improve short-term survival, but long-term prognosis is poor (< 5% survive > 5 years from diagnosis).

Hematology/Oncology

Clotting Cascade

Hemostasis requires the interaction of blood vessels, platelets, monocytes, and coagulation factors. This activates the clotting cascade, as shown in Figure 2.7-1.

- **Heparin:** ↑ PTT, affects the **intrinsic pathway,** and ↓ fibrinogen levels; safe in pregnancy.
- **Warfarin:** ↑ PT, affects the **extrinsic pathway,** and ↓ vitamin K; teratogenic.

Hemophilias

X-linked recessive coagulopathies that are due to ↓ factor VIII (hemophilia A) or factor IX (hemophilia B).

History/PE

- Bleeding severity is proportional to factor VIII or IX levels and is defined as follows:

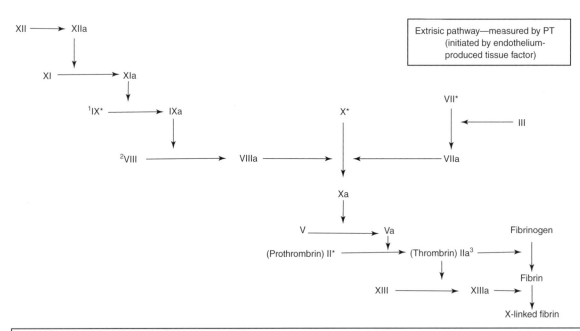

Intrinsic pathway—measured by PTT (initiated by exposure of collagen following vascular trauma)

Extrisic pathway—measured by PT (initiated by endothelium-produced tissue factor)

[1] Hemophilia B is characterized by factor IX deficiency.
[2] Hemophilia A is characterized by factor VIII deficiency.
[3] Thrombin is inactivated by antithrombin III. The rate of inactivation in creases in the presence of hepatin.
* Vitamin K–dependent clotting factors (II, VII, IX, X). Their synthesis is inhibited by warfarin.

FIGURE 2.7-1. **Coagulation cascade.**

- **Mild (5–25% normal activity):** Bleeding that occurs only after major trauma or surgery.
- **Moderate (1–5%):** Bleeding with mild trauma or surgery.
- **Severe (< 1%):** Spontaneous bleeding.
- Also presents with soft tissue hemorrhages, **hemarthroses** (blood in joints), IM bleeding, or GI bleeding.

DIAGNOSIS

- **Prolonged aPTT.** See Table 2.7-1 for other laboratory findings.
- ↓ factor VIII or IX levels.
- PT, bleeding time, von Willebrand's factor (vWF), and serum fibrinogen levels are normal.

TREATMENT

- Factor VIII (A) or IX (B) concentrate is given during bleeding episodes and as prophylaxis before surgical and dental procedures.
- In mild hemophilia A, desmopressin (DDAVP) may be administered before minor surgical procedures to ↑ endogenous factor VIII activity.

Unlike vWD, bleeding time in hemophilia A and B is normal because no platelet function abnormality is present.

von Willebrand's disease (vWD)

The **most common hereditary bleeding disorder (autosomal dominant).** Due to deficient or abnormal vWF, which stabilizes factor VIII and enhances platelet aggregation/attachment to injured vascular endothelium.

TABLE 2.7-1. **Lab Findings with Bleeding Disorders**

DISEASE	PT	PTT	BLEEDING TIME	PLATELET COUNT	RBC COUNT
Hemophilia A/B	Normal	↑	Normal	Normal	Normal
von Willebrand's disease (vWD)	Normal	↑	Normal/↑	Normal	Normal
DIC	↑	↑	↑	↓	Normal/↓
Liver failure	↑	Normal/↑	Normal	Normal/↓	Normal
Heparin	Normal	↑	Normal	Normal/↓	Normal
Warfarin	↑	Normal	Normal	Normal	Normal
Idiopathic thrombocytopenic purpura (ITP)	Normal	Normal	↑	↓	Normal
Thrombotic thrombocytopenic purpura (TTP)	Normal	Normal	↑	↓	↓

149

HISTORY/PE

- Generally presents with mild bleeding. Spontaneous hemarthroses do not occur.
- Mucosal bleeding (epistaxis, gingival bleeding, and menorrhagia) predominates, but GI bleeding may also occur. Incisional bleeding is seen after surgery or dental procedures.
- Symptoms worsen with aspirin use.

DIAGNOSIS

- ↓ levels of activated factor VIII; low levels of immunoreactive vWF.
- **Prolonged bleeding time.** See Table 2.7-1 for other laboratory findings.
- Abnormal platelet aggregation in response to ristocetin.

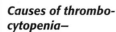

Ristocetin cofactor assay measures the ability of vWF to agglutinate platelets in the presence of ristocetin.

TREATMENT

- FFP or cryoprecipitate for major bleeding.
- **DDAVP is effective in mild disease.**
- OCPs for menorrhagia.
- ε-aminocaproic acid is a useful addition to dental or minor surgery.
- Avoid aspirin and aspirin-containing products.

Idiopathic Thrombocytopenic Purpura (ITP)

An autoimmune platelet disorder in which IgG autoantibody binds to platelets → lysis by splenic macrophages. **Evans' syndrome** is ITP with autoimmune hemolytic anemia. Peak incidence is between 20 and 50 years of age, and the female-to-male ratio is 2:1.

Causes of thrombocytopenia—

PLATELETS

Platelet disorders: TTP, ITP, DIC
Leukemia
Anemia
Trauma
Enlarged spleen
Liver disease
EtOH
Toxins (benzene, heparin, aspirin, chemotherapy)
Sepsis

HISTORY/PE

- Presents in **pediatric patients** with **acute onset following viral illness.**
- In **adults,** it has a gradual onset and typically follows viral infection, although it can also be drug related (e.g., sulfa drugs).
- There are no systemic symptoms, and patients are generally **afebrile** (vs. TTP).
- Mucosal or skin bleeding includes epistaxis, oral bleeding or hemorrhagic bullae, menorrhagia, and **purpura** or **petechiae.**
- If splenomegaly is present, consider an alternative diagnosis.

DIAGNOSIS

- A diagnosis of exclusion.
- CBC shows **thrombocytopenia** (< 150,000/μL) and possibly anemia.
- PT and PTT are normal; bleeding time is prolonged; DIC panel is normal.
- ⊕ **platelet-associated IgG test.**
- Peripheral blood smear reveals **megathrombocytes without schistocytes.**
- Bone marrow aspiration is normal or shows ↑ megakaryocytes.

Petechiae suggest Platelet deficiency.

TREATMENT

- **Pediatric patients:** The disease is self-limited, and 70% of patients recover in 4–6 weeks.
- **Adults:**
  - Observation if platelet count > 50,000/μL and the patient is asymptomatic.

- **Prednisone** (may mask a leukemia masquerading as ITP, so consider bone marrow aspiration before treatment).
- **IV gamma globulin anti-Rho(D)** (for Rh-⊕ patients) for life-threatening hemorrhage or severe thrombocytopenia (< 10,000/μL).
- **Platelets** should be given for severe, uncontrollable bleeding.
- **Splenectomy** provides effective treatment for two-thirds of patients who are refractory to medical treatment.

Bleeding into body Cavities or joints suggests Clotting factor deficiency.

Hypercoagulable State

Associated with an ↑ risk of **thromboembolic disease,** including DVT, pulmonary embolus, and cerebrovascular accidents.

HISTORY/PE

- Patients with congenital hypercoagulability often present with venous thrombosis or recurrent thromboembolism in adolescence or early adult life.
- Most patients with their first DVT do not need workup for hypercoagulable state. Maintain a high level of suspicion in patients with venous thrombosis in unusual locations (e.g., mesenteric, hepatic, and splenic venous beds) as well as those with recurrent thromboses.
- Arterial thrombosis may manifest as large-vessel occlusion (stroke, MI) or as microvascular events (**erythromelalgia,** or painful redness and burning of the hands; seen in myeloproliferative disorders).
- Look for a history of recurrent miscarriages.
- Major causes of hypercoagulable states are listed in Table 2.7-2.

Suspect pulmonary embolism in a patient with rapid onset of tachypnea, tachycardia, hypoxia, hypocapnia, and an ↑ A-a gradient without another obvious explanation.

TABLE 2.7-2. **Causes of Hypercoagulable State**

INHERITED	ACQUIRED
Factor V Leiden (or activated protein C resistance)	Cancer (Trousseau's syndrome)
	MI
Protein C or S deficiency	Prolonged bed rest or immobilization
Antithrombin III deficiency	**Pregnancy,** estrogens
Homocystinemia	Tissue damage (surgery, fracture)
Fibrinolysis defects	Hyperlipidemia
Prothrombin gene mutation	Vasculitis
	Multiple myeloma
	Lupus anticoagulant (antiphospholipid syndrome)
	Nephrotic syndrome
	Smoking
	Warfarin (on initiation of therapy)
	Myeloproliferative disorders (essential thrombocytosis, polycythemia vera)
	Paroxysmal nocturnal hemoglobinuria
	Heparin-induced thrombocytopenia/thrombosis
	TTP

Factor V Leiden mutation is the most common inherited cause of hypercoagulability.

DIAGNOSIS

- **Inherited:** Factor V Leiden, prothrombin gene mutation, antithrombin III, protein S and protein C assays.
- **Acquired:** Look for an underlying cause.

TREATMENT

- If surgery is needed, preoperative minidose heparin (5000 U q 8–12 h) should be given to ↓ perioperative thrombosis.
- In congenital biochemical defects, warfarin is effective if given indefinitely.
- The patient's family members should be screened for the defect.

LEUKEMIA

Malignant proliferations of hematopoietic cells. Categorization is based on cellular origin and on the level of differentiation of neoplastic cells. Figure 2.7-2 shows the different blood cell lineages. Subtypes are as follows:

- **Acute leukemias:** Proliferations of minimally differentiated **blast** cells.
- **Chronic leukemias:** Proliferations of more mature, differentiated cells.
- **Lymphocytic leukemias:** Neoplasms of lymphoid cells (B and T lymphocytes).
- **Myelogenous leukemias:** Neoplasms of myeloid cells (granulocytes, monocytes, platelets, erythrocytes).

Acute Lymphocytic Leukemia (ALL)

HISTORY/PE

- **Most common in children;** occurs more frequently in whites than in blacks.
- Acute onset of symptoms, typically within a few weeks of diagnosis.

Signs of **LEUKEMIA:**

Light skin (pallor)
Energy ↓
Underweight
Kidney failure
Excess heat (fever)
Mottled skin (hemorrhage)
Infections
Anemia

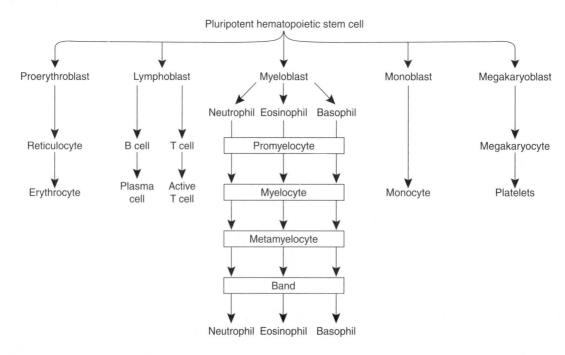

FIGURE 2.7-2. **Blood cell differentiation.**

- Presents with malaise, fever, lethargy, and weight loss.
- **Bone pain,** infection, and hemorrhage are also seen.
- Examination reveals lymphadenopathy and hepatosplenomegaly.

DIAGNOSIS

- CBC shows depression of bone marrow elements (anemia, thrombocytopenia) and high or low leukocyte count.
- LDH and uric acid are ↑.
- Marrow biopsy reveals ↑ blasts (**PAS** ⊕, **TdT** ⊕, **CALLA** ⊕).
- **Cytogenetics:**
  - Approximately **25–30%** of patients have **t(9;22)** (also known as the **Philadelphia chrosome**) or **t(4;11);** associated with an **unfavorable prognosis.**
  - Roughly 80% of cases are of B-cell lineage and express CD10 (CALLA antigen) and CD19 +/– CD20.
  - Some 15–20% of cases are of T-cell lineage and express CD2, CD5, and CD7.
- Chest CT to rule out mediastinal involvement; LP to rule out leptomeningeal involvement; head CT to rule out parenchymal brain involvement.

TREATMENT

- **Chemotherapy:** Vincristine, prednisone, daunorubicin, L-asparaginase, and cyclophosphamide are used.
- Roughly 99% of children achieve complete remission with chemotherapy, and 80% achieve long-term leukemia-free survival. For adults, these numbers are 80% and 30%, respectively.
- Patients with the Philadelphia chromosome often need bone marrow transplant.

Acute Myelogenous Leukemia (AML)

Subdivided into eight different types, M0 through M7, based on the neoplastic cell type and cytogenetics (FAB classification).

HISTORY/PE

- Most commonly occurs in adults (median age 60); incidence ↑ with age.
- Presents with fatigue, hemorrhage, or bruising.
- Skin and lung infections are common.
- **Symptoms of bone marrow failure** are also seen (anemia, neutropenia, and thrombocytopenia).
- Splenomegaly, hepatomegaly, and lymphadenopathy are present in < 25% of patients.
- AML type M3 (acute promyelocytic leukemia) is associated with DIC; AML type M5 is associated with gingival hyperplasia.
- Patients with a high WBC count may present with symptoms of **leukostasis,** which arises from the sludging of circulating leukemic blast in tissue microvasculature. Symptoms include the following:
  - **Neurologic:** Range from mild confusion and somnolence to stupor and coma.
  - **Pulmonary:** Exertional dyspnea to respiratory distress.
  - **Vascular:** DIC, retinal hemorrhage, MI, acute limb ischemia, renal vein thrombosis.

The most common leukemias

by age:

Up to age 15: ALL

Age 15–59: AML and CML

Age 60 and over: CLL

Association of ALL and Down

syndrome:

*"We will **ALL** go **DOWN***

together."

Association of ALL and Down syndrome:

"We will **ALL** go **DOWN** together."

Diagnosis

- CBC count with differential shows varying levels of anemia and thrombocytopenia.
- WBC count may be high, normal, or low.
- DIC panel (with AML type M3) shows ↑ PT, ↓ fibrinogen level, and ⊕ fibrin split products.
- Peripheral blood smear and marrow biopsy reveal ↑ blasts, **Auer rods,** and ⊕ **Sudan black** and **myeloperoxidase stains (10%).**
- Cytogenetics:
    - t(8;21), t(15;17), and inv(16)(p13;q22) have a favorable prognosis.
    - Monosomy 5 and 7 and complex abnormalities have an unfavorable prognosis.
    - **AML type M3:** t(15;17) is a translocation involving the retinoic acid receptor alpha and promyelocytic leukemia (PML) genes.

Auer rods are eosinophilic, needle-like cytoplasmic inclusions that are found in blast cells and are pathognomonic of AML.

Treatment

- **Chemotherapy:** Cytarabine plus an anthracycline (e.g., daunorubicin).
- Stem cell transplantation for those who do not achieve remission or have unfavorable cytogenetics.
- **AML type M3** is treated with **all-*trans*-retinoic acid** in addition to chemotherapy.
- In patients with a **high WBC count,** leukapheresis or immediate chemotherapy may be needed.
- Do **not** transfuse RBCs if the WBC count > 50,000 until the issue has been discussed with an oncologist, even in the presence of a very low hematocrit.

Chronic Lymphocytic Leukemia (CLL)

A clonal malignancy of B lymphocytes (> 98%) and T lymphocytes (1–2%). Has an indolent course with slowly progressive accumulation of long-lived small lymphocytes that are immunocompetent. **Median age is 65.**

History/PE

- Most patients are asymptomatic at presentation. **May present with fatigue,** lymphadenopathy, and splenomegaly.
- ↑ infections occur 2° to neutropenia and hypogammaglobulinemia.
- At later stages, patients may have fever, night sweats, and weight loss.

Diagnosis

- CBC: Incidental finding of **isolated lymphocytosis (lymphocyte count > 5000).**
    - WBC count is usually > 20,000/μL and may be > 100,000/μL.
    - Hematocrit and platelet count are often normal.
- Peripheral blood smear shows small, mature cells with condensed nuclear chromatin as well as **smudge cells**—leukocytes that have been damaged during the smear preparation as a result of cell fragility.
- Bone marrow is infiltrated with small lymphocytes.
- **Coexpression of CD19 and CD5 on flow cytometry.**
- **Hypogammaglobulinemia** is found in 50% of cases and is more common in advanced disease.

Treatment

- **Supportive** therapy is appropriate for cases of early indolent CLL.

- Indications for chemotherapy include progressive fatigue, symptomatic lymphadenopathy, or anemia/thrombocytopenia.
  - **Fludarabine:** First-line therapy, but avoid in autoimmune hemolytic anemia.
  - **Chlorambucil:** Usually well tolerated and effective in older patients.
  - **Rituximab:** Well tolerated in the elderly, and can be used to treat autoimmune hemolytic anemia.
- Associated autoimmune hemolytic anemia and immune thrombocytopenia are treated with prednisone and splenectomy.

COMPLICATIONS

- **Autoimmune hemolytic anemia or autoimmune thrombocytopenia** is found in **5–10%** of cases.
- **Richter's syndrome:** Involves isolated lymph node transformation into aggressive large cell lymphoma.

Chronic Myelogenous Leukemia (CML)

A clonal stem cell disorder with proliferation of myeloid cells at all stages of differentiation. Median age at presentation is 42 years.

HISTORY/PE

- Presents with fatigue, night sweats, and low-grade fever.
- Examination reveals abdominal fullness from **splenomegaly.**
- Presentation varies according to phase:
  - **Chronic phase:** ↑ WBC count; spleen and liver enlargement.
  - **Accelerated phase:** ↓ RBCs and platelets; bone pain; fever, night sweats, and weight loss.
  - **Blast phase:** Peripheral blood and marrow are filled with rapidly proliferating leukemic blast cells.

DIAGNOSIS

- CBC:
  - Markedly ↑ WBC count (median WBC count at diagnosis is 150,000/μL).
  - Basophilia and eosinophilia may be present.
  - Hematocrit is normal; platelet count is normal or ↑ (anemia and thrombocytopenia in accelerated and blast phases).
- **Peripheral blood smear:** Myeloid series is left shifted with mature forms dominating; blasts are usually < 5%.
- Approximately **90% of patients have the Philadelphia chromosome t(9;22)** → bcr-abl gene.
- ↓ leukocyte alkaline phosphatase.
- **Bone marrow:** Hypercellular with left-shifted myelopoiesis. The blast phase is diagnosed when blasts comprise > 20% of bone marrow.

TREATMENT

- Not emergent even with a WBC > 200,000/μL.
- Chemotherapy:
  - Imatinib mesylate (**Gleevec**) inhibits tyrosine kinase activity of the bcr-abl oncogene.
  - Interferon-α has a 10–20% durable complete remission rate but has many side effects.
  - Hydroxyurea for patients who cannot tolerate other therapies.

The bcr-abl gene encodes a chimeric protein with strong tyrosine kinase activity. The expression of this protein leads to the development of the CML phenotype.

■ Allogeneic bone marrow transplant is indicated for patients < 60 years of age or if there is no cytogenetic response to Gleevec after six months.

COMPLICATIONS

Leukostasis clinical syndrome, which may present with neurologic, respiratory, or vascular symptoms.

LYMPHOMAS

Neoplasms of cells from lymphoid tissue (e.g., lymphocytes, histiocytes, and their precursors and derivates). Hodgkin's lymphomas are distinguished pathologically from non-Hodgkin's lymphomas by the presence of **Reed-Sternberg giant cells** (see Figure 2.7-3). Other differences are summarized in Table 2.7-3.

PLASMA CELL DISORDERS

Neoplastic or potentially neoplastic disorders with proliferation of monoclonal plasma cells of B-cell series. Each immunoglobulin is composed of two heavy and two light chains.

Multiple Myeloma

Neoplastic proliferation of plasma cells → a monoclonal immunoglobulin or light chain. Those > 50 years of age are most commonly affected. Blacks are affected more frequently than whites, and women are affected more than men.

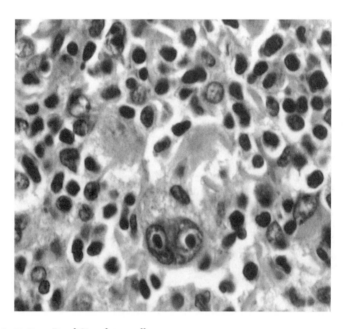

FIGURE 2.7-3.   Reed-Sternberg cells.

Binucleate Reed-Sternberg cells displaying prominent inclusion-like nucleoli surrounded by lymphocytes. The Reed-Sternberg cell is a necessary but insufficient pathologic finding for the diagnosis of Hodgkin's disease.

TABLE 2.7-3. Non-Hodgkin's vs. Hodgkin's Lymphomas

	NON-HODGKIN'S	HODGKIN'S
Description	Monoclonal proliferation of B or T lymphocytes.	Lymph malignancy of proliferating germinal center cell.
Risk factors	EBV (Burkitt's), HIV.	EBV. **Bimodal age distribution,** with the first peak at 20–30 years and the second peak at > 50 years.
Histology	Varies.	**Reed-Sternberg cells.**
Distribution	**Noncontiguous** lymph node spread.	**Contiguous** lymph node spread.
Variants	The largest group of hematologic neoplasms. Separated into low, intermediate, and high grade.	**Nodular sclerosis** (60–75% of cases; primarily affects young females); mixed cellularity; lymphocyte predominant; lymphocyte depleted.
History	Painless adenopathy; **B symptoms** (fever > 38.5°C, night sweats, or 10% weight loss over six months).	Same plus pruritus.
PE	**Systemic adenopathy, hepatosplenomegaly.**	**Regional** adenopathy, hepatosplenomegaly.
Diagnosis	Biopsy for diagnosis; CXR; whole-body CT; consider bone marrow biopsy and LP.	Biopsy the largest node for diagnosis, then obtain a CXR. Consider bone marrow biopsy and LP.
Treatment	Radiation and chemotherapy (CHOP).[a]	Radiation for localized disease; chemotherapy for advanced/widespread disease (ABVD).[b]
Complications	Tumor lysis syndrome—rapid tumor cell death releases intracellular contents → ↑ K⁺, ↑ phosphate, ↑ uric acid, and ↓ Ca²⁺.	

[a] CHOP = Cytoxan, Adriamycin, Oncovin (vincristine), and prednisone.

[b] ABVD = Adriamycin, bleomycin, vincristine, and dacarbazine.

HISTORY/PE

- Presents with symptoms of **anemia.**
- Frequent infections with encapsulated organisms (*Streptococcus pneumoniae* and *Haemophilus influenzae*) are seen.
- **Bone pain** in the back or ribs is common, as are pathologic fractures (especially of the femoral neck).
- Symptoms of **renal failure** and hypercalcemia ("stones, bones, abdominal moans, and psychiatric overtones") are seen.
- Also presents with neuropathy or spinal cord compression as well as with pallor, fever, bone tenderness, soft tissue masses, bone deformities, and lethargy.

Multiple myeloma presents with the triad of back pain, anemia, and renal insufficiency.

DIAGNOSIS

- Anemia, ↑ Ca²⁺, proteinuria, ↑ ESR, narrow anion gap.
- On peripheral blood smear, plasma cells are rarely visible.
- UA may reveal proteinuria.

- Serum and urine protein electrophoresis (SPEP/UPEP) reveals monoclonal gammopathy, most commonly **IgG**, and free kappa and lambda light chains (**Bence Jones proteinuria**).
- X-rays reveal **lytic lesions**, especially in the axial skeleton, as well as osteoporosis and fractures.
- Bone marrow biopsy shows 10–20% plasma cells (normal is < 5%).

TREATMENT

- **Thalidomide** is used for those who have few symptoms at the time of presentation.
- Patients who are refractory to thalidomide or are acutely symptomatic may receive **chemotherapy** in the form of an alkylating agent (melphalan or cyclophosphamide) + prednisone or vincristine, doxorubicin (Adriamycin), and dexamethasone (VAD).
- **Hypercalcemia:** Treat with hydration, bisphosphonates, prednisone, and calcitonin.
- **Renal failure:** Allopurinol; hemodialysis or plasmapheresis if symptomatic.
- Autologous stem cell transplantation for young patients.

Monoclonal Gammopathy of Undetermined Significance (MGUS)

- Also known as benign monoclonal gammopathy.
- Some 25% of patients go on to develop myeloma, macroglobulinemia, amyloidosis, or lymphoma.
- **Dx: M protein in serum without evidence of systemic disease.**

Waldenström's Macroglobulinemia

- Affects patients > 40 years of age.
- **Dx: IgM spike,** hyperviscosity, cold agglutinins (Raynaud's phenomenon with cold sensitivity).

RED BLOOD CELL DISORDERS

Anemia

Defined as a hemoglobin level < 13.5 g/dL in men or < 12.0 g/dL in women. Etiologies are categorized by ↓ RBC production, ↑ RBC destruction, and/or blood loss. Risk factors include a history of bleeding, a past history of anemia, and a ⊕ family history.

HISTORY/PE

- Presents with fatigue, dyspnea, and dizziness, including orthostatic blood pressure/pulse.
- **Iron deficiency:** Atrophic glossitis, angular cheilitis (scaling of the corners of the mouth), and koilonychias ("spoon nails") are seen.
- **B$_{12}$ deficiency:** Glossitis, peripheral neuropathy.
- Perform a rectal exam with stool guaiac.

DIAGNOSIS

- Initial laboratory studies for the classification of anemia are as follows (see also Figure 2.7-4 and Table 2.7-4):

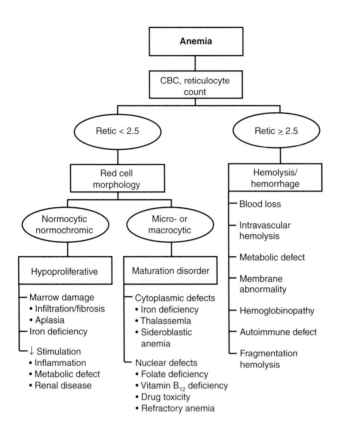

FIGURE 2.7-4. Anemia algorithm.

- CBC with red cell indices (MCV, MCHC, RDW).
- Peripheral blood smear may show characteristic cell types (see Table 2.7-5).
- Reticulocyte count (↑ if anemia due to blood loss or RBC destruction; ↓ if due to marrow failure).
- Etiology-specific studies include the following:
  - **Iron panel:** Iron, ferritin, transferrin, TIBC. Characteristic results are displayed in Table 2.7-6.
  - Haptoglobin, vitamin B_{12} and folate levels, bilirubin, LDH.
  - Coombs' test, LFTs, TSH, renal function tests.

Causes of microcytic anemia—

TICS

Thalassemia
Iron deficiency
Chronic disease
Sideroblastic anemia

TABLE 2.7-4. Anemia Classification

MICROCYTIC (MCV < 80)	NORMOCYTIC (MCV 80–100)	MACROCYTIC (MCV > 100)
Iron deficiency	Anemia of chronic disease	Vitamin B_{12} deficiency
Thalassemia	Uremia	Folate deficiency
Anemia of chronic disease	Hypothyroidism	Myelodysplasia
Sideroblastic anemia	Bone marrow failure (aplastic anemia)	Drug induced
		Hepatic dysfunction
		Alcohol use

TABLE 2.7-5. Blood Cell Morphologies and Associated Diseases

CELL TYPE	ASSOCIATED DISEASE
Spherocytes	G6PD deficiency, membranopathy (immune and nonimmune)
Blister cell	G6PD deficiency
Burr cell	Acute renal failure (ARF), uremia
Heinz body	Thalassemia, hemoglobinopathies, and enzymopathies (G6PD)
Schistocyte	Artificial heart valves and microangiopathic hemolytic anemias
Target cell	Splenectomy

Features of iron deficiency anemia—

Fe *(iron)* **KAP**

Fatigue
Exercise tolerance ↓
Koilonychia
Angular cheilitis
Pica, **P**allor

TREATMENT

- Identify and treat the underlying disease.
- **Iron deficiency:** Identify the site of blood loss or the reason for poor intake; give iron supplements. **Suspect colorectal cancer in male patients > 50 years of age with anemia.**
- **Vitamin B$_{12}$ deficiency:** Monthly B$_{12}$ shots.
- **Anemia due to chronic renal disease and anemia of chronic disease:** Erythropoietin.
- Transfusions are indicated for patients with severe symptoms.

Glucose-6-Phosphate Dehydrogenase (G6PD) Deficiency

An X-linked enzyme deficiency → hemolysis that is triggered by the release of oxidants by macrophages. It is the **most common metabolic disorder of RBCs.** Precipitating causes of acute hemolysis include the following:

- **Infection, DKA,** low pH (acidosis).
- **Drugs:** Antimalarials, quinolones, sulfa drugs, NSAIDs, nitrofurantoin, fava beans, vitamin C (acids).

TABLE 2.7-6. Iron Studies in Patients with Microcytic Anemia

	SERUM FE	TIBC (TRANSFERRIN)	FERRITIN	OTHER
Iron deficiency	↓	↑	↓	Most common; look for blood loss.
Anemia of chronic disease	↓	↓	Normal/↑	May be microcytic or normocytic.
Sideroblastic anemia	↑	Normal/↑	↑	Give pyridoxine (vitamin B$_6$) to see if patients are responsive.
Thalassemia	Normal/↑	Normal/↑	Normal/↑	Check HbA$_2$, HbF levels.

- **Acute hemolysis:**
    - Presents with jaundice, dark urine, and acute tubular necrosis (ATN) 1–3 days after exposure.
    - **Anemia:** Pallor, tachycardia, systolic ejection murmur.
    - Mesenteric and renal ischemia → abdominal and/or back pain.
- **Chronic hemolysis:** Hepatosplenomegaly.

DIAGNOSIS

- **G6PD assay** (cannot assess during acute hemolytic episodes or after transfusion).
- **Hemolysis:**
    - Peripheral smear reveals **Heinz bodies,** microcytosis, and schistocytosis.
    - CBC shows anemia and ↑ reticulocyte count.
    - UA shows hemoglobinuria, ↑ urobilinogen, and ATN.
    - ↓ haptoglobin.
    - ⊖ direct and indirect Coombs' tests.
    - ↑ direct and indirect bilirubin.

TREATMENT

- Volume loading with IV fluids for renal protection.
- Remove the oxidative stressor if possible (discontinue the drug; treat infection).
- RBC replacement if necessary.
- Acute crises resolve spontaneously after approximately one week owing to new erythrocytes with ↑ G6PD activity.

Microangiopathic Hemolytic Anemia

- A group of disorders in which a coagulopathy is associated with a platelet deficiency and RBC hemolysis.
- Includes TTP, hemolytic-uremic syndrome (HUS), and DIC.
- **Dx:** Characteristics of these disorders are summarized in Table 2.7-7. Peripheral blood smear shows **schistocytes** (fragmented RBCs).

Sickle Cell Disease

An autosomal-recessive disease. Carriers are common and are typically asymptomatic (8% of African-Americans).

HISTORY/PE

- Identified during neonatal screening.
- Sickle cell crises are precipitated by infection, dehydration, and hypoxia. Specific symptoms are as follows:
    - **Acute crisis:** Symptoms include arthralgias and pain. Caused by vascular sludging and thrombosis. Vaso-occlusive crisis may → organ failure (2° to infarction) as well as dehydration, fever, and leukocytosis.
    - **Acute chest syndrome:** Chest pain, pulmonary infiltrate, ↑ WBC, hypoxia; indistinguishable from pneumonia.
    - **Aplastic crisis:** Often due to parvovirus B19 infection.
    - **Hemolytic crisis:** Associated with G6PD deficiency.

> **Pentad of TTP—**
>
> **FAT RN**
>
> **F**ever
> **A**nemia
> **T**hrombocytopenia
> **R**enal dysfunction
> **N**eurologic abnormalities

> In DIC, activation of the clotting cascade leads to ↑ PT/PTT; in TTP and HUS, platelet aggregation plays a larger role and PT/PTT are often normal.

> **Signs of sickle cell disease—**
>
> **SICKLE**
>
> **S**plenomegaly, **S**ludging
> **I**nfection
> **C**holelithiasis
> **K**idney—hematuria
> **L**iver congestion, leg ulcers
> **E**ye changes

HIGH-YIELD FACTS

HEMATOLOGY/ONCOLOGY

TABLE 2.7-7. **Microangiopathic Hemolytic Anemia**

	HUS	TTP	DIC
Causes	Mild viral illness or gastroenteritis with *E. coli* O157:H7.	HIV infection, pregnancy, OCP use.	Sepsis, transfusion reaction, neoplasia, trauma, obstetric complications.[a]
History/PE	Triad of anemia, thrombocytopenia, and acute renal failure (ARF).	Pentad of fever, anemia/splenomegaly, thrombocytopenia, ARF, and **neurologic abnormalities.**[b]	**Bleeding:** Venipuncture sites, epistaxis. **Thrombosis:** Digital gangrene, hypotension.
CBC/electrolytes	Anemia, thrombocytopenia.	Anemia, thrombocytopenia.	Anemia, thrombocytopenia.
Coagulation	Normal PT/PTT.	Normal PT/PTT, ↑ bleeding time.	↑ **PT/PTT,** ↑ bleeding time.
Other labs	↑ **LDH,** Coombs' test ⊖.	↑ indirect bilirubin, ↑ **LDH,** Coombs' test ⊖.	↑ D-dimer, ↑ fibrin split products, ↓ **fibrinogen.**
Pathology	Blood smear shows **schistocytes.**	Hyaline thrombi in small vessels without inflammatory changes; blood smear reveals **schistocytes.**	Blood smear reveals **schistocytes.**
Treatment	Dialysis for ARF.	Large-volume **plasmapheresis,** corticosteroids, ASA, splenectomy.	Treat the underlying condition; transfuse with platelets and cryoprecipitate.

[a] Obstetric complications include amniotic embolus and septic abortion.

[b] Neurologic abnormalities vary and include confusion, headache, photophobia seizures, and focal abnormalities.

Sickle cell crises are precipitated by infection, dehydration, and hypoxia.

- **Sequestration crisis:** RBCs pool in the spleen and may → shock and death.
- **Splenic crisis:** Autoinfarction of the spleen → ↑ risk of osteomyelitis and infections by encapsulated organisms.

DIAGNOSIS

- Blood smear shows sickled cells and **Howell-Jolly bodies** (cytoplasmic remnants of nuclear chromatin normally removed by the spleen).
- Blood tests show anemia, ↑ reticulocyte count, and ↑ indirect bilirubin.
- Hemoglobin electrophoresis shows HbS.

TREATMENT

Sickle cell disease—a defect in the β-globin chain.

Thalassemia—↓ quantity of an α- or β-globin chain.

Porphyria—a defect in heme synthesis.

- **Acute crisis:** Analgesia and hydration.
- Hydroxyurea to ↑ the amount of fetal hemoglobin.
- *H. influenzae* and pneumococcal vaccines; prophylactic penicillin for children < 5 years of age.
- **Acute chest syndrome:** Respiratory support and exchange transfusion.

Thalassemia

A group of disorders resulting from ↓ synthesis of α- or β-globin protein subunits. There are four α and two β genes.

α-THALASSEMIA

↓ α-globin chain synthesis. Most common in Asians (αα/--) and African-Americans (α-/α-).

HISTORY/PE

Symptoms depend on how many of the four foci are deleted or mutated:

- **1/4 foci:** Silent thalassemia; asymptomatic.
- **2/4 foci:** Thalassemia trait; mild anemia.
- **3/4 foci:** Hemoglobin H disease; splenomegaly.
- **4/4 foci:** Hemoglobin Barts, **hydrops fetalis;** incompatible with life.

DIAGNOSIS

- Blood smear demonstrates microcytic anemia, hypochromia, target cells, and Heinz bodies.
- HbH inclusion bodies are seen on brilliant cresyl blue stain.

TREATMENT

Periodic transfusions.

β-THALASSEMIA

↓ β-globin chain synthesis. Most common in people of Mediterranean origin, those of Asian ethnicity, and African-Americans.

HISTORY/PE

- **β-thalassemia major (Cooley's anemia):**
  - Has no β-globin production.
  - Presents with anemia at six months due to the switch from fetal γ to adult β.
  - Jaundice, splenomegaly.
- **β-thalassemia minor:** Mild or no anemia; asymptomatic carriers.

DIAGNOSIS

Electrophoresis shows ↑ **HbF,** ↓ HbA, and ↑ HbA_2 measurements.

TREATMENT

- **β-thalassemia major:**
  - Aggressive transfusions; **splenectomy** to enhance the survival of RBCs; bone marrow transplant.
  - Give **deferoxamine,** which ↑ urinary excretion of iron to prevent iron overload complications (e.g., cardiac toxicity).
- **β-thalassemia minor:** Avoid oxidative stress.

Polycythemia

↑ RBC count and hematocrit. May be a physiologic adaptation to low O_2 conditions.

- **1°:** Idiopathic; polycythemia vera.
- **2°: Hypoxemia.**
  - COPD, lung disease, high altitude, smoking (↑ carboxyhemoglobin).
  - If blood O_2 saturation is normal, consider renal cell carcinoma.

HISTORY/PE

- Presents with general malaise, fever, **plethora** ("red-faced"), and pruritus **(especially after a warm shower).**
- **Vascular sludging** → stroke, angina, MI, claudication, hepatic vein thrombosis, headache, and blurred vision.
- Examination reveals **splenomegaly.**

DIAGNOSIS

- Hematocrit > 50%, ↑ RBC mass, ↓ ESR.
- Erythropoietin is ↓ in 1° cases and ↑ in 2° cases.
- WBCs and platelets are normal, or there may be an ↑ of all blood cell lines.

TREATMENT

- Serial phlebotomy to ↓ blood volume and ↓ the risk of vascular events.
- Consider hydroxyurea for myelosuppression.
- Aspirin to prevent thromboses.
- Polycythemia vera ↑ **the risk of conversion to CML,** myelofibrosis, or AML.

Transfusion Reactions

Acute hemolysis during RBC transfusion occurs as a result of preformed recipient antibodies → lysis of donor RBCs. The most frequent cause is **ABO incompatibilities due to clerical errors.**

HISTORY/PE

Hemoglobinuria may → ATN and subsequent renal failure.

- **Febrile reaction (fever,** chills, headache, back pain) from preformed antibodies to donor WBCs.
- **Hemolytic reaction** (anxiety or discomfort, dyspnea, chest pain, hypotension, jaundice) from preformed antibodies to donor RBCs.
- **Allergic reaction** (urticaria, edema, dizziness, wheezing, anaphylaxis) to an unknown component.
- **Hemoglobinuria** within minutes of ABO blood group–incompatible transfusion → ATN, oliguria, and renal failure.
- Patients with **IgA deficiency** may have an anaphylactic reaction to donor IgA.

DIAGNOSIS

- Retype the patient's blood type against that of the donor to confirm a cross-match.
- Culture donor blood and check DIC labs.
- Evaluate for free hemoglobin in blood and urine.

TREATMENT

- **Stop the transfusion.**
- In the setting of a hemolytic reaction, administer IV fluid and mannitol in efforts to prevent oliguric renal failure.
- For allergic reaction, treat with diphenhydramine or, if severe, steroids.
- For febrile reaction, premedicate for future transfusions with acetaminophen.

Transplant rejection remains a risk despite immunosuppressive drugs. Patients may present with fever, pain, lethargy, and **dysfunction of the transplanted organ.**

- **Kidney:** ↑ BP and ↑ BUN/creatinine and proteinuria may indicate chronic kidney rejection.
- **Liver:** ↑ GGT, alkaline phosphatase, and bilirubin may be seen.

Hyperacute Rejection

- **Hx/PE:** Occurs within **minutes.** Immediate vascular thrombi result from preformed antidonor antibodies.
- **Dx:** Prevent by checking ABO compatibility.
- **Rx: Remove the transplanted organ.**

Acute Rejection

- **Hx/PE:** Occurs between five **days** and three **months** after transplant. Cytotoxic T lymphocytes react against foreign MHCs.
- **Dx:** Biopsy of transplanted organ reveals lymphocyte- and antibody-induced reaction with T-cell graft tissue injury.
- **Rx:** Steroids and antilymphocyte antibodies (OKT3).

Chronic Rejection

- **Hx/PE:** Gradual, irreversible loss of organ function occurs **months to years** after transplant.
- **Dx:** Associated with antibody-mediated vascular damage (fibrinoid necrosis).
- **Rx:** No effective treatment.

Graft-Versus-Host Disease (GVHD) in Bone Marrow Transplant

- Donor-engrafted immunocompetent T cells proliferate in the host and attack host proteins recognized as "foreign."
- **Hx/PE:**
  - **Acute:** Presents with a painful, pruritic maculopapular rash as well as with hepatic dysfunction (jaundice, hepatosplenomegaly) and diarrhea.
  - **Chronic:** An autoimmune disorder with protean manifestations that may include keratoconjunctivitis sicca and lichenoid changes of buccal mucosa.
- **Dx:**
  - **Acute:** Clinical presentation within the first 100 days of transplantation.
  - **Chronic:** Occurs 100 days after transplant.
- **Rx:** Prophylaxis with cyclosporine, tacrolimus, or methotrexate.

GVHD may manifest as a pruritic, painful rash.

Diseases Associated with Neoplasms

Table 2.7-8 outlines common hematologic disorders that are associated with neoplasia.

TABLE 2.7-8. Diseases Associated with Neoplasms

CONDITION	NEOPLASM
1. **Down** syndrome	1. **A**cute **L**ymphoblastic **L**eukemia—"We will **ALL** go **DOWN** together"
2. Xeroderma pigmentosum	2. Squamous cell and basal cell carcinomas of skin
3. Chronic atrophic gastritis, pernicious anemia, postsurgical gastric remnants	3. Gastric adenocarcinoma
4. Tuberous sclerosis (facial angiofibroma, seizures, mental retardation)	4. Astrocytoma and cardiac rhabdomyoma
5. Actinic keratosis	5. Squamous cell carcinoma
6. Barrett's esophagus (chronic GI reflux)	6. Esophageal adenocarcinoma
7. Plummer-Vinson syndrome (atrophic glossitis, esophageal webs, anemia; all due to iron deficiency)	7. Squamous cell carcinoma of esophagus
8. Cirrhosis (alcoholic, hepatitis B or C)	8. Hepatocellular carcinoma
9. Ulcerative colitis	9. Colonic adenocarcinoma
10. Paget's disease of bone	10. 2° osteosarcoma and fibrosarcoma
11. Immunodeficiency states	11. Malignant lymphomas
12. AIDS	12. Aggressive malignant lymphomas (non-Hodgkin's) and Kaposi's sarcoma
13. Autoimmune diseases (e.g., Hashimoto's thyroiditis, myasthenia gravis)	13. Benign and malignant thymomas
14. Acanthosis nigricans (hyperpigmentation and epidermal thickening)	14. Visceral malignancy (stomach, lung, breast, uterus)
15. Dysplastic nevus	15. Malignant melanoma

Neutropenia

- Neutropenia = neutrophils < 2000 /mm^3. Clinical problems arise when neutrophils < 1000/mm^3.
- Etiologies are as follows:
  - **Marrow failure:** Many cases are drug induced (e.g., sulfonamides, penicillin, chlorpromazine, chemotherapy).
  - **Marrow invasion:** Results from cancer or infection.
  - **Maturation arrest:** Results from folate or B$_{12}$ deficiency.
- Hx/PE: Variable; ranges from asymptomatic to signs of severe infection.
- Dx: Bone marrow aspiration and biopsy if no obvious cause.
- Rx: Treat the underlying cause. **G-CSF,** empiric antibiotics, glucocorticoids, and bone marrow transplant.

Infectious Disease

Pneumonia

Some common causes of pneumonia are outlined in Table 2.8-1.

HISTORY/PE

- **Classic symptoms:** Sudden onset, fever, productive cough (purulent yellow-green sputum or hemoptysis), dyspnea, night sweats, pleuritic chest pain.
- **Atypical symptoms:** Gradual onset, dry cough, headaches, myalgias, sore throat.
- Lung exam may show ↓ or bronchial breath sounds, rales, wheezing, dullness to percussion, egophony, and tactile fremitus.
- Elderly patients as well as those with COPD, diabetes, or immunocompromised status may have minimal signs on physical exam.

DIAGNOSIS

- Workup includes physical exam, **CXR,** CBC, sputum Gram stain and culture (see Figures 2.8-1 and 2.8-2), blood culture, and ABG.
- Tests for specific pathogens include the following:
  - *Legionella:* Urine *Legionella* antigen test, sputum staining with direct fluorescent antibody, culture.
  - *Chlamydia pneumoniae:* Serologic testing, culture, PCR.
  - *Mycoplasma:* Usually clinical. Serum cold agglutinins and serum *Mycoplasma* antigen may also be used.

An adequate sputum Gram stain sample has many PMNs (> 25 cells/hpf) and few epithelial cells (< 25 cells/hpf).

TABLE 2.8-1. Common causes of pneumonia

CHILDREN (6 WKS–18 YR)	ADULTS (18–40 YR)	ADULTS (40–65 YR)	ELDERLY
Viruses (RSV)	Mycoplasma	S. pneumoniae	S. pneumoniae
Mycoplasma	C. pneumoniae	Haemophilus influenzae	Viruses
Chlamydia pneumoniae	S. pneumoniae	Anaerobes	Anaerobes
Streptococcus pneumoniae		Viruses	H. influenzae
		Mycoplasma	Gram-⊕ rods

Special groups:	
Atypical	Mycoplasma, Legionella, Chlamydia
Nosocomial (hospital acquired)	Staphylococcus, gram-⊕ rods, anaerobes, gram-⊖ rods
Immunocompromised	Staphylococcus, gram-⊕ rods, fungi, viruses, Pneumocystis carinii (with HIV)
Aspiration	Anaerobes
Alcoholic/IV drug user	S. pneumoniae, Klebsiella, Staphylococcus
CF	Pseudomonas, S. aureus
COPD	H. influenzae, Moraxella catarrhalis, S. pneumoniae
Postviral	Staphylococcus, H. influenzae
Neonate	Group B streptococci (GBS), E. coli
Recurrent	Obstruction, bronchogenic carcinoma, lymphoma, Wegener's granulomatosis, immunodeficiency, unusual organisms (e.g., Nocardia, Coxiella burnetii, Aspergillus, Pseudomonas)

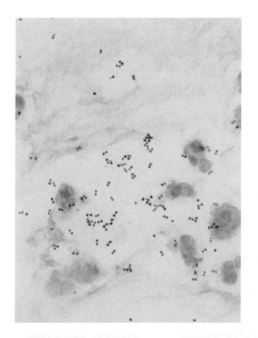

FIGURE 2.8-1. *S. aureus.*

These clusters of gram-⊕ cocci were isolated from the sputum of a patient who developed pneumonia while hospitalized. (Reproduced courtesy of Vinnie Piscitelli, Yale Microbiology Lab.)

TREATMENT

- Table 2.8-2 summarizes the recommended initial treatment for pneumonia.
- Outpatient treatment with oral antibiotics is recommended only in uncomplicated cases.

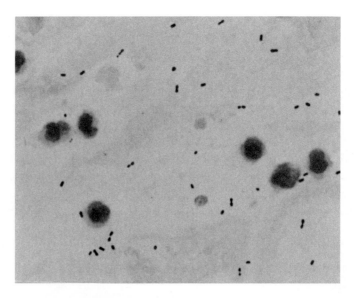

FIGURE 2.8-2. *S. pneumoniae.*

Sputum sample from a patient with pneumonia. Note the characteristic lancet-shaped gram-⊕ diplococci. (Reproduced courtesy of Vinnie Piscitelli, Yale Microbiology Lab.)

170

TABLE 2.8-2. **Treatment of Pneumonia**

PATIENT TYPE	SUSPECTED PATHOGENS	EMPIRIC COVERAGE
Outpatient community-acquired pneumonia, ≤ 65 years of age, otherwise healthy	*S. pneumoniae, Mycoplasma pneumoniae, C. pneumoniae, H. influenzae,* viral.	Macrolide (azithromycin), doxycycline, or fluoroquinolone.
> 65 years of age or with comorbidity (COPD, heart failure, renal failure, diabetes, liver disease, EtOH abuse)	*S. pneumoniae, H. influenzae,* aerobic gram-⊝ rods (GNR = *E. coli, Enterobacter, Klebsiella*), *S. aureus, Legionella,* viruses.	Macrolide or fluoroquinolone. May need to add a second-generation cephalosporin or β-lactam.
Community-acquired pneumonia requiring hospitalization	*S. pneumoniae, H. influenzae,* anaerobes, aerobic GNRs, *Legionella, Chlamydia.*	Extended-spectrum cephalosporin, β-lactam/β-lactamase inhibitor, or fluoroquinolone. Add a macrolide if atypical organisms are suspected.
Community-acquired pneumonia requiring hospitalization (needing ICU care)	*S. pneumoniae, H. influenzae,* anaerobes, aerobic GNRs, *Mycoplasma, Legionella, Pseudomonas.*	Fluoroquinolone or extended-spectrum cephalosporin or β-lactam/β-lactamase inhibitor + macrolide.
Institution-/hospital-acquired pneumonia—patient hospitalized > 48 hours or in a long-term care facility > 14 days	GNRs (including *Pseudomonas*), *S. aureus, Legionella,* mixed flora.	Extended-spectrum cephalosporin or β-lactam with antipseudomonal activity. Add aminoglycoside or fluoroquinolone for double coverage against *Pseudomonas.*

Adapted, with permission, from Mandell LA et al. Update of practice guidelines for the management of community-acquired pneumonia in immunocompetent adults. *Clin Infect Dis* 37(11):1405–1433, 2003.

- **In-hospital treatment with IV antibiotics** is recommended for patients > 65 years of age and in those with comorbidity (alcoholism, COPD, diabetes, malnutrition), immunosuppression, unstable vitals or signs of respiratory failure, altered mental status, and/or multilobar involvement.
- For patients with obstructive diseases (e.g., CF or bronchiectasis), consider adding pseudomonal coverage.

Tuberculosis (TB)

Infection due to *Mycobacterium tuberculosis*. Most symptomatic cases remain confined to the lung and are due to reactivation of old infection rather than to new 1° disease. Risk factors include immunosuppression, alcoholism, preexisting lung disease, diabetes, advancing age, homelessness, and crowded living conditions (e.g., prison). Also at risk are immigrants from developing nations, health care workers, and persons with "sick contacts."

HISTORY/PE

Cough, hemoptysis, dyspnea, **weight loss, fatigue, night sweats, fever,** cachexia, hypoxia, tachycardia, lymphadenopathy, abnormal lung sounds. TB is a common cause of fever of unknown origin (FUO).

Rifampin turns body fluids orange. Ethambutol can cause optic neuritis. INH causes peripheral neuritis and hepatitis.

Drugs for TB—

RIPE

Rifampin
INH
Pyrazinamide
Ethambutol

DIAGNOSIS

- ⊕ sputum **acid-fast stain** (see Figure 2.8-3).
- CXR may show lower lobe infiltrates (in 1° TB) or apical fibronodular infiltrates with or without cavitation (in reactivated pulmonary TB).
- A ⊕ PPD test (see Figure 2.8-4) indicates previous exposure (not necessarily active infection). Exposed immunocompromised individuals may not mount a ⊕ PPD (anergy).

TREATMENT

All cases should be reported to local and state health departments. Respiratory isolation should be instituted if TB is suspected. Treatment is as follows:

- Directly observed multidrug therapy with a four-drug regimen (**INH, pyrazinamide, rifampin, ethambutol**) until drug susceptibility tests are finalized. Administer **vitamin B$_6$** (pyridoxine) with INH to prevent peripheral neuritis.
- Therapy on at least rifampin and INH should continue for six months.
- Initiate prophylactic therapy (INH × 9 months) for PPD conversion without active symptoms in patients with a CXR suggestive of old TB infection, recent new conversion (< 2 years), or the risk factors mentioned above.

Acute Pharyngitis

Viral causes are more common, but it is important to identify streptococcal pharyngitis (**group A β-hemolytic *Streptococcus pyogenes***). Etiologies are as follows:

- **Bacterial:** Group A streptococci (GAS), *Neisseria gonorrhoeae, Corynebacterium diphtheriae, M. pneumoniae.*
- **Viral:** Rhinovirus, coronavirus, adenovirus, HSV, EBV, CMV, influenza virus, coxsackievirus.

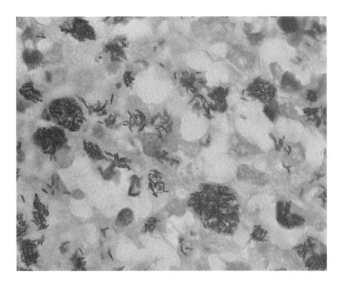

FIGURE 2.8-3. **TB organisms are identified by their red color ("red snappers") on acid-fast staining.**

(Reproduced courtesy of the Pathology Education Instructional Resource Digital Library [http://peir.net] at the University of Alabama, Birmingham.)

172

PPD is injected intradermally on the volar surface of the forearm. The diameter of induration is measured at 48–72 hours. BCG vaccination typically renders a patient PPD ⊕ but should not preclude prophylaxis as recommended for unvaccinated individuals. The size of induration that indicates a ⊕ test is interpreted as follows:

- **≥ 5 mm:** HIV or risk factors, close TB contacts, CXR evidence of TB.
- **≥ 10 mm:** Indigent/homeless, developing nations, IV drug use, chronic illness, residents of health and correctional institutions.
- **≥ 15 mm:** Everyone else, including those with no known risk factors.

A ⊖ reaction with ⊖ controls implies anergy from immunosuppression, old age, or malnutrition and thus does not rule out TB.

FIGURE 2.8-4. **PPD interpretation.**

HISTORY/PE

- **Typical of streptococcal pharyngitis: Fever, sore throat, pharyngeal erythema, tonsillar exudate,** cervical lymphadenopathy, soft palate petechiae, headache, vomiting, scarlatiniform rash (indicates scarlet fever).
- **Atypical of streptococcal pharyngitis:** Coryza, hoarseness, rhinorrhea, **cough,** conjunctivitis, anterior stomatitis, ulcerative lesions, GI symptoms.

DIAGNOSIS

Clinical evaluation, rapid GAS antigen detection, throat culture.

TREATMENT

If GAS is suspected, begin empiric antibiotic therapy with penicillin × 10 days. Amoxicillin or azithromycin are alternative options. Symptom relief can be attained with fluids, rest, antipyretics, and salt-water gargles.

COMPLICATIONS

- **Nonsuppurative:** Acute rheumatic fever (see Cardiology section), poststreptococcal glomerulonephritis.
- **Suppurative:** Cervical lymphadenitis, mastoiditis, sinusitis, otitis media, retropharyngeal or peritonsillar abscess.
- **Peritonsillar abscess** may present with odynophagia, trismus ("lockjaw"), muffled voice, unilateral tonsillar enlargement, and erythema with the uvula and soft palate deviated away from the affected side. Culture abscess fluid and localize the abscess via intraoral ultrasound or CT. Treat with antibiotics and surgical drainage.

Signs suggestive of streptococcal pharyngitis include fever, pharyngeal erythema, exudate, cervical lymphadenopathy, and lack of cough.

Sinusitis

Infection of the sinuses due to a collection of pus. The maxillary sinuses are most commonly infected. Subtypes are as follows:

- **Acute sinusitis (symptoms lasting < 1 month):** Most commonly associated with *S. pneumoniae, H. influenzae, M. catarrhalis,* and viral infection.
- **Chronic sinusitis (symptoms persisting > 3 months):** Often due to obstruction of sinus drainage and ongoing low-grade anaerobic infections. In diabetic patients, mucormycosis infection may develop.

HISTORY/PE

- **Fever, facial pain, headache,** nasal congestion, discharge.
- Exam may reveal tenderness, erythema, and swelling over the affected area.
- High fever, leukocytosis, and purulent nasal discharge are suggestive of acute bacterial sinusitis.

DIAGNOSIS

Always consider occult sinusitis in febrile ICU patients.

- A clinical diagnosis. Culture is generally not required.
- Transillumination shows opacification of the sinuses (low sensitivity).
- Maxillary sinus radiographs may show air-fluid levels or opacification (see Figure 2.8-5) but are helpful only if symptoms persist after therapy. Obtain a CT if complications are suspected.

TREATMENT

- Amoxicillin/clavulanate 500 mg PO TID × 10 days (for acute sinusitis only).
- Alternative therapies include clarithromycin, azithromycin, TMP-SMX, or second-generation cephalosporin × 10 days.
- Symptomatic therapy (e.g., nasal decongestants, antihistamines, pain relief) can be used for acute or chronic sinusitis.

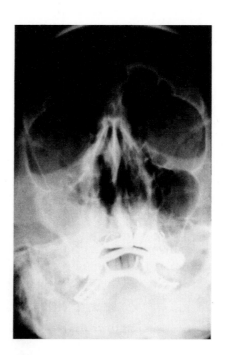

FIGURE 2.8-5. Sinusitis.

Compare the opacified right maxillary sinus and normal air-filled left sinus on this sinus x-ray. (Reproduced, with permission, from Saunders CE. *Current Emergency Diagnosis & Treatment*, 4th ed. Stamford, CT: Appleton & Lange, 1992:443.)

Meningitis

Risk factors include recent ear infection, sinusitis, immunodeficiencies, recent neurosurgical procedures, and sick contacts. Causes are listed in Table 2.8-3.

HISTORY/PE

Patients present with **fever,** malaise, **headache, neck stiffness, photophobia,** altered mental status, **nausea/vomiting,** seizures, or signs of meningeal irritation (⊕ Kernig's and Brudzinski's signs).

DIAGNOSIS

 Blood cultures.
- **LP** for **CSF Gram stain and culture;** obtain glucose, protein, WBC count plus differential, RBC, and O&P (in the absence of papilledema or focal neurologic deficits).
- **CT or MRI** to rule out other diagnoses. CBC may reveal leukocytosis; CSF findings vary (see Table 2.8-4).

Check for papilledema or focal neurologic deficits before performing an LP!

TREATMENT

Antibiotics should be administered rapidly (see Table 2.8-5) and may be empirically given prior to performing a LP. Viral disease can be treated with supportive care and close follow-up. Close contacts of patients with meningococcal meningitis should receive rifampin, ciprofloxacin, or ceftriaxone prophylaxis.

COMPLICATIONS

- **Cerebral edema:** Visible on CT/MRI. Presents with loss of oculocephalic reflex. Treat with IV mannitol.
- **Subdural effusions:** May be seen on CT scan. Occur in 50% of infants with *H. influenzae* meningitis. No treatment is necessary.
- **Ventriculitis/hydrocephalus:** Presents as a worsening clinical picture with improved CSF findings. Requires ventriculostomy and possibly intraventricular antibiotics.

TABLE 2.8-3. Causes of Meningitis[a,b]

NEWBORN (0–6 MOS)	CHILDREN (6 MOS–6 YRS)	6–60 YRS	60 YRS +
GBS	*S. pneumoniae*	*N. meningitidis*	*S. pneumoniae*
E. coli/GNR	*Neisseria meningitidis*	Enteroviruses	GNR
Listeria	*H. influenzae* B	*S. pneumoniae*	*Listeria*
	Enteroviruses	HSV	*N. meningitidis*

[a] Causes in HIV include *Cryptococcus,* CMV, toxoplasmosis (brain abscess), and JC virus (PML).

[b] Note: The incidence of *H. influenzae* meningitis has ↓ greatly with the introduction of *H. influenzae* vaccine in the last 10–15 years.

TABLE 2.8-4. CSF Profiles

	RBCs (PER mm³)	WBCs (PER mm³)	GLUCOSE (mg/dL)	PROTEIN (mg/dL)	OPENING PRESSURE (cm H₂O)	APPEARANCE	GAMMA GLOBULIN (% PROTEIN)
Normal	< 10	< 5	~2/3 of serum	15–45	10–20	Clear	3–12
Bacterial meningitis	↔	↑ (> 1000 PMN)	↓	↑	↑	Cloudy	↔ or ↑
Viral meningitis	↔	↑ (monos/ lymphs)	↔	↔ or ↑	↔ or ↑	Most often clear	↔ or ↑
Aseptic meningitis	↔	↑	↔	↔ or ↑	↔	Clear	↔
SAH	↑↑	↑	↔	↑	↔ or ↑	Yellow/red	↔ or ↑
Guillain-Barré syndrome	↔	↔	↔ or ↑	↑↑	↔	Clear or yellow (high protein)	↔
MS	↔	↔ or ↑	↔	↔	↔	Clear	↑↑
Pseudotumor cerebri	↔	↔	↔	↔	↑↑↑	Clear	↔

- **Seizures:** Benzodiazepines and phenytoin.
- **Hyponatremia:** Administer fluids and monitor sodium concentration.
- **Subdural empyema:** Presents with intractable seizures. Requires surgical evacuation.
- **Other:** Cranial nerve palsies, sensorineural hearing loss, coma, death.

TABLE 2.8-5. Empiric Treatment of Bacterial Meningitis

AGE	CAUSATIVE ORGANISM	TREATMENT
< 1 month	GBS, *E. coli*/gram-⊖ rods, *Listeria*.	Ampicillin + cefotaxime or gentamicin.
1–3 months	Pneumococci, meningococci, *H. influenzae*.	Vancomycin IV + ceftriaxone or cefotaxime.
3 months – adulthood	Pneumococci, meningococci.	Vancomycin IV + ceftriaxone or cefotaxime.
> 60 years/alcoholism/ chronic illness	Pneumococci, gram-⊖ bacilli, *Listeria*, meningococci.	Ampicillin + vancomycin + cefotaxime or ceftriaxone.

Encephalitis

HSV and **arboviruses** are the most common etiologies. Rarer etiologies include CMV, toxoplasmosis, West Nile virus, VZV, *Borrelia*, *Rickettsia*, *Legionella*, enterovirus, *Mycoplasma*, and cerebral malaria. Children and the elderly are the most vulnerable.

HISTORY/PE

Altered consciousness, headache, fever, seizures. Lethargy, confusion, coma, and focal neurologic deficits (cranial nerve deficits, accentuated DTRs) may also be present. The differential includes brain abscess or malignancy, toxic-metabolic encephalopathy, subdural hematoma, and SAH.

DIAGNOSIS

- **CSF:** Lymphocytic pleocytosis and moderately ↑ protein. RBCs without evidence of trauma suggest HSV encephalitis. Glucose level is low in tuberculous, fungal, bacterial, and amebic infections.
- CSF Gram stain (bacteria), acid-fast stain (mycobacteria), India ink (*Cryptococcus*), wet preparation (free-living amebae), and Giemsa stain (trypanosomes). PCR for HSV, CMV, EBV, VZV, and enterovirus.
- **MRI** may demonstrate a **contrast-enhancing lesion** in the **temporal** lobe (in HSV).

TREATMENT

HSV encephalitis requires immediate IV acyclovir. CMV encephalitis is treated with IV ganciclovir +/− foscarnet.

HUMAN IMMUNODEFICIENCY VIRUS (HIV)

A retrovirus that targets and destroys CD4+ T lymphocytes. Infection is characterized by a progressively high rate of viral replication → progressive decline in the CD4+ count.

- **CD4+ count** indicates **degree of immunosuppression,** guides therapy, and helps determine prognosis.
- **Viral load** indicates the **rate** of disease progression, indications for treatment, and response to antiretroviral therapy.
- Figure 2.8-6 illustrates the typical time course of HIV infection.

HISTORY/PE

- 1° infection is often **asymptomatic;** patients may also present with **flulike symptoms** (e.g., fever, lymphadenopathy, maculopapular rash, pharyngitis, diarrhea, nausea/vomiting, weight loss, headache).
- HIV may later present as night sweats, weight loss, thrush, recurrent infections, or opportunistic infections. Complications correlate with CD4+ count.

DIAGNOSIS

- **ELISA test** (high sensitivity, moderate specificity) detects anti-HIV antibodies in the bloodstream (can take up to six months to appear after exposure).
- **Western blot** (low sensitivity, high specificity) is confirmatory.
- **Rapid HIV tests.**

The presence of RBCs in CSF without a history of trauma indicates HSV encephalitis.

HSV encephalitis requires immediate IV acyclovir even before labs confirm the diagnosis.

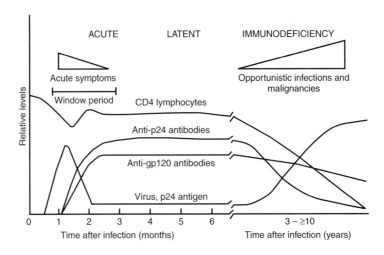

FIGURE 2.8-6. **Time course of HIV infection.**

(Adapted, with permission, from Levinson W, Jawetz E. *Medical Microbiology and Immunology: Examination & Board Review*, 6th ed. New York: McGraw-Hill, 2000:276.)

- Baseline evaluation should include HIV RNA PCR (viral load), CD4+ cell count, CXR, PPD skin testing, Pap smear, VDRL/RPR, and serologies for CMV, hepatitis, toxoplasmosis, and VZV.

TREATMENT

- Currently, **antiretroviral therapy** is initiated for patients with a CD4+ count < 350.
- **Starting regimen:** Two **nucleoside analogs** + a **non-nucleoside reverse transcriptase inhibitor** or a **protease inhibitor.**
- The choice of regimen depends on drug–drug interactions, drug tolerance, and patient adherence. Do not use monotherapy or dual therapy.
- See Table 2.8-6 for an outline of prophylactic measures against opportunistic infections.

OPPORTUNISTIC INFECTIONS

Figure 2.8-7 illustrates the microscopic appearance of some common opportunistic organisms.

Candidal Thrush

- Risk factors include xerostomia and immunosuppressed states (e.g., HIV, leukemias, lymphomas, cancer, diabetes, corticosteroid inhaler use, immunosuppressive treatment).
- **Hx/PE:** Presents with **soft white plaques that can be rubbed off,** with an erythematous base and possible mucosal burning. The differential includes oral hairy leukoplakia (lateral borders of the tongue; not easily rubbed off).
- **Dx:** Usually clinical. KOH or Gram stain shows budding yeast and/or pseudohyphae.
- **Rx:** Treat with oral **nystatin** suspension QID. Clotrimazole is another option. If topical therapy is not effective or odynophagia/dysphagia is present (suggestive of esophagitis), oral fluconazole may be used.

TABLE 2.8-6. **Prophylaxis for HIV-Related Opportunistic Infections**

PATHOGEN	INDICATION FOR PROPHYLAXIS	MEDICATION	COMMENTS
Pneumocystis carinii pneumonia (PCP)	CD4+ < 200/mm³, prior PCP, unexplained fever × 2 weeks, or HIV-related oral candidiasis.	TMP-SMX SS[a] or dapsone +/– pyrimethamine.	Discontinue prophylaxis when CD4+ > 200/mm³ for ≥ 3 months.
Mycobacterium avium complex (MAC)	CD4+ < 50–100/mm³.	Weekly azithromycin or daily clarithromycin.	Discontinue prophylaxis when CD4+ > 100/mm³ for > 6 months.
Toxoplasma gondii	CD4+ < 100/mm³ + ⊕ IgG serologies.	TMP-SMX DS.[a]	–
M. tuberculosis	PPD > 5 mm or "high risk" (see TB section).	**Sensitive:** INH × 9 months (+ pyridoxine) or rifampin +/– pyrazinamide × 2 months.	Include pyridoxine with INH-containing regimens.
Candida	Multiple recurrences.	**Esophagitis:** Fluconazole. **Oral:** Nystatin swish and swallow.	–
HSV	Multiple recurrences.	Acyclovir or famciclovir or valacyclovir.	–
S. pneumoniae	All patients.	Pneumovax.	Give every five years or when CD4+ > 200.
Influenza	All patients.	Influenza vaccine annually.	–

[a] SS = single strength; DS = double strength.

(Adapted, with permission, from Mandell GL. *Principles and Practice of Infectious Diseases,* 5th ed. London: Churchill Livingstone, 2000:1507. Also adapted, with permission, from Bartlett JG, Gallant JE. *2003 Medical Management of HIV Infection.* Baltimore, MD: Johns Hopkins University Division of Infectious Diseases and AIDS Services, 2003:40–45.)

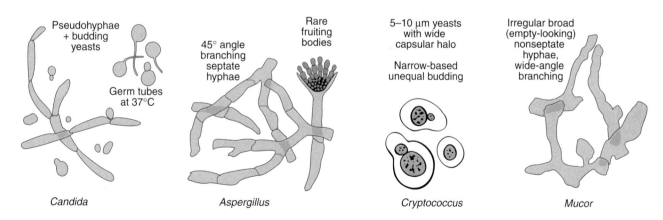

FIGURE 2.8-7. **Common opportunistic organisms.**

HIGH-YIELD FACTS

INFECTIOUS DISEASE

Cryptococcal Meningitis

- Risk factors include AIDS and exposure to pigeon droppings.
- **Hx/PE:** Headache, fever, impaired mentation, absent meningismus. The differential includes toxoplasmosis, lymphoma, TB meningitis, AIDS dementia complex, PML, HSV encephalitis, and other fungal disease.
- **Dx: LP** ($\downarrow$ CSF glucose; $\uparrow$ protein; $\uparrow$ leukocyte count with monocytic predominance); $\oplus$ CSF cryptococcal antigen test, India ink stain, and fungal culture.
- **Rx:**
  - **IV amphotericin B** + flucytosine $\times$ 2 weeks; then give fluconazole 400 mg $\times$ 8 weeks. Lifelong **maintenance therapy** with fluconazole 200 mg QD.
  - $\uparrow$ opening pressure may require serial LPs.

Histoplasmosis

- Risk factors include AIDS, spelunking, and exposure to bird or bat excrement.
- **Hx/PE:** 1° exposure is often asymptomatic or causes a flulike illness. Fever, weight loss, hepatosplenomegaly, lymphadenopathy, nonproductive cough, and pancytopenia indicate disseminated infection (often within 14 days and in immunocompromised hosts). The differential includes atypical bacterial pneumonias, blastomycosis, coccidioidomycosis, TB, sarcoidosis, pneumoconiosis, and lymphoma.
- **Dx: CXR** shows diffuse nodular densities, focal infiltrate, cavity, or hilar lymphadenopathy (chronic infection is usually cavitary). The **urine and serum polysaccharide antigen test** is the most sensitive test for initial diagnosis, monitoring response to therapy, and diagnosing relapse. Culture is also diagnostic (blood, sputum, bone marrow, CSF). The yeast form is seen with **silver stain** on biopsy (bone marrow, lymph node, liver) or bronchoalveolar lavage.
- **Rx:** Amphotericin B or amphotericin B liposomal $\times$ 3–10 days, followed by itraconazole $\times$ 12 weeks. Maintenance therapy with daily itraconazole.

Pneumocystis carinii Pneumonia (PCP)

- Risk factors include impaired cellular immunity and AIDS.
- **Hx/PE:** Presents with dyspnea on exertion, fever, nonproductive cough, tachypnea, weight loss, fatigue, and impaired oxygenation. CXR shows diffuse, bilateral interstitial infiltrates with ground-glass appearance, but any presentation is possible. The differential includes TB, histoplasmosis, and coccidioidomycosis.
- **Dx:** Cytology of induced sputum or bronchoscopy specimen with silver stain and immunofluorescence. Obtain an ABG to check PaO_2.
- **Rx:** Treat with TMP-SMX $\times$ 21 days. Prednisone taper should be used in patients with moderate to severe hypoxemia ($PaO_2 < 70$ mm).

> **AIDS pathogens—**
>
> **The Major Pathogens Concerning Complete T-Cell Collapse**
>
> **T**oxoplasma gondii
> **M**ycobacterium avium-intracellulare
> **P**neumocystis carinii
> **C**andida albicans
> **C**ryptococcus neoformans
> **T**uberculosis
> **C**MV
> **C**ryptosporidium parvum

SEXUALLY TRANSMITTED DISEASES (STDs)

Chlamydia

- The most common bacterial STD in the United States. Caused by *Chlamydia trachomatis*, which can infect the genital tract, urethra, anus, and eye. Often coexists with or mimics *N. gonorrhoeae* infection (non-gonococcal urethritis).

- **Hx/PE:** Infection is often asymptomatic but may present with **urethritis, mucopurulent cervicitis,** or **PID.** Exam may reveal cervical/adnexal tenderness in women or penile discharge and testicular tenderness in men. The differential includes gonorrhea, endometriosis, PID, orchitis, vaginitis, and UTI.
- **Dx:** Usually clinical. Urine tests (PCR or ligase chain reaction) are a rapid means of detection, while DNA probes and immunofluorescence (for gonorrhea/chlamydia) take 48–72 hours. Gram stain of urethral or genital discharge may show PMNs but no bacteria (intracellular).
- **Rx:** Doxycycline 100 mg PO BID × 7 days or azithromycin 1 g PO × 1 day. Use erythromycin in pregnant patients. **Treat sexual partners.**
- **Complications:** Chronic infection and pelvic pain, Reiter's syndrome (urethritis, conjunctivitis, arthritis), Fitz-Hugh–Curtis syndrome (perihepatic inflammation and fibrosis). Ectopic pregnancy/infertility can result from PID (in women) and epididymitis (in men).

Chlamydia is a common cause of nongonococcal urethritis in men.

Chlamydia species cause arthritis, neonatal conjunctivitis, pneumonia, nongonococcal urethritis/PID, and lymphogranuloma venereum.

Gonorrhea

- This gram-⊖ intracellular diplococcus can infect almost any site in the female reproductive tract, whereas infection in men tends to be limited to the urethra.
- **Hx/PE: Greenish-yellow discharge,** pelvic or **adnexal pain,** swollen Bartholin's glands. Men experience **purulent urethral discharge,** dysuria, and erythema of the urethral meatus. The differential includes chlamydia, endometriosis, pharyngitis, PID, vaginitis, UTI, salpingitis, and tubo-ovarian abscess.
- **Dx:** Swab the pharynx, cervix, urethra, or anus as appropriate. Conduct urine and probe tests as with chlamydia. Obtain a Gram stain of cervical discharge. Disseminated disease may present with monoarticular septic arthritis, rash, and/or tenosynovitis.
- **Rx:** Ceftriaxone IM. Also treat for presumptive chlamydia coinfection (doxycycline × 7 days or macrolide × 1 dose). Condoms are effective prophylaxis. Treat the sexual partner or partners if possible.
- **Complications:** Persistent infection with pain; infertility; tubo-ovarian abscess with rupture; disseminated gonococcal infection (see Figure 2.8-8).

Treat for gonorrhea and chlamydia in light of the high prevalence of coinfection.

Syphilis

Caused by *Treponema pallidum*, a spirochete.

HISTORY/PE

- **1° (10–90 days after infection):** Presents with a **painless ulcer (chancre;** see Figure 2.8-9).
- **2° (4–8 weeks after chancre):** Low-grade fever, headache, malaise, and generalized lymphadenopathy with a diffuse, symmetric, asymptomatic (nonpruritic) **maculopapular rash on the soles and palms.** Highly infective 2° eruptions include mucous patches or **condylomata lata** (see Figure 2.8-10). Meningitis, hepatitis, nephropathy, and eye involvement may also be seen.
- **Early latent:** No symptoms; ⊕ serology; first year of infection.
- **Late latent:** No symptoms; ⊕ or ⊖ serology; > 1 year infection. One-third progress to 3° syphilis.

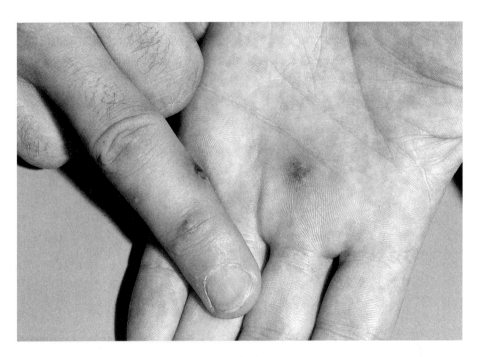

FIGURE 2.8-8. **Disseminated gonococcal infection.**

Hemorrhagic, painful pustules on erythematous bases. (Reproduced, with permission, from Wolff K, Johnson RA, Suurmond D. *Fitzpatrick's Color Atlas & Synopsis of Clinical Dermatology*, 5th ed. New York: McGraw-Hill, 2005:910.)

- **3° (1–20 years after initial infection):** Destructive, granulomatous **gummas.** Neurologic findings include **tabes dorsalis** (posterior column degeneration), meningitis, and **Argyll Robertson pupil** (constricts with accommodation but not reactive to light). Cardiovascular findings include dilated aortic root, aortitis, aortic root aneurysms, and aortic regurgitation.

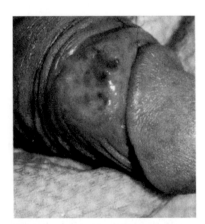

FIGURE 2.8-9. **1° syphilis.**

The chancre is an ulcerated papule with a smooth, clean base; raised, indurated borders; and scant discharge. (Reproduced, with permission, from Bondi EE. *Dermatology: Diagnosis and Therapy*, 1st ed. Stamford, CT: Appleton & Lange, 1991:394.)

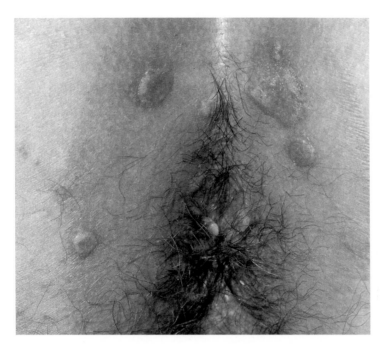

FIGURE 2.8-10. **Condylomata lata.**

Typical appearance of the verrucous heaped-up lesions of condylomata lata. (Reproduced, with permission, from Wolff K, Johnson RA, Suurmond D. *Fitzpatrick's Color Atlas & Synopsis of Clinical Dermatology*, 5th ed. New York: McGraw-Hill, 2005:921.)

DIAGNOSIS

See Table 2.8-7. **VDRL false positives** are seen with **V**iruses (mononucleosis, HSV, HIV, hepatitis), **D**rugs/IV drug use, **R**heumatic fever/**R**heumatoid arthritis, and SLE/**L**eprosy.

TREATMENT

- 1°/2°: Benzathine penicillin IM. Tetracycline or doxycycline × 14 days may be used for patients with penicillin allergies.
- Latent infection should be treated with penicillin once weekly × 3 weeks.
- Neurosyphilis should be treated with penicillin IV; penicillin-allergic patients should be desensitized prior to therapy.

Syphilis is the "great imitator" because the dermatologic findings resemble those of many other diseases.

TABLE 2.8-7. **Diagnostic Tests for Syphilis**

TEST	COMMENTS
Dark-field microscopy	Identifies motile spirochetes (only 1° and 2° lesions).
VDRL/RPR	Rapid and cheap, but sensitivity is only 60–75% in 1° disease. Reverts to negative with successful treatment.
FTA-ABS	Sensitive, specific. Used as a 2° diagnostic test. ⊕ for life.

TABLE 2.8-8. **Sexually Transmitted Genital Lesions**[a]

	CALYMMATOBACTERIUM GRANULOMATIS (GRANULOMA INGUINALE-DONOVANOSIS)	*HAEMOPHILUS DUCREYI* (CHANCROID)	HSV-1 OR -2[a]	HPV[b]	*TREPONEMA PALLIDUM*
Lesion	Papule becomes beefy-red ulcer	Papule or pustule (chancroid; see Figure 2.8-11)	Vesicle	Papule (condylomata acuminata; warts)	Papule (chancre)
Appearance	Raised red lesions with white border	Irregular, deep, well demarcated, necrotic	Regular, red, shallow ulcer	Irregular, pink or white, raised; cauliflower	Regular, red, round, raised
Number	1 or multiple	1–3	Multiple	Multiple	Single
Size	5–10 mm	10–20 mm	1–3 mm	1–5 mm	1 cm
Pain	No	Yes	Yes	No	No
Concurrent signs and symptoms	Granulomatous ulcers	Inguinal lymphadenopathy	Vulvar pain and pruritus	Pruritus	Regional adenopathy
Diagnosis	Clinical exam, biopsy	Difficult to culture; diagnosis made on clinical grounds	Tzanck smear or viral cultures	Clinical exam; biopsy for confirmation	Spirochetes seen under dark-field microscopy; *T. pallidum* identified by serum antibody test
Treatment[c]	Doxycycline (100 mg BID × 3 weeks)	Ceftriaxone, IM erythromycin, or azithromycin	Acyclovir for 1° infection	Cryotherapy, topical agents such as podophyllin, trichloroacetic acid, or 5-FU cream	Penicillin IM

[a] Some 85% of genital herpes lesions are caused by HSV-2.

[b] HPV serotypes 6 and 11 are associated with genital warts; types 16, 18, and 31 are associated with cervical cancer.

[c] For all, treat sexual partners.

Genital Lesions

See Table 2.8-8 for a description of common sexually transmitted genital lesions along with an outline of their diagnosis and treatment.

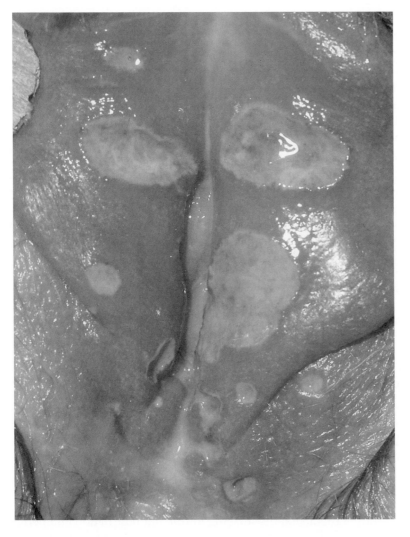

FIGURE 2.8-11. Chancroid.

Multiple, painful ulcers. (Reproduced, with permission, from Wolff K, Johnson RA, Suurmond D. *Fitzpatrick's Color Atlas & Synopsis of Clinical Dermatology*, 5th ed. New York: McGraw-Hill, 2005:927.)

GENITOURINARY INFECTIONS

Urinary Tract Infections (UTIs)

Affect women more frequently than men, and ⊕ **E. coli** cultures are obtained in 80% of cases. See the mnemonic **SEEKS PP** for other pathogens. Risk factors include catheters or other urologic instrumentation, anatomic abnormalities (e.g., BPH, vesicoureteral reflux), previous UTIs or pyelonephritis, diabetes mellitus (DM), recent antibiotic use, immunosuppression, and pregnancy.

HISTORY/PE

Dysuria, urgency, frequency, suprapubic pain, and possibly hematuria. Children may present with bed-wetting, poor feeding, recurrent fevers, and foul-smelling urine. The differential includes vaginitis, STDs, urethritis or acute urethral syndrome, and prostatitis.

DIAGNOSIS

- **Urine dipstick/UA:** ↑ **leukocyte esterase** (marker of WBCs) is 75% sensitive and up to 95% specific (good to rule out UTI). ↑ **nitrites** (marker of bacteria), ↑ urine pH (*Proteus* infections), and hematuria (seen with cystitis).
- **Microscopic analysis: Pyuria** (> 5 WBCs/hpf) and **bacteriuria** (1 organism/hpf = 10^6 organisms/mL) are seen.
- **Urine culture** (gold standard: > 10^5 **CFU/mL**).

TREATMENT

- Treat healthy young females on an outpatient basis with oral **TMP-SMX** or a **fluoroquinolone** × 3 days.
- Treat with fluoroquinolone or TMP-SMX for at least 7–10 days in high-risk patients (immunosuppressed, DM, pregnancy) and in cases of complicated UTI (urinary obstruction, men, renal transplant, catheters, instrumentation).
- Patients with urosepsis should be hospitalized and treated with **IV antibiotics** (ciprofloxacin or ampicillin/sulbactam + gentamicin to cover enterococcus).
- Prophylactic antibiotics may be given to women with uncomplicated recurrent UTIs. Check for prostatitis in men.

Pyelonephritis

- Nearly 85% of community-acquired cases result from the same pathogens that cause cystitis. Cystitis and pyelonephritis have similar risk factors.
- **Hx/PE: Flank pain, fever/chills,** nausea/vomiting. Dysuria, frequency, and urgency are possible.
- **Dx:**
  - **UA and culture:** Similar to cystitis plus **WBC casts.**
  - **CBC:** Leukocytosis.
  - Consider radiographic imaging to rule out obstruction and perinephric abscess. **IVP** is the initial study of choice in nonpregnant patients with adequate renal function, but **ultrasound** is the test of choice in all other patients. **CT** is recommended for patients who do not respond to adequate therapy after three days of treatment or who have had nondiagnostic IVP and ultrasound evaluations.
- **Rx:**
  - **Fluoroquinolone** or other antibiotics with similar coverage based on culture results; administer fluids and reevaluate in 72 hours.
  - If patients are improving, they may continue treatment on an outpatient basis for 14 days.
  - Patients with high fever, hypotension, and/or severe nausea/vomiting should be hospitalized and treated with IV antibiotics.

BLOOD AND SOFT TISSUE INFECTIONS

Sepsis

Systemic inflammatory response syndrome (**SIRS**) with a **documented infection,** induced by microbial invasion or toxins in the bloodstream. **Septic shock** refers to sepsis-induced hypotension and organ dysfunction due to poor perfusion. Etiologies include the following:

- **Gram-⊕ shock** (e.g., staphylococci and streptococci) 2° to fluid loss caused by exotoxins.
- **Gram-⊖ shock** (e.g., *E. coli*, *Klebsiella*, *Proteus*, and *Pseudomonas*) 2° to vasodilation caused by endotoxins (lipopolysaccharide).
- **Neonates:** GBS, *E. coli*, *Listeria monocytogenes*, *H. influenzae*.
- **Children:** *H. influenzae*, pneumococcus, meningococcus.
- **Adults:** Gram-⊕ cocci, aerobic gram-⊖ bacilli, anaerobes (dependent on the presumed site of infection).
- **IV drug users/indwelling lines:** *S. aureus*, coagulase-⊖ *Staphylococcus* spp.
- **Asplenic patients:** Pneumococcus, *H. influenzae*, meningococcus (encapsulated organisms).

HISTORY/PE

- Abrupt onset of fever and chills, altered mental status, tachycardia, and tachypnea. **Hypotension** and shock occur in severe cases.
- Septic shock is typically a warm shock with **warm skin and extremities.** Cold shock with **cool skin and extremities** is possible with other underlying factors (e.g., CHF).
- Petechiae or ecchymoses suggest DIC (2–3% of cases).

DIAGNOSIS

- A clinical diagnosis.
- Leukocytosis or leukopenia with ↑ bands, thrombocytopenia (50% of cases), and evidence of ↓ tissue perfusion (↑ creatinine, ↑ LFTs). Blood, sputum, and urine cultures may be ⊕ (sepsis may also result from toxins in the bloodstream); CXR may show an infiltrate. Obtain coagulation studies and consider a DIC panel (fibrinogen, fibrin split products, D-dimer).

TREATMENT

- May require ICU admission. Treat aggressively with IV fluids, pressors, and empiric antibiotics (based on the likely source of infection).
- Treat underlying factors (e.g., remove Foley catheter or infected lines).
- The 1° goal is to **maintain BP and perfusion** to end organs.

Osteomyelitis

- Bone infection 2° to **direct spread** from a soft tissue infection (80% of cases) is most common in adults, whereas infection due to **hematogenous seeding** (20% of cases) is more common in children (metaphyses of the long bones) and IV drug users (vertebral bodies). Common pathogens are outlined in Table 2.8-9.
- Hx/PE: **Localized bone pain and tenderness;** warmth, swelling, erythema, and limited motion of the adjacent joint. Systemic symptoms (fevers, chills) and purulent drainage may be present.
- Dx:
  - ↑ WBC count, **ESR** (> 100), and **CRP** levels. Blood cultures may be ⊕.
  - X-rays are often ⊖ initially but may show periosteal elevation within 10–14 days. Bone scans are sensitive for osteomyelitis but lack specificity.
  - **MRI** (test of choice) will show ↑ signal in the bone marrow and associated soft tissue infection.

TABLE 2.8-9. **Common Pathogens in Osteomyelitis**

IF	THINK
Most people	*S. aureus*
IV drug user	*S. aureus* or *Pseudomonas*
Sickle cell disease	*Salmonella*
Hip replacement	*S. epidermidis*
Foot puncture wound	*Pseudomonas*
Chronic	*S. aureus, Pseudomonas,* Enterobacteriaceae
Diabetic	Polymicrobial, *Pseudomonas, S. aureus,* streptococci, anaerobes

- Definitive diagnosis is made by bone aspiration with Gram stain and culture.
- **Rx:** Treat with **surgical debridement** of necrotic, infected bone and then with **IV antibiotics** × 4–6 weeks. Empiric antibiotic selection is based on the suspected organism and Gram stain. Consider clindamycin + ciprofloxacin, ampicillin/sulbactam, or oxacillin/nafcillin (for methicillin-sensitive *S. aureus*); vancomycin (for methicillin-resistant *S. aureus*); or ceftriaxone or ciprofloxacin (for gram-⊖ bacteria).
- **Complications:** Chronic osteomyelitis, sepsis, septic arthritis. Long-standing chronic osteomyelitis with a draining sinus tract may eventually → **squamous cell carcinoma** (Marjolin's ulcer).

FEVER

Fever of Unknown Origin (FUO)

FUO patients without other symptoms do not require empiric antibiotic therapy.

- A temperature of > 38.3°C of at least three weeks' duration that remains undiagnosed following three outpatient visits or three days of hospitalization. In adults, infections and cancer account for > 60% of cases of FUO, while autoimmune diseases account for approximately 15%.
- **Hx/PE:** Fever, headache, myalgia, malaise. The differential includes the following:
  - **Infectious:** TB, endocarditis (e.g., HACEK organisms; see the discussion of infective endocarditis), occult abscess, osteomyelitis, catheter infections.
  - **Neoplastic:** Lymphomas, leukemias, hepatic and renal cell carcinomas.
  - **Autoimmune:** Still's disease, SLE, cryoglobulinemia, polyarteritis nodosa, connective tissue disease, granulomatous disease (including sarcoidosis).
  - **Miscellaneous:** Pulmonary emboli, alcoholic hepatitis, drug fever, familial Mediterranean fever, factitious fever.
  - Undiagnosed (10–15%).
- **Dx:** Confirm fever; obtain CXR, CBC with differential, ESR, multiple blood cultures, sputum Gram stain and culture, UA, and PPD. CT and

MRI scans should be done if malignancy or abscess is suspected. Specific tests (ANA, RF, viral cultures, viral serologies/antigen tests) can be obtained if an infectious or autoimmune etiology is suspected.

- **Rx: Stop unnecessary medications.** Give empiric antibiotics to severely ill patients until the etiology has been determined. Stop antibiotics if there is no response.

Neutropenic Fever

- Defined as a single oral temperature of ≥ 38.3°C (101°F) or a temperature of ≥ 38.0°C (100.4°F) for ≥ 1 hour in a neutropenic patient (i.e., a neutrophil count of < 500 cells/mm³).
- **Hx/PE:** Common in cancer patients undergoing chemotherapy (neutropenic nadir 7–10 days postchemotherapy). Inflammation may be minimal or absent.
- **Dx:** Thorough physical examination, but **avoid rectal examination** because of the bleeding risk. CBC with differential, serum creatinine, BUN, and transaminases; blood, urine, lesion, and stool cultures. CXR for patients with respiratory symptoms; CT scan to evaluate for abscess.
- **Rx:** Empiric antibiotic therapy (see Figure 2.8-12). Routine use of colony-stimulating factors is not indicated. If fevers persist after 72 hours despite antibiotic therapy, start antifungal treatment.

Avoid doing a rectal exam on a neutropenic patient.

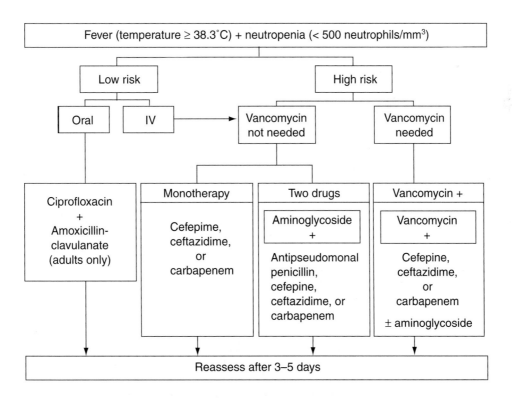

FIGURE 2.8-12. Empiric treatment algorithm for a neutropenic fever patient.

(Reproduced, with permission, from Hughes WT. 2002 guidelines for the use of antimicrobial agents in neutropenic patients with cancer. *Clin Infec Dis* 34:730–751, 2002.)

Lyme Disease

Lyme disease is the most common vector-borne disease in North America.

- A tick-borne disease caused by the spirochete *Borrelia burgdorferi*. Usually seen during the **summer months** and carried by *Ixodes* ticks on white-tailed deer and white-footed mice. Endemic to the **Northeast**, northern Midwest, and Pacific coast.
- Hx/PE: Onset of rash with fever, malaise, fatigue, headache, myalgias, and/or arthralgias. Infection usually occurs after a tick feeds for > 18 hours.
    - 1°: **Erythema migrans** begins as a small erythematous macule or papule that is found at the tick-feeding site and expands slowly over days to weeks. The border may be macular or raised, often with central clearing ("bull's eye").
    - 2°: Migratory polyarthropathies, neurologic phenomena (e.g., Bell's palsy), meningitis and/or myocarditis, conduction abnormalities (third-degree heart block).
    - 3°: Arthritis and subacute encephalitis (memory loss and mood change).
- Dx—erythema migrans:
    - **ELISA** and **Western blot.** Use the Western blot to confirm a ⊕ or indeterminate ELISA. A ⊕ ELISA denotes **exposure** but is not specific for active disease.
    - Tissue culture/PCR.
- Rx: Treat early disease with **doxycycline** and later disease with **ceftriaxone.** Consider empiric therapy for patients with characteristic rash, arthralgias, or a tick bite acquired in an endemic area. Prevent with tick bite avoidance.

Rocky Mountain Spotted Fever

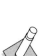

Rocky Mountain spotted fever starts on the wrists and ankles and then spreads centrally.

- A disease caused by *Rickettsia rickettsii* and carried by the American dog tick (*Dermacentor variabilis*). The organism invades the endothelial lining of capillaries and causes **small vessel vasculitis.**
- Hx/PE: Headache, fever, malaise, rash. The characteristic rash is initially macular (beginning on the wrists and ankles) but becomes petechial/purpuric as it spreads centrally (see Figure 2.8-13). Altered mental status or DIC may develop in severe cases.
- Dx: Clinical diagnosis should be confirmed with indirect immunofluorescence of rash biopsy.
- Rx: Doxycycline or chloramphenicol. The condition can be rapidly fatal if left untreated. Prevent by avoiding tick bites.

CONGENITAL INFECTIONS

May occur at any time during pregnancy, labor, and delivery. Common sequelae include **premature delivery, CNS abnormalities,** anemia, **jaundice,** hepatosplenomegaly, and growth retardation. The most common pathogens can be remembered through use of the mnemonic **TORCHeS** (see also Table 2.8-10):

- Toxoplasmosis: Transplacental transmission, with 1° infection occurring via consumption of **raw meat** or contact with **cat feces.** Specific findings include hydrocephalus, **intracranial calcifications,** chorioretinitis, and **ring-enhancing lesions** on head CT.
- Other: **HIV,** parvovirus, varicella, *Listeria*, TB, malaria, fungi.
- Rubella: Transplacental transmission in the first trimester. Specific findings include a purpuric **"blueberry muffin"** rash, cataracts, mental retardation, hearing loss, and **PDA.**
- CMV: The **most common congenital infection,** primarily transmitted transplacentally. Specific findings include petechial rash (similar to "blueberry muffin" rash) and **periventricular calcifications.**

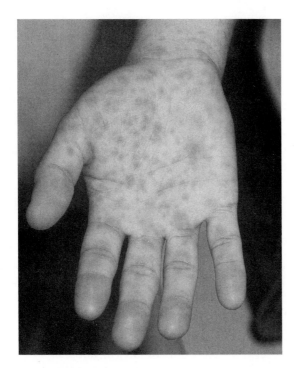

FIGURE 2.8-13. **Rocky Mountain spotted fever.**

These erythematous macular lesions will evolve into a petechial rash that will spread centrally. (Courtesy of Daniel Noltkamper, MD; reproduced, with permission, from Knoop KJ, Stack LB, Storrow AB. *Atlas of Emergency Medicine*, 2nd ed. New York: McGraw-Hill, 2002:382.)

TABLE 2.8-10. **Diagnosis and Treatment of Common Congenital Infections**

DISEASE	DIAGNOSIS	TREATMENT	PREVENTION
Toxoplasmosis	Serologic testing.	Pyrimethamine + sulfadiazine; spiramycin prophylaxis (for pregnant women).	Avoid exposure to cats and cat feces (e.g., changing litter or gardening) during pregnancy. Treat the mother during the third trimester.
Rubella	Serologic testing.		Immunize before pregnancy; otherwise, consider abortion if infected or exposed (≤ 20 weeks' gestation). Vaccinate the mother after delivery if serologic titers remain ⊖.
CMV	Urine culture, PCR of amniotic fluid.	Ganciclovir.	
HSV	Serologic testing.	Acyclovir.	Perform a C-section if lesions are present at delivery.
HIV	ELISA, Western blot.		AZT or nevirapine in pregnant women with HIV; perform a C-section; treat infants with prophylactic AZT; avoid breast-feeding.
Syphilis	Dark-field microscopy, VDRL/RPR, FTA-ABS.	Penicillin.	Penicillin in pregnant women who test ⊕.

- Herpes: Intrapartum transmission if mom has **active lesions.** Can cause skin, eye, and mouth infections or life-threatening CNS/systemic infection.
- Syphilis: Primarily intrapartum transmission. Specific findings include **maculopapular skin rash,** lymphadenopathy, hepatomegaly, "snuffles" (mucopurulent rhinitis), and osteitis. In childhood, late congenital syphilis is characterized by saber shins, saddle nose, CNS involvement, and Hutchinson's triad: **peg-shaped upper central incisors, deafness,** and **interstitial keratitis** (photophobia, lacrimation).

MISCELLANEOUS INFECTIONS

Infective Endocarditis

Infection of the endocardium, usually 2° to bacterial or other infectious causes. Most commonly affects the heart valves, especially the mitral valve. Risk factors include rheumatic, congenital, or valvular heart disease; prosthetic heart valves; IV drug abuse; and immunosuppression. Etiologies are as follows:

- **S. aureus** is the causative agent in > 80% of cases of acute bacterial endocarditis in patients with a history of IV drug abuse.
- **Viridans streptococci** are the most common pathogens for left-sided subacute bacterial endocarditis.
- Coagulase-⊖ *Staphylococcus* is the most common infecting organism in prosthetic valve endocarditis.
- *Streptococcus bovis* endocarditis is associated with coexisting GI malignancy.
- *Candida* and *Aspergillus* species account for most cases of fungal endocarditis. Predisposing factors include long-term indwelling IV catheters, malignancy, AIDS, organ transplantation, and IV drug use. Table 2.8-11 lists the causes of endocarditis.

HISTORY/PE

- Fever, chills, weakness, dyspnea, sweats, anorexia, skin lesions, IV drug use, FUO.
- Exam reveals **heart murmur.** Affects the mitral valve more than the aortic valve in non–IV drug users; more right-sided involvement is found in IV drug users (tricuspid valve > mitral valve > aortic valve).

TABLE 2.8-11. Causes of Endocarditis

ACUTE	SUBACUTE
S. aureus (IV drug abuse)	Viridans streptococci
S. pneumoniae	Enterococcus
N. gonorrhoeae	Staphylococcus epidermidis
	Fungi

MARANTIC	HACEK (CULTURE-NEGATIVE)	SLE
Cancer (poor prognosis). Mets seed valves; emboli can cause cerebral infarcts.	Haemophilus parainfluenzae	Libman-Sacks (autoantibody to valve)
	Actinobacillus	
	Cardiobacterium	
	Eikenella	
	Kingella	

Pregnant women should not change the cat's litterbox. First-trimester toxoplasmosis infection is less common and more severe. Third-trimester infection is more common and less severe.

Endocarditis: indications for surgery—

PUS RIVER

Prosthetic valve endocarditis (most cases)

Uncontrolled infection

Suppurative local complications with conduction abnormalities

Resection of mycotic aneurysm

Ineffective antimicrobial therapy (e.g., vs. fungi)

Valvular damage (significant)

Embolization (repeated systemic)

Refractory CHF (or sudden onset)

- **Osler's nodes** (small, tender nodules on the finger and toe pads) **Janeway lesions** (small, peripheral hemorrhages; see Figure 2.8-14), **splinter hemorrhages** (subungual petechiae; see Figure 2.8-15), **Roth's spots** (retinal hemorrhages), and other embolic phenomena are also seen.

DIAGNOSIS

- Diagnosis is guided by risk factors, clinical symptoms, and the **Duke criteria** (see Table 2.8-12).
- CBC with leukocytosis and left shift; ↑ **ESR** and CRP.

TREATMENT

Early empiric IV antibiotic treatment includes vancomycin or ceftriaxone + gentamicin. Acute valve replacement is sometimes necessary. See the mnemonic **PUS RIVER** for indications for surgery. Give antibiotic prophylaxis before dental work in patients with valvular disease.

Anthrax

Caused by the spore-forming gram-⊕ bacterium *Bacillus anthracis.* Its natural incidence is rare, but infection is an occupational hazard for veterinarians, farmers, and individuals who handle **animal wool, hair, hides,** or bone meal products. Also a biological weapon. *B. anthracis* can cause cutaneous (most common), inhalation (most deadly), or GI anthrax.

HISTORY/PE

- **Cutaneous:** Presents 1–7 days after skin exposure and penetration of spores. The lesion begins as a **pruritic papule** that enlarges to form an ulcer surrounded by a satellite bulbus/lesion with an edematous halo and a

The anthrax-associated pruritic papule forms an ulcer with an edematous halo and then a black eschar.

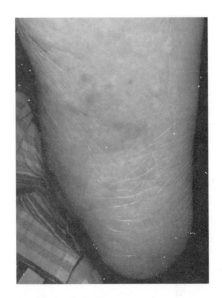

FIGURE 2.8-14.   Janeway lesions.

Peripheral embolization to the sole → a cluster of erythematous macules known as Janeway lesions. (Courtesy of the Department of Dermatology, Wilford Hall USAF Medical Center and Brooke Army Medical Center, San Antonio, TX.)

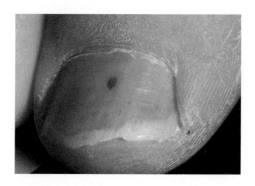

FIGURE 2.8-15. **Splinter hemorrhages.**

Note the splinter hemorrhages along the distal aspect of the nail plate, due to emboli from sub-acute bacterial endocarditis. (Courtesy of the Armed Forces Institute of Pathology, Bethesda, MD.)

round, regular, and raised edge. **Regional lymphadenopathy** is also characteristic. The lesion evolves into a **black eschar** within 7–10 days.

- **Inhalational:** Fever, dyspnea, hypoxia, hypotension, or symptoms of pneumonia (1–3 days after exposure). CXR may show a widened mediastinum.
- **GI:** Occurs after the ingestion of poorly cooked, contaminated meat; can present with dysphagia, nausea/vomiting, bloody diarrhea, and abdominal pain.

DIAGNOSIS

Aerobic culture and Gram stain of ulcer exudate show nonmotile short chains of bacilli. Antibody tests are also useful in confirming the diagnosis.

TREATMENT

Penicillin G, ciprofloxacin, erythromycin, tetracycline, or chloramphenicol × 7–10 days for cutaneous anthrax; high-dose penicillin for inhalational and GI anthrax. Postexposure prophylaxis (ciprofloxacin) to prevent inhalation anthrax should be continued for 60 days.

TABLE 2.8-12. **Duke Criteria for the Diagnosis of Endocarditis**

CRITERIA	COMPONENTS
Major	1. At least two separate ⊕ blood cultures for typical organism or persistent bacteremia with any organism.
	2. Evidence of endocardial involvement (via transesophageal echocardiography [TEE] or new murmur).
Minor	1. Predisposing risk factors.
	2. Fever ≥ 38.3°C.
	3. **Vascular phenomena:** Septic emboli, septic infarcts, mycotic aneurysm, Janeway lesions.
	4. **Immunologic phenomena:** Glomerulonephritis, Osler's nodes, Roth's spots.
	5. Microbiological evidence that does not meet major criteria.

Coccidioidomycosis

- A pulmonary fungal infection endemic to the **southwestern United States** (e.g., San Joaquin Valley, California). Can present as a flulike illness or as acute pneumonia and may involve extrapulmonary sites, including bone, CNS, and skin. The incubation period is 1–4 weeks after exposure.
- **Hx/PE:** Patients present with **fever,** anorexia, headache, chest pain, **cough,** dyspnea, arthralgias, and **night sweats.**
- **Dx:**
  - **Serology:** Precipitin antibodies (IgM) ↑ within two weeks and disappear after two months; complement fixation antibodies (IgG) ↑ at 1–3 months.
  - Culture of sputum, wound exudate, joint aspirate.
  - CXR findings may be normal or may show infiltrate(s), nodule(s), cavity, mediastinal or hilar adenopathy, or pleural effusion.
  - Consider bronchoscopy, fine-needle biopsy, open lung biopsy, or pleural biopsy.
- **Rx:** Amphotericin B for severe or protracted 1° pulmonary infection and disseminated disease. Itraconazole is an alternate treatment option.

Otitis media should not cause pain with movement of the tragus/pinna.

Otitis Externa

- An inflammation of the external auditory canal, also known as "swimmer's ear." *Pseudomonas* (from poorly chlorinated pools) and Enterobacteriaceae are the most common etiologic agents. Both grow in the presence of excess moisture.
- **Hx/PE:** Presents with pain, pruritus, and possible purulent discharge. Exam reveals pain with movement of the tragus/pinna (unlike otitis media) and an edematous and erythematous ear canal.
- **Dx:** A clinical diagnosis. Gram stain and culture are helpful if a fungal etiology is suspected. CT scan if the patient is toxic appearing.
- **Rx:** Eardrops with polymyxin B or neomycin. Use systemic antibiotics in patients with severe disease. Diabetics are at risk for malignant otitis externa and osteomyelitis of the skull base and thus require hospitalization and IV antibiotics.

Diabetics are at risk for malignant otitis externa.

Musculoskeletal

COMPARTMENT SYNDROME

- ↑ **pressure** within a confined space that compromises nerve, muscle, and soft tissue perfusion. Occurs primarily in the anterior compartment of the lower leg and forearm.
- **Hx/PE:** Pain out of proportion to physical findings; **pain with passive motion** of the fingers and toes; paresthesias, pallor, poikilothermia, pulselessness, and paralysis.
- **Dx:** Measure compartment pressures (usually ≥ 30 mmHg); measure delta pressures (diastolic pressure − compartment pressure).
- **Rx: Immediate fasciotomy** to ↓ pressures and ↑ tissue perfusion.

LOW BACK PAIN (LBP)

May arise from paraspinous muscles, ligaments, facet joints, disks, or nerve roots (see Table 2.9-1); typically resolves within four weeks. Prolonged bed rest is contraindicated. Risk factors for malignancy include age > 50, a previous history of cancer, pain not relieved by lying down, symptoms > 1 month, pain that worsens at night, and constitutional symptoms.

Herniated Disk

Causes include degenerative changes, trauma, or neck/back strain or sprain. Most common in the lumbar region, especially at **L4–L5** and **L5–S1.**

HISTORY/PE

- Sudden onset of severe, electricity-like LBP, usually preceded by several months of aching, "discogenic" pain.
- Common among middle-aged and older men.
- Exacerbated by straining (e.g., coughing).
- Associated with **sciatica,** paresthesias, muscle weakness, atrophy, contractions, or spasms.
- **Passive straight leg raise** ↑ **pain** (highly sensitive but not specific).
- Large midline herniations can cause **cauda equina syndrome.**

DIAGNOSIS

- Obtain a plain radiograph if other causes of back pain are suspected (e.g., infection, fracture).

TABLE 2.9-1. **Motor and Sensory Deficits in Back Pain**

| NERVE ROOT | ASSOCIATED DEFICIT | | |
	MOTOR	REFLEX	SENSORY
L4	Foot dorsiflexion (tibialis anterior).	Patellar	Medial aspect of the lower leg.
L5	Big toe dorsiflexion (extensor hallucis longus), foot eversion (peroneus muscles).	None	Dorsum of the foot and lateral aspect of the lower leg.
S1	Plantar flexion (gastrocnemius/soleus), gluteus maximus (hip extension).	Achilles	Plantar and lateral aspects of the foot.

- Order an MRI if symptoms are refractory to conservative management. May show disk herniation (see Figure 2.9-1).

TREATMENT

- NSAIDs, physical therapy, and local heat → resolution within four weeks.
- Severe or rapidly evolving neurologic deficits and cauda equina syndrome are indications for discectomy.

Spinal Stenosis

A narrowing of the lumbar or cervical spinal canal that can → compression of the nerve roots. Most commonly due to degenerative joint disease; typically occurs in middle-aged or elderly patients.

HISTORY/PE

- Neck pain; back pain that radiates to the buttocks and legs; leg numbness and weakness.
- Leg cramping is worse **at rest, with standing,** and **with walking (pseudo- or neurogenic claudication).**
- Symptoms **improve** with **flexion at the hips.**

DIAGNOSIS

- Radiographs show degenerative changes and a narrowed spinal canal.
- MRI or CT shows spinal stenosis.

TREATMENT

- **Mild to moderate:** NSAIDs and abdominal muscle strengthening.
- **Advanced:** Epidural steroid injections can provide relief.
- **Refractory:** Surgical laminectomy may achieve significant short-term success, but many patients will have a recurrence of symptoms.

Lung, breast, and prostate cancer can metastasize to vertebrae and cause back pain.

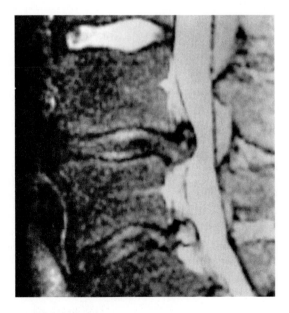

FIGURE 2.9-1.   Disk herniation.

MRI reveals herniations od L4–L5 and L5–S1 (arrows). (Reproduced, with permission, from Skinner HB. *Current Diagnosis & Treatment in Orthopedics,* 1st ed. Stamford, CT: Appleton & Lange, 1995:186.)

A chronic inflammatory disease of the spine and pelvis that causes sacroiliitis and, eventually, fusion of the affected joints. Strongly associated with **HLA-B27**. Risk factors include male gender and a ⊕ family history.

History/PE

- Typical onset is in the late teens and early 20s. Presents with intermittent hip pain and LBP that **worsen with inactivity and in the mornings** but improve with activity.
- ↓ spine flexion (⊕ Schober test), loss of lumbar lordosis, hip pain and stiffness, and ↓ chest expansion are seen as the disease progresses.
- Anterior **uveitis** and **third-degree heart block** may occur.
- Other seronegative spondyloarthropathies must be ruled out, including the following:
  - **Reactive arthritis (aka Reiter's syndrome):** A disease of young men. The characteristic arthritis, uveitis, conjunctivitis, and urethritis usually follow an infection with *Campylobacter, Shigella, Salmonella, Chlamydia,* or *Ureaplasma.*
  - **Psoriatic arthritis:** An oligoarthritis of the **DIP joints.** Associated with psoriatic skin changes and **sausage-shaped digits.**

Diagnosis

- ⊕ HLA-B27.
- Radiographs show **bamboo spine and fused sacroiliac joints.**
- ESR is often ↑.
- ⊖ **RF**; ⊖ ANA.

Treatment

- **NSAIDs** (e.g., indomethacin) for pain; exercise to improve posture and breathing.
- **Tumor necrosis factor (TNF) inhibitors** are used in refractory cases.

An **X-linked recessive disorder** resulting from a deficiency of **dystrophin,** a cytoskeletal protein. Onset is usually at 3–5 years of age.

History/PE

- Affects axial and proximal muscles more than distal muscles.
- May present with progressive **clumsiness, fatigability,** difficulty standing or walking, difficulty walking on toes (gastrocnemius shortening), **Gowers' maneuver** (using the hands to push off the thighs when rising from the floor), and waddling gait.
- **Pseudohypertrophy of the gastrocnemius muscles** is also seen.
- Mental retardation is common.
- Table 2.9-2 outlines the differential diagnosis of DMD and Becker muscular dystrophy.

Diagnosis

- ⊖ **dystrophin** immunostain; ↑ CK.
- EMG shows polyphasic potentials and ↑ recruitment.

TABLE 2.9-2. **DMD vs. Becker Muscular Dystrophy**

	DMD	BECKER MUSCULAR DYSTROPHY
Onset	3–5 years.	5–15 years and beyond.
Life expectancy	Teens.	30s–40s.
Mental retardation	Common.	Uncommon.
Western blot	Dystrophin is markedly ↓ or absent.	Dystrophin levels are normal, but protein is abnormal.

- Dystrophin mutation is sometimes seen.
- **Muscle biopsy** shows degeneration and variation in fiber size with fibrosis.

TREATMENT

- Physical therapy is necessary to maintain ambulation and to prevent contractures.
- Perform Achilles tendon release if necessary.

FIBROMYALGIA

- A connective tissue disorder characterized by myalgias, weakness, and fatigability. Inflammation is notably absent.
- Hx/PE: Most common in **women 30–50 years of age;** associated with depression, anxiety, sleep disorders, and IBS.
- Dx: Multiple (≥ 11 of 18), diffuse tender points are seen (see Figure 2.9-2). The presence of < 11 of 18 tender points or non-fibromyalgia-associated tender points is known as **myofascial pain syndrome.**
- Rx: **Antidepressants**, stretching, heat application, hydrotherapy, transcutaneous electrical nerve stimulation (TENS).

GOUT

Recurrent attacks of **acute monoarticular arthritis** resulting from intra-articular deposition of **monosodium urate crystals.** Risk factors include male gender, obesity, and Pacific Islander heritage.

HISTORY/PE

- Presents with excruciating joint pain of sudden onset that awakens the patient from sleep.
- Most commonly affects the **first MTP joint** (podagra) and the midfoot, knees, ankles, and wrists; the hips and shoulders are generally spared.
- Joints are erythematous, swollen, and exquisitely tender.
- **Tophi** (urate crystals deposits → deformed joints) may be seen with chronic disease.

DIAGNOSIS

- Joint fluid aspirate shows **needle-shaped, negatively birefringent crystals** (see Table 2.9-3 and Clinical Images).
- Elevated WBC count during flares may be seen.

Gout crystals appear yeLLow when paraLLel to the condenser.

Colchicine inhibits chemotaxis and is most effective when used early, during a gout flare.

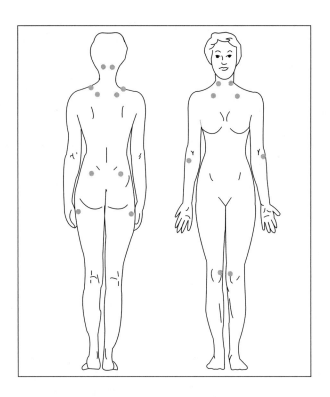

FIGURE 2.9-2. Tender points characteristic of fibromyalgia.

(From the brochure "Fibromyalgia," Arthritis Information, Advice and Guidance, Disease Series. Reprinted with permission of the Arthritis Foundation.)

Causes of hyperuricemia:

↑ cell turnover (hemolysis, blast crisis, tumor lysis)
Cyclosporine
Diabetes insipidus
Diet (e.g., ↑ red meat, alcohol)
Diuretics
Lead poisoning
Lesch-Nyhan syndrome
Salicylates

- Serum uric acid is usually ↑ (≥ 7.5), but some patients have normal levels.
- Punched-out erosions with overhanging cortical bone ("**rat-bite**" **erosions**) are seen in advanced gout.

TREATMENT

- **Acute attacks:** High-dose **NSAIDs** (e.g., indomethacin), colchicine, and/or **steroids.**
- Weight loss and avoidance of triggers of hyperuricemia will prevent recurrent attacks in many patients.
- **Maintenance therapy: Allopurinol** for overproducers and refractory cases; **probenecid** for undersecretors.

TABLE 2.9-3. Gout vs. Pseudogout

DISORDER	CRYSTAL SHAPE	CRYSTAL BIREFRINGENCE
Gout	Needle shaped	⊖
Pseudogout	Rhomboid	⊕

- A chronic, noninflammatory arthritis of movable joints (e.g., **DIP** joints). Characterized by deterioration of the articular cartilage and osteophyte formation at joint surfaces.
- Risk factors include a ⊕ family history, **obesity**, and a **history of joint trauma.**
- Hx/PE: **Crepitus;** ↓ range of motion (ROM); **pain that worsens with activity and weight bearing but improves with rest.**
- Dx:
  - Radiographs show **joint space narrowing,** osteophytes, subchondral sclerosis, and subchondral bone cysts.
  - Synovial fluid shows straw-colored fluid, normal viscosity, and a WBC count < 3000 cells/μL.
- Rx: Physical therapy, **weight reduction, NSAIDs.** Intra-articular corticosteroid injections may provide temporary relief. **Consider joint replacement** (e.g., total hip/knee arthroplasty) in advanced cases.

POLYMYOSITIS AND DERMATOMYOSITIS

Polymyositis is a progressive, systemic connective tissue disease characterized by striated muscle inflammation. **Dermatomyositis** presents with symptoms of polymyositis plus cutaneous involvement, although the pathogenesis is different. Most often affect patients 50–70 years of age; the male-to-female ratio is 1:2. African-Americans are affected more often than Caucasians.

HISTORY/PE

- Distinguished as follows:
  - **Polymyositis:** Presents with **symmetric,** progressive **proximal** muscle weakness; pain; and difficulty breathing or swallowing (advanced disease).
  - **Dermatomyositis:** Patients may have **heliotrope rash** (a violaceous periorbital rash), **"shawl sign"** (a rash involving the shoulders, upper chest, and back), and/or **Gottron's papules** (a papular rash with scales located on the dorsa of the hands, over bony prominences).
- Patients may also develop myocarditis, cardiac conduction deficits, or malignancy.

DIAGNOSIS

- ↑ serum CK, aldolase, and **CPK.**
- **EMG** shows fibrillations.
- **Muscle biopsy** reveals inflammation and muscle fibers in varying stages of necrosis and regeneration.

TREATMENT

- High-dose corticosteroids with taper after 4–6 weeks to ↓ the maintenance dose.
- Azathioprine and/or methotrexate can be used as an adjunct.

RHEUMATOID ARTHRITIS (RA)

A chronic, destructive, systemic inflammatory arthritis characterized by **symmetric** involvement of both large and small joints that → synovial hypertrophy and pannus formation → erosion of adjacent cartilage, bone, and tendons. Risk factors include female gender, age 35–50, and **HLA-DR4.**

HISTORY/PE

- **Insidious onset of morning stiffness** for > 1 hour along with painful, warm swelling of multiple symmetric joints (**wrists, MCP** and **PIP joints,** ankles, knees, shoulders, hips, elbows, and cervical spine) for > 6 weeks.
- Fever, fatigue, malaise, anorexia, and weight loss may also be seen.
- Ulnar deviation of the fingers is seen with MCP joint hypertrophy (see Figure 2.9-3).
- Also presents with ligament and tendon deformations (e.g., swan-neck and boutonnière deformities), **Baker's cysts,** vasculitis, atlantoaxial subluxation, carpal tunnel syndrome, and Felty's syndrome.

DIAGNOSIS

- **Labs:**
    - ↑ **RF** (anti-Fc IgG antibody) in > 75% of cases.
    - ↑ ESR may also be seen.
- Synovial fluid aspirate shows turbid fluid, ↓ viscosity, and an ↑ WBC count (3000–50,000 cells/µL).
- **Radiographs:**
    - **Early:** Soft tissue swelling and juxta-articular demineralization.
    - **Late:** Joint space narrowing and erosions.

TREATMENT

- **NSAIDs.**
- **Disease-modifying antirheumatic drugs (DMARDs)** should be started early. First-line drugs are methotrexate, hydroxychloroquine, and TNF inhibitors. Second-line agents include penicillamine and cyclosporine.

JUVENILE RHEUMATOID ARTHRITIS (JRA)

A nonmigratory, nonsuppurative mono- and polyarthropathy with bony destruction that occurs in patients ≤ 16 years of age and lasts > 6 weeks. Approximately 95% of cases resolve by puberty.

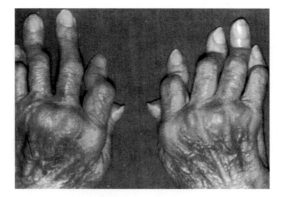

FIGURE 2.9-3.   Rheumatoid arthritis.

Note the boutonnière deformities of the digits, ulnar deviation of the fingers, MCP joint hypertrophy, and severe involvement of the PIP joints. (Reproduced, with permission, from Chandrasoma P. *Concise Pathology*, 3rd ed. Stamford, CT: Appleton & Lange, 1998:978.)

HISTORY/PE

- Can be accompanied by **fever, nodules, erythematous rashes, pericarditis,** and **fatigue.**
- Subtypes are as follows:
    - **Pauciarticular:** An asymmetric arthritis that involves weight-bearing joints. Associated with an ↑ risk of **iridocyclitis** that → blindness if left untreated.
    - **Polyarticular:** Resembles RA with symmetric involvement of multiple (≥ 5) small joints. Systemic features are less prominent; carries a ↓ risk of iridocyclitis.
    - **Acute febrile:** The least common subtype; manifests as arthritis with **daily high, spiking fevers** and an **evanescent, salmon-colored rash.** Hepatosplenomegaly and serositis may also be seen. No iridocyclitis is present; remission occurs within one year.

DIAGNOSIS

- There is **no diagnostic test for JRA.**
- **Labs:**
    - ⊕ RF in 15% of cases.
    - ANA may be ⊕, especially in the pauciarticular subtype.
    - ↑ ESR, WBC count, and platelets.
- **Imaging:** Soft tissue swelling and osteoporosis may be seen.

TREATMENT

- **NSAIDs** or corticosteroids; methotrexate is second-line therapy.
- ROM and strengthening exercises.

SCLERODERMA

Also called systemic sclerosis; characterized by excessive deposition of collagen. Commonly manifests as **CREST syndrome** but can also occur in a diffuse form. Risk factors include female gender and age 35–50.

HISTORY/PE

- Exam may reveal symmetric thickening of the skin of face and/or distal extremities.
- **CREST syndrome** involves Calcinosis, Raynaud's phenomenon, Esophageal dysmotility, Sclerodactyly, and Telangiectasias.
- The diffuse form can → **pulmonary fibrosis,** cor pulmonale, acute renal failure, and malignant hypertension.

DIAGNOSIS

- RF and ANA may be ⊕.
- **Anticentromere antibodies** are specific for CREST syndrome.
- **Anti-Scl-70** (antitopoisomerase 1) **antibodies** are associated with a poor prognosis.
- Eosinophilia may be seen.

TREATMENT

- Steroids for acute flares; penicillamine can be used for skin changes.
- Calcium channel blockers for Raynaud's.
- ACEIs for renal disease and malignant hypertension.

> **CREST** *syndrome*
>
> **C**alcinosis
> **R**aynaud's phenomenon
> **E**sophageal dysmotility
> **S**clerodactyly
> **T**elangiectasias

HIGH-YIELD FACTS

MUSCULOSKELETAL

205

Discoid rash
Oral ulcers
Photosensitivity
Arthritis
Malar rash
Immunologic criteria
Neurologic symptoms
   (lupus cerebritis,
   seizures)
Elevated ESR
Renal disease
ANA +
Serositis
Hematologic
   abnormalities

Drugs that can cause a lupus syndrome:

Chlorpromazine
Hydralazine
INH
Methyldopa
Penicillamine
Procainamide
Quinidine

SYSTEMIC LUPUS ERYTHEMATOSUS (SLE)

A multisystem autoimmune disorder related to antibody-mediated cellular attack and deposition of antigen-antibody complexes. African-American women are at highest risk.

HISTORY/PE

- Presents with nonspecific symptoms such as fever, anorexia, weight loss, and symmetric joint pain.
- The mnemonic **DOPAMINE RASH** summarizes the criteria for diagnosing SLE (see also Figure 2.9-4 and Clinical Images). Patients with four of the criteria are likely to have SLE.

DIAGNOSIS

- A ⊕ ANA is highly sensitive.
- **Anti-dsDNA** and **anti-Sm antibodies** are highly specific but not as sensitive.
- **Drug-induced SLE:** ⊕ antihistone antibodies are seen **in 100% of cases** but are nonspecific.
- **Neonatal SLE:** ⊕ anti-Ro antibodies.
- The following may also be seen:
  - Antiphospholipid antibodies.
  - Anemia, leukopenia, and/or thrombocytopenia.
  - Proteinuria and/or casts.

TREATMENT

- Treat with **NSAIDs** for mild joint symptoms.
- **Steroids** for **acute exacerbations.**
- Steroids, hydroxychloroquine, cyclophosphamide, and azathioprine for progressive or refractory cases.

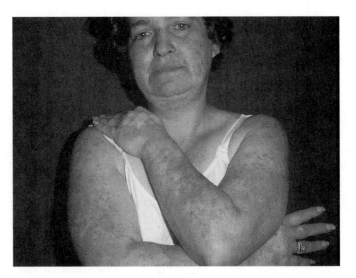

FIGURE 2.9-4. Systemic lupus erythematosus.

Erythematous patches and plaques of SLE, predominantly in sun-exposed areas. Note the malar rash across the bridge of the nose. (Reproduced, with permission, from Hurwitz RM. *Pathology of the Skin: Atlas of Clinical-Pathological Correlation*, 2nd ed. Stamford, CT: Appleton & Lange, 1998:39.)

TEMPORAL ARTERITIS (TA)

Also called giant cell arteritis; due to subacute granulomatous inflammation of the large vessels, including the aorta, external carotid (especially the **temporal** branch), and vertebral arteries. The most feared manifestation is **blindness** 2° to occlusion of the **central retinal artery** (a branch of the internal carotid artery). Risk factors include polymyalgia rheumatica (affects almost half of TA patients), age > 50, and female gender.

HISTORY/PE

- New headache (unilateral or bilateral); scalp pain and **temporal tenderness; jaw claudication.**
- Fever; transient or permanent **monocular blindness;** weight loss; myalgias/arthralgias (especially of the shoulders and hips).

DIAGNOSIS

- **ESR** > 50 (usually > 100).
- Ophthalmologic evaluation.
- **Temporal artery biopsy:** Look for thrombosis; necrosis of the media; and lymphocytes, plasma cells, and giant cells.

TREATMENT

High-dose prednisone for 1–2 months before tapering. Obtain a biopsy, but do not delay treatment; follow-up eye exam.

POLYMYALGIA RHEUMATICA

- Risk factors include female gender and age > 50.
- Hx/PE:
    - **Pain and stiffness of the shoulder and pelvic girdle** areas with difficulty getting out of a chair or lifting the arms above the head.
    - Other symptoms include **fever,** malaise, and weight loss. Weakness is generally not appreciated on exam.
- Dx: Markedly ↑ ESR, often associated with anemia.
- Rx: **Low-dose prednisone** (10–20 mg/day).

COMMON ADULT ORTHOPEDIC INJURIES

Table 2.9-4 outlines the presentation and treatment of orthopedic injuries that commonly affect adults.

COMMON PEDIATRIC ORTHOPEDIC INJURIES

Table 2.9-5 outlines the presentation and treatment of common pediatric orthopedic injuries.

DEVELOPMENTAL DYSPLASIA OF THE HIP

Also called congenital hip dislocation; can result in subluxed, dislocatable, or dislocated femoral heads. Dislocations result from poor development of the acetabulum and hip due to lax musculature and **excessive uterine packing** in

TABLE 2.9-4. Common Adult Orthopedic Injuries

INJURY	MECHANICS	TREATMENT
Shoulder dislocation	**Anterior dislocation:** Most common; the axillary artery and nerve are at risk. Patients hold the arm in external rotation. **Posterior dislocation:** Associated with seizure and electrocutions; can injure the radial artery. Patients hold the arm in internal rotation.	Reduction followed by a sling and swath. Recurrent dislocations may need surgical repair.
Hip dislocation	**Posterior dislocation:** Most common; occurs via a posteriorly directed force on an internally rotated, flexed, adducted hip ("dashboard injury"). Associated with a risk of sciatic nerve injury and avascular necrosis (AVN). **Anterior dislocation:** Can injure the obturator nerve.	Closed reduction followed by abduction pillow/bracing. Evaluate with CT scan after reduction.
Colles' fracture	Involves the distal radius. Often results from a fall onto an outstretched hand → a dorsally displaced, dorsally angulated fracture. Commonly seen in the elderly (osteoporosis) and children.	Closed reduction followed by application of a long-arm cast; open reduction if the fracture is intra-articular.
Scaphoid (carpal navicular) fracture	The **most commonly fractured carpal bone.** May take two weeks for radiographs to show the fracture. Assume a fracture if there is tenderness in the anatomical snuff box.	Thumb spica cast. If displacement or navicular nonunion is present, treat with open reduction. With proximal third scaphoid fractures, AVN may result from disruption of blood flow.
Boxer's fracture	Fracture of the fifth metacarpal neck. Due to forward trauma of a closed fist (e.g., punching a wall).	Closed reduction and ulnar gutter splint; percutaneous pinning if the fracture is excessively angulated. If skin is broken, assume infection by human oral pathogens → surgical irrigation, debridement, and IV antibiotics (covering *Eikenella*).
Humerus fracture	Direct trauma. May have radial nerve palsy → wrist drop and loss of thumb abduction (see Figure 2.9-5).	Hanging-arm cast vs. coaptation splint and sling. Functional bracing.
"Nightstick fracture"	Ulnar shaft fracture resulting from self-defense with the arm against a blunt object.	Open reduction and internal fixation (ORIF) if significantly displaced.
Monteggia's fracture	Diaphyseal fracture of the proximal ulna with subluxation of the radial head.	ORIF of the shaft fracture (due to poor fracture diaphyseal blood supply) and closed reduction of the radial head.
Galeazzi's fracture	Diaphyseal fracture of the radius with dislocation of the distal radioulnar joint. Results from a direct blow to the radius.	ORIF of the radius and casting of the fracture forearm in supination to reduce the distal radioulnar joint.

HIGH-YIELD FACTS

MUSCULOSKELETAL

TABLE 2.9-4. **Common Adult Orthopedic Injuries** (continued)

INJURY	MECHANICS	TREATMENT
Hip fracture	↑ risk with osteoporosis. Presents with a shortened and externally rotated leg. **Displaced femoral neck fractures:** Associated with an ↑ risk of AVN, nonunion, and DVTs.	ORIF with parallel pinning of the femoral neck. Displaced fractures in elderly patients may require a hip hemiarthroplasty. Anticoagulate to ↓ the likelihood of DVTs.
Femoral fracture	Direct trauma. Beware of fat emboli, which present with fever, change in mental status, dyspnea, hypoxia, petechiae, and ↓ platelets.	Intramedullary nailing of the femur. Irrigate and debride open fractures.
Tibial fracture	Direct trauma. Watch for compartment syndrome.	Casting vs. intramedullary nailing.
Open fractures	An orthopedic emergency; patients must be taken to the OR in < 6 hours owing to ↑ infection risk.	OR emergently to repair fracture. Treat with antibiotics.
Achilles tendon rupture	Presents with a sudden "pop" like a rifle shot. More likely with ↓ physical conditioning. Exam shows limited plantar flexion and a ⊕ Thompson's test (pressure on the gastrocnemius → absent foot plantar flexion).	Treat surgically followed by long leg cast for six weeks.
Knee injuries	Present with knee instability, edema, and hematoma. **ACL:** ■ Results from forced hyperflexion or impact to an extended knee. ■ ⊕ anterior drawer and Lachman's tests. ■ Rule out a meniscal or MCL injury. **PCL:** ■ Results from forced hyperextension. ■ ⊕ posterior drawer test. **Meniscal tears:** ■ Clicking or locking may be present. ■ Exam shows joint line tenderness and a ⊕ McMurray's test.	Treatment of MCL/LCL and meniscal tears is usually conservative. Treatment of ACL injuries is generally surgical with graft from the patellar or hamstring tendons. Operative PCL repair is reserved for highly competitive athletes.

the flexed and adducted position (e.g., breech presentation) → excessive stretching of the posterior hip capsule and adductor muscle contracture.

HISTORY/PE

■ Most commonly found in **first-born females** born in the **breech position.**
■ **Barlow's maneuver:** Pressure is placed on the inner aspect of the abducted thigh, and the hip is then adducted → posterior dislocation.
■ **Ortolani's maneuver:** The thighs are gently abducted from the midline with anterior pressure on the greater trochanter. A **soft click** signifies reduction of the femoral head into the acetabulum.

TABLE 2.9-5.   Orthopedic Injuries in Children

INJURY	MECHANICS	TREATMENT
Clavicular	The most commonly fractured long bone in children. May be birth related (especially in large infants) and can be associated with brachial nerve palsies. Usually involve the middle third of the clavicle, with the proximal fracture end displaced superiorly owing to the pull of the sternocleidomastoid.	Figure-of-eight sling vs. arm sling.
Greenstick fracture	Incomplete fracture involving the cortex of only one side of the bone.	Reduction with casting. Order films at 10–14 days.
Nursemaid's elbow	Radial head subluxation that typically occurs as a result of being pulled or lifted by the hand. Presents with pain and refusal to bend the elbow.	Manual reduction by gentle supination of the elbow at 90 degrees of flexion. No immobilization.
Torus fracture	Buckling of the cortex of a long bone 2° to trauma. Usually occurs in the distal radius or ulna.	Cast immobilization for 3–5 weeks.
Supracondylar humerus fractures	Tends to occur at 5–8 years of age. Proximity to the brachial artery ↑ the risk of Volkmann's contracture (results from compartment syndrome of the forearm).	Cast immobilization; closed reduction with percutaneous pinning if significantly displaced.
Osgood-Schlatter disease	Overuse apophysitis of the tibial tubercle. Causes localized pain, especially with quadriceps contraction, in active young boys.	↓ activity for 1–2 years. A neoprene brace may provide symptomatic relief.
Salter-Harris fractures 	Fractures of the growth plate in children. Classified by fracture location: ■ I: Physis (growth plate). ■ II: Metaphysis and physis. ■ III: Epiphysis and physis. ■ IV: Epiphysis, metaphysis, and physis. ■ V: Crush injury of the physis.	**Types I and II:** Conservative. **Types III–V:** Surgical repair to prevent complications such as leg length inequality.

■ **Allis' (Galeazzi's) sign:** The knees are at unequal heights when the hips and knees are flexed (the dislocated side is lower).
■ **Asymmetric skin folds** and limited abduction of the affected hip.

DIAGNOSIS

■ **Early detection is critical** to allow for proper hip development.
■ Ultrasound may be helpful, especially after 10 weeks of age.

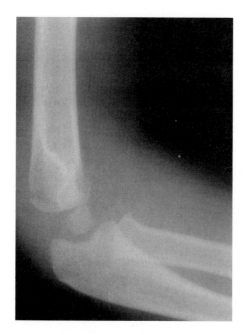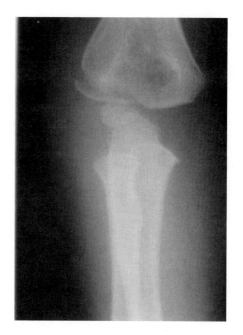

FIGURE 2.9-5. **Lateral condyle fracture of the humerus.**

(Reproduced, with permission, from Skinner HB. *Current Diagnosis & Treatment in Orthopedics*, 2nd ed. Stamford, CT: Appleton & Lange, 2000:572.)

- Radiographs are unreliable until patients are > 4 months of age because of the radiolucency of the neonatal femoral head.

TREATMENT

Begin treatment early.

- **< 6 months:** Splint with a **Pavlik harness** (maintains hip flexed and abducted).
- **6–15 months:** Spica cast.
- **15–24 months:** Open reduction.

COMPLICATIONS

- Joint contractures and AVN of the femoral head.
- Without treatment, a significant defect is likely in patients < 2 years of age.

LIMP

One of the most common musculoskeletal disorders of childhood. There are multiple etiologies, but trauma remains the most common cause.

HISTORY/PE

- Presents with abnormal gait (e.g., Trendelenburg, antalgic gaits) and pain.
- **Trauma-associated limp:** Characterized by point tenderness.
- **Infection:** Consider septic joint, osteomyelitis, toxic synovitis, or infection acquired during contact with TB-⊕ patients. Presents with fever, erythema, edema, and limited ROM.
- Look for neurologic involvement (e.g., reflexes, muscle atrophy, changes in sensation, bowel and bladder function).

> **Differential diagnosis of limp—**
>
> **STARTSS HOTT**
>
> **S**eptic joint
> **T**umor
> **A**vascular necrosis
>   (Legg-Calvé-Perthes)
> **R**heumatoid
>   arthritis/JRA
> **T**uberculosis
> **S**ickle cell disease
> **S**CFE
> **H**enoch-Schönlein
>   purpura
> **O**steomyelitis
> **T**rauma
> **T**oxic synovitis

- Young children and toddlers are more likely to have an infected joint.
- Adolescents are more likely to develop JRA, slipped capital femoral epiphyses (SCFEs), and Legg-Calvé-Perthes disease.
- The **STARTSS HOTT** mnemonic summarizes the differential for limp.

DIAGNOSIS

- Obtain a thorough H&P.
- Radiograph the affected joint as well as the joint above and that below.
- CBC, ESR, and CRP may reveal inflammation.
- Additional tests include bone scan, nerve conduction studies, and joint aspiration and culture.

TREATMENT

Depends on the etiology. Immediate treatment for emergent causes (e.g., septic joint).

Legg-Calvé-Perthes Disease

AVN of the femoral head of unknown etiology (see Figure 2.9-6). Most commonly found in boys 4–10 years of age. Usually a self-limited disease, with symptoms lasting < 18 months.

HISTORY/PE

- Usually asymptomatic at first, but patients can develop a painless limp.
- If pain is present, it can be referred to the knee.

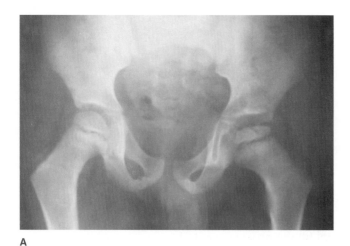
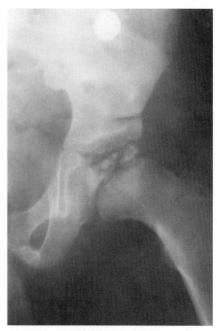

A   B

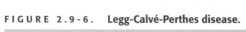

FIGURE 2.9-6. Legg-Calvé-Perthes disease.

AVN of the femoral head. (Reproduced, with permission, from Skinner HB. *Current Diagnosis & Treatment in Orthopedics*, 2nd ed. Stamford, CT: Appleton & Lange, 2000:543.)

- **Limited abduction and internal rotation;** atrophy of the affected leg.
- Usually unilateral.

TREATMENT

- **Observation** if there is limited femoral head involvement or if full ROM is present.
- If extensive or if there is ↓ ROM, consider bracing, hip abduction with a Petrie cast, or an osteotomy.
- The prognosis is good if the patient is < 5 years of age and has full ROM, ↓ femoral head involvement, and a stable joint.

Slipped Capital Femoral Epiphysis (SCFE)

Separation of the proximal femoral epiphysis through the growth plate → medial and posterior displacement of the femoral head (relative to the femoral neck). May be due to an imbalance between growth hormone and sex hormones. Risk factors include obesity, age 11–13, male gender, and African-American ethnicity. Associated with hypothyroidism and other endocrinopathies.

HISTORY/PE

- Typically presents with acute or insidious **thigh** or **knee pain** and a **painful limp.**
- Acute cases present with restricted ROM and, commonly, **inability to bear weight.**
- Bilateral in 30% of cases.
- Limited internal rotation and abduction of the hip. Flexion of the hip → an obligatory external rotation 2° to physical displacement.

DIAGNOSIS

- Radiographs of **both** hips in **AP and frog-leg lateral views** reveal **posterior and medial displacement** of the femoral head (see Figure 2.9-7).
- Rule out hypothyroidism with TSH.

TREATMENT

- The disease is progressive, so treatment should begin promptly.
- **No weight bearing** should be allowed until the defect is surgically stabilized.
- **Gentle closed reduction** only in acute slips.

COMPLICATIONS

Chondrolysis, AVN of the femoral head, and premature hip osteoarthritis → hip arthroplasty.

OSTEOSARCOMA

The second most common 1° malignant tumor of bone (after multiple myeloma). Tends to occur in the **metaphyseal** regions of the **distal femur, proximal tibia,** and proximal humerus; often metastasizes to the lungs. Some cases are preceded by Paget's disease. Risk factors include male gender and age 20–30.

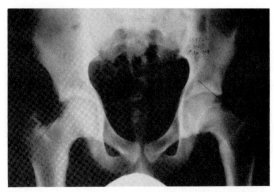

A

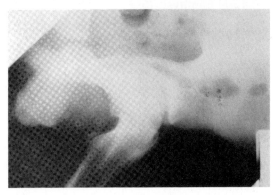

B

FIGURE 2.9-7. **Slipped capital femoral epiphysis.**

(A) AP x-ray. The medial displacement of the left femoral epiphysis is best seen with a line drawn up the lateral femoral neck. The abnormal epiphysis does not protrude beyond this line. (B) Frog-leg lateral x-ray. Posterior displacement of the femoral epiphysis is characteristic. (Reproduced, with permission, from Skinner HB. *Current Diagnosis & Treatment in Orthopedics*, 2nd ed. Stamford, CT: Appleton & Lange, 2000:546.)

HISTORY/PE

- Progressive and eventually intractable **pain that is worse at night.**
- Constitutional symptoms such as fever, weight loss, and night sweats may be present.
- Erythema and enlargement over the site of the tumor may be seen.

DIAGNOSIS

- Radiographs show **Codman's triangle** (periosteal new bone formation at the diaphyseal end of the lesion) or **"sunburst pattern"** of the osteosarcoma (see Figure 2.9-8)—in contrast to multilayered **"onion skinning,"** which is classic for Ewing's sarcoma.
- MRI and CT for staging (soft tissue and bony invasion) and to plan for surgery.

TREATMENT

- Limb-sparing surgical procedures and pre- and postoperative chemotherapy (e.g., methotrexate, doxorubicin, cisplatin, ifosfamide).
- Amputation may be necessary.

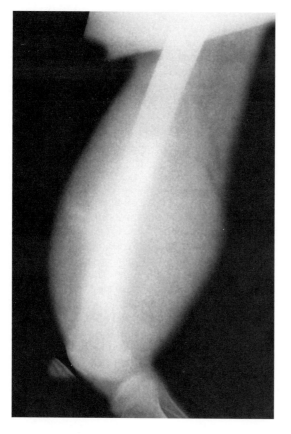

FIGURE 2.9-8. **Osteosarcoma.**

"Sunburst" appearance of neoplastic bone formation in the femur of a 15-year-old girl. Amputation was required owing to the size of the tumor. (Reproduced, with permission, from Skinner HB. *Current Diagnosis & Treatment in Orthopedics*, 2nd ed. Stamford, CT: Appleton & Lange, 2000:272.)

Neurology

Stroke

Acute onset of focal neurologic deficits resulting from disruption of cerebral circulation. **Nonmodifiable risk factors** include **age, male** gender, genetics, and ethnicity (African-American, Hispanic, Asian). **Modifiable risk factors** include **hypertension, diabetes mellitus, obesity, smoking, hypercholesterolemia,** carotid stenosis, heavy alcohol intake, cocaine use, IV drug use, and **atrial fibrillation (AF).** Etiologies are as follows:

- Atherosclerosis of the extracranial vessels (internal/common carotid, basilar, vertebral arteries).
- Lacunar infarcts in regions supplied by perforating vessels (result from hypertension, atherosclerosis, or diabetes).
- **Cardiac:** Emboli from mural thrombi, diseased or prosthetic valves, arrhythmias, endocarditis.
- **Fibromuscular dysplasia** (young females), inflammatory diseases, arterial dissection, migraine, venous thrombosis.
- **Hypercoagulable states:** Malignancy, pregnancy, venous stasis.

HISTORY/PE

Symptoms are dependent on the vascular territory affected:

- **Middle cerebral artery (MCA):** Aphasia (dominant hemisphere), neglect (nondominant hemisphere), contralateral hemiparesis, gaze preference, homonymous hemianopsia.
- **Anterior cerebral artery (ACA):** Leg paresis, amnesia, personality changes, foot drop, gait dysfunction, cognitive changes.
- **Posterior cerebral artery (PCA):** Homonymous hemianopsia, memory deficits, dyslexia/alexia.
- **Basilar artery:** Coma, "locked-in" syndrome, cranial nerve palsies, apnea, visual symptoms, drop attacks, dysphagia.
- **Lacunar stroke:** Pure motor or sensory stroke, dysarthria–clumsy hand syndrome, ataxic hemiparesis.
- **TIA:** A transient neurologic deficit that lasts < 24 hours (most last < 1 hour).

DIAGNOSIS

- **CT without contrast:** To differentiate ischemic from hemorrhagic stroke (see Figure 2.10-1).
- **MRI:** To identify early ischemic changes (e.g., diffusion-weighted MRI is specific for acute stroke).
- ECG and an echocardiogram if embolic stroke is suspected.
- **Vascular studies:** For extracranial disease (carotid ultrasound, MRA, or traditional angiography) and for intracranial disease (transcranial Doppler or MRA) (see Figure 2.10-2A).
- **Screen for hypercoagulable states** with a history of bleeding, first stroke, or patients < 50 years of age.

TREATMENT

- **Acute:**
  - Monitor for signs and symptoms of brain swelling, ↑ ICP, and herniation.
  - For ischemic stroke, **tPA** is indicated if administered within **three hours** of symptom onset. Patients must first be screened for contraindications.

Contraindications to tPA therapy:

- Systolic BP > 185 or diastolic BP > 110
- Prior intracranial hemorrhage
- Stroke or head trauma within the last three months
- Recent MI
- Current anticoagulation with INR > 1.7 or prolonged PTT
- A platelet count < 100,000/mm³
- Major surgery in the past 14 days
- GI or urinary bleeding in the past 21 days
- Seizures present at the onset of stroke
- Blood glucose < 50 or > 400 mg/dL
- Age < 18

A

B

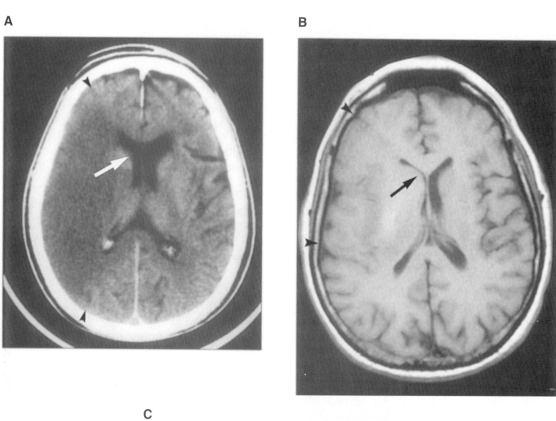

C

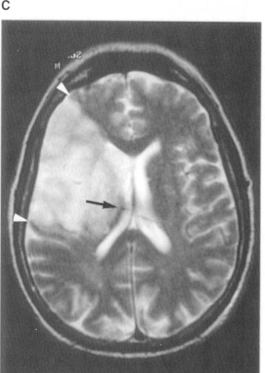

FIGURE 2.10-1. **CT-MRI findings in ischemic stroke in the right MCA territory.**

(A) CT shows low density and effacement of cortical sulci (between arrowheads) and compression of the anterior horn of the lateral ventricle (arrow). (B) T1-weighted MRI shows loss of sulcal markings (between arrowheads) and compression of the anterior horn of the lateral ventricle (arrow). (C) T2-weighted MRI scan shows increased signal intensity (between arrowheads) and ventricular compression (arrow). (Reproduced, with permission, from Aminoff MJ. *Clinical Neurology*, 3rd ed. Stamford, CT: Appleton & Lange, 1996:275.)

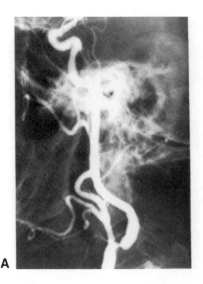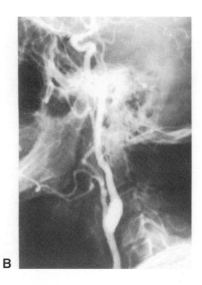

FIGURE 2.10-2. Pre- and postendarterectomy.

(A) Cartoid arteriogram showing stenosis of the proximal internal carotid artery. (B) Postoperative arteriogram with restoration of the normal luminal size following endarterectomy. (Reproduced, with permission, from Way LW. *Current Surgical Diagnosis & Treatment*, 10th ed. Stamford, CT: Appleton & Lange, 1994: 763.)

- **ASA:** Associated with ↓ morbidity and mortality in acute ischemic stroke presenting ≤ 48 hours from onset.
- **Prevent hypotension and hypoxemia.** Maintain systolic BP at 20 mmHg above the patient's normal BP.
- Treat poststroke complications (aspiration pneumonia, UTI, DVT).
- **Prevention and long-term treatment:**
  - **ASA, clopidogrel:** If stroke is 2° to small vessel disease or thrombosis or if anticoagulation is contraindicated.
  - **Carotid endarterectomy:** If stenosis is > 70% in symptomatic patients or > 60% in asymptomatic patients (contraindicated in 100% occlusion).
  - **Anticoagulation:** In cases of emboli, new AF, or hypercoagulable states (target INR = 2–3).
  - **Management of hypertension, hypercholesterolemia,** and **diabetes** (hypertension is the single biggest risk factor for stroke).

Subarachnoid Hemorrhage (SAH)

Etiologies include **trauma,** aneurysms, AVM, or trauma to the circle of Willis (often at the MCA).

HISTORY/PE

Acute-onset, intensely painful headache, often with **neck stiffness** and other signs of meningeal irritation, as well as fever, nausea/vomiting, and a fluctuating level of consciousness.

DIAGNOSIS

- Immediate head **CT without contrast** (see Figure 2.10-3) to look for blood in the subarachnoid space.
- Immediate **LP if CT is** ⊖ to look for RBCs, xanthochromia (yellowish CSF due to breakdown of RBCs), and ↑ ICP.

SAH will give the patient the "the worst headache of my life."

CN III palsy with pupil involvement is associated with berry aneurysms.

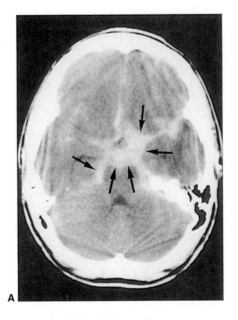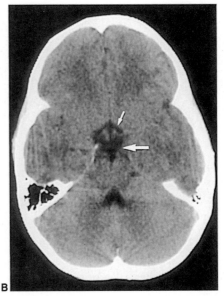

FIGURE 2.10-3. Subarachnoid hemorrhage.

(A) CT scan without contrast reveals blood in the subarachnoid space at the base of the brain (arrows). (B) A normal CT scan without contrast shows no density in this region (arrows). (Reproduced, with permission, from Aminoff MJ. *Clinical Neurology*, 3rd ed. Stamford, CT: Appleton & Lange, 1996:78.)

The three most common cerebral aneurysms are ACA (30%), PCA (25%), and MCA (20%).

- **Four-vessel angiography** should be performed once SAH is confirmed.
- Call neurosurgery.

TREATMENT

- **Prevent rebleeding** (most likely to occur in the first 48 hours).
- Calcium channel blockers and IV fluids; maintain BP to **prevent vasospasm** and further neurologic deterioration.
- **Seizure prophylaxis.**
- ↓ ICP by raising the head of the bed and instituting hyperventilation.
- Surgical treatment involves open clipping or endovascular coiling of vascular abnormalities.

Subdural Hematoma

- Typically occurs after head trauma → rupture of **bridging veins;** common in the elderly and alcoholics.
- Hx/PE: Headache, changes in mental status, contralateral hemiparesis, or other focal changes (subacute or chronic); may present as dementia in the elderly.
- Dx: CT demonstrates a **crescent-shaped, concave hyperdensity** that does **not cross the midline** (see Figure 2.10-4A).
- Rx: **Surgical evacuation if symptomatic.** Subdural blood may regress spontaneously if it is chronic.

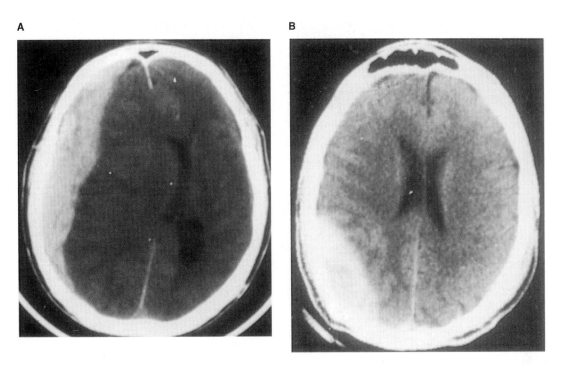

FIGURE 2.10-4.   Head CT scans.

(A) Subdural hematoma. Note the crescent shape and the mass effect with midline shift. (B) Epidural hematoma with classic bi-convex lens shape. (Reproduced, with permission, from Aminoff MJ. *Clinical Neurology*, 3rd ed. Stamford, CT: Appleton & Lange, 1996:296.)

Epidural Hematoma

- Usually a result of a **lateral skull fracture** → tear of the **middle meningeal artery.**
- Hx/PE: **Lucid interval (minutes to hours)** followed by headache, progressive obtundation, hemiparesis, and ultimately a **"blown pupil"** (fixed and dilated).
- **Dx:** CT shows a **lens-shaped, convex hyperdensity limited by the sutures** (see Figure 2.10-4B).
- **Rx:** Emergent neurosurgical evacuation.

Parenchymal Hemorrhage

- Risk factors include hypertension, tumor, amyloid angiopathy (in the elderly), and vascular malformations (AVMs, cavernous hemangiomas).
- **Hx/PE: Lethargy and headache; focal motor and sensory deficits;** obtundation is possible.
- **Dx:** Immediate noncontrast head CT (see Figure 2.10-5). Look for mass effect or edema that may predict herniation.
- **Rx:** Similar to that of SAH. Elevate the head of the bed and institute antiseizure prophylaxis. Surgical evacuation may be necessary if mass effect is present. Several types of herniation may occur, including central, **uncal,** subfalcine, and tonsillar (see Figure 2.10-6).

With an epidural hematoma, mental status changes occur within minutes to hours and have a classic lucid interval. With a subdural hematoma, mental status changes can occur within days to weeks.

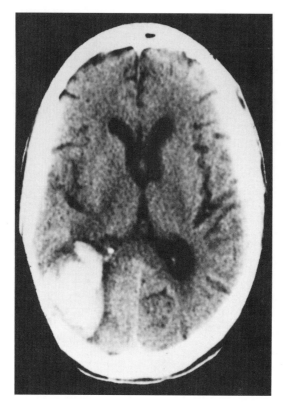

FIGURE 2.10-5. Intraparenchymal hematoma.

Head CT without contrast reveals the irregularly shaped hyperdensity with midline shift of the choroid plexus. (Reproduced, with permission, from Saunders CE. *Current Emergency Diagnosis & Treatment*, 4th Ed. Stamford, CT: Appleton & Lange, 1992: 248.)

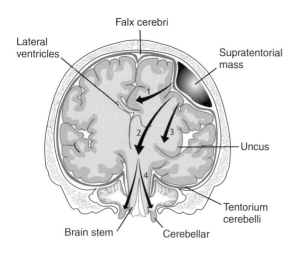

1. Cingulate herniation under falx cerebri
2. Downward transtentorial (central) herniation
3. Uncal herniation
4. Cerebellar tonsillar herniation into the foramen magnum

Coma and death result when these herniations compress the brain stem

FIGURE 2.10-6. Herniation syndromes.

(Adapted, with permission, from Simon RP et al. *Clinical Neurology*, 4th ed. Stamford, CT: Appleton & Lange, 1999:314.)

1° headache is generally classified into three categories: **migraine, tension, and cluster.** The causes of headache include the following:

- **Acute:** SAH, hemorrhagic stroke, meningitis, seizure, acutely ↑ ICP, hypertensive encephalopathy, post-LP, ocular disease (glaucoma, iritis), new migraine.
- **Subacute:** Temporal arteritis (TA), intracranial tumor, subdural hematoma, pseudotumor cerebri, trigeminal/glossopharyngeal neuralgia, postherpetic neuralgia, hypertension.
- **Chronic/episodic:** Migraine, cluster headache, tension headache, rebound headaches from NSAID use, sinusitis, dental disease, neck pain, caffeine withdrawal.

DIAGNOSIS

Evaluate the following:

- **Is the headache new or old?** Recent or sudden-onset, severe headaches (e.g., those that awaken the patient from sleep) warrant immediate workup (e.g., for tumor, TA, and meningitis).
- **What are its characteristics?** Assess intensity, quality, location, and duration.
- **Are there associated symptoms?** Look for associated jaw claudication, fever, nausea, vomiting, and weight loss.
- **Are there neurologic symptoms?** Look for paresthesias, numbness, ataxia, visual disturbances, photophobia, and neck stiffness. Focal neurologic deficits and papilledema warrant immediate workup for more serious causes.
- **If an SAH is suspected with a ⊖ head CT, LP is mandatory.**
- **Labs:** Obtain a CBC, ESR, and CT/MRI for suspected SAH, ↑ ICP, or focal neurologic findings. Use **CT without contrast** to evaluate acute hemorrhage.

Recent-onset headaches warrant immediate workup! If headache is associated with focal neurologic deficits, rule out more serious etiologies with CT or MRI. Also rule out meningitis or SAH with an LP if symptoms are acute in onset.

Migraine Headache

- Affects **women** more often than men; may be familial; associated with **vascular** and brain neurotransmitter (**serotonin**) abnormalities.
- **Triggers** include certain foods (e.g., chocolate), fasting, stress, menses, OCPs, and bright light.
- **Hx/PE:** Throbbing headache (> 2 hours but usually < 24 hours). Associated with **nausea, vomiting, photophobia,** and noise sensitivity. **Classic migraines** are often **unilateral** and are preceded by a visual **aura** in the form of either scintillating scotomas (bright light or flashing lights) or visual field cuts. **Common migraines** may be **bilateral** and periorbital and may have **no associated symptoms.**
- **Dx:** Based on history.
- **Rx:**
  - **Avoid known triggers.**
  - **Abortive therapy:** ASA/NSAIDs and triptans (sumatriptan).
  - **Prophylaxis** (frequent/severe migraines): β-blockers (propranolol), **TCAs** (amitriptyline), calcium channel blockers, valproic acid.

Cluster Headache

- **Men** are affected more often than women; average age of onset is 25. Risk factors include recent alcohol use or vasodilating drugs.

- **Hx/PE:** A brief, severe, **unilateral periorbital headache** lasting 30 minutes to three hours. Attacks tend to occur in **clusters,** affecting the same part of the head at the same time of day and in a certain season of the year. Associated symptoms include **ipsilateral tearing** of the eye, conjunctival injection, Horner's syndrome, and nasal stuffiness.
- **Dx:** Classic presentations require no evaluation.
- **Rx:**
  - **Acute therapy:** High-flow O_2 (100% nonrebreather), ergots, sumatriptan, intranasal lidocaine, corticosteroids.
  - **Prophylactic therapy:** Ergots, calcium channel blockers, prednisone, lithium, valproic acid, topiramate.

Tension Headache

- **Hx/PE: Tight, bandlike pain** that is exacerbated by noise, bright lights, fatigue, and stress. Nonspecific symptoms (e.g., anxiety, poor concentration, difficulty sleeping) may also be seen. May be generalized or most intense in the **occipital and neck region.** Usually occurs at the end of the day.
- **Dx:** A diagnosis of exclusion. There are no focal neurologic signs.
- **Rx:** Relaxation, massage, hot baths, **avoidance of exacerbating factors. NSAIDs** are first-line abortive therapy, but triptans and ergots may also be considered.

SEIZURE DISORDERS

Due to **excessive or hypersynchronous discharge by cortical neurons** → a change in neurologic perception or behavior. An aura is experienced by 50–60% patients with epilepsy. See Table 2.10-1 for common etiologies by age.

DIAGNOSIS

Assess the following:

- **Was the seizure epileptic?** Use the history to differentiate. ↑ serum prolactin levels are consistent with an epileptic seizure in the immediate postictal period.
- **Was the seizure provoked by a systemic process?** Non-neurologic etiologies include **hypoglycemia, hyponatremia, hypocalcemia, hyperosmolar states, hepatic encephalopathy,** uremia, porphyria, **drug overdose** (cocaine, antidepressants, neuroleptics, methylxanthines, lidocaine), **drug withdrawal** (alcohol and other sedatives), eclampsia, hyperthermia, hypertensive encephalopathy, and cerebral hypoperfusion.

Table 2.10-1. **Causes of Seizures**

INFANT	CHILD (2–10)	ADOLESCENT	ADULT (18–35)	ADULT (35+)
Perinatal injury	Idiopathic	Idiopathic	Trauma	Trauma
Infection	Infection	Trauma	Alcoholism	Stroke
Metabolic	Trauma	Drug withdrawal	Brain tumor	Metabolic disorder
Congenital	Febrile seizure	AVM		Alcoholism
				Brain tumor

- **Was the seizure caused by an underlying neurologic disorder?** Seizures with focal onset (or focal postictal deficit) suggest focal CNS pathology. They may be the presenting sign of a tumor, stroke, AVM, infection, hemorrhage, or developmental abnormality.
- **Is anticonvulsant therapy indicated?** First seizures that resolve after a single episode are frequently left untreated when the underlying cause is unknown.

Partial Seizures

- Arise from a **discrete region** in one cerebral hemisphere and **do not lead to loss of consciousness** unless they secondarily generalize.
- Hx/PE:
    - **Simple partial seizures** may include motor features (e.g., jacksonian march, or the progressive jerking of successive body regions) as well as sensory, autonomic, or psychic features (e.g., fear, déjà vu) **without alteration of consciousness.** Postictal focal neurologic deficit (e.g., hemiplegia/hemiparesis = Todd's paralysis) is possible and usually resolves within 24 hours. Often confused with acute stroke (ruled out by MRI).
    - **Complex partial seizures** typically involve the temporal lobe (70–80%) and are characterized by **impaired level of consciousness,** auditory or visual hallucinations, déjà vu, automatisms (e.g., lip smacking, chewing, or even walking), and postictal confusion/disorientation and amnesia.
- Dx:
    - Obtain an **EEG.**
    - Rule out systemic causes with CBC, electrolytes, calcium, fasting glucose, LFTs, renal panel, RPR, ESR, and toxicology screen.
    - A focal seizure implies a focal brain lesion. Rule out a mass by MRI or CT with contrast.
- Rx:
    - **Treat the underlying cause.**
    - **Recurrent partial seizures:** Phenytoin, oxcarbazepine, carbamazepine (Tegretol), phenobarbital, and valproic acid can be administered as monotherapy. In **children, phenobarbital** is the first-line anticonvulsant.
    - **Intractable temporal lobe seizures:** Consider **anterior temporal lobectomy.**

Both simple partial and complex partial seizures may evolve into 2° generalized tonic-clonic (grand mal) seizures.

Tonic-Clonic (Grand Mal) Seizures

- Primarily idiopathic. Partial seizures can evolve into secondarily generalized tonic-clonic seizures.
- Hx/PE: Sudden onset of tonic extension of the back and extremities, continuing with 1–2 minutes of repetitive, symmetric clonic movements. Marked by **incontinence** and **tongue biting.** Patients may appear **cyanotic** during the ictal period. Consciousness is slowly regained in the postictal period; muscle aches and headaches may be present.
- Dx: EEG typically shows 10-Hz activity during the tonic phase and slow waves during the clonic phase.
- Rx:
    - **Protect the airway.**
    - Treat the underlying cause if known.

- **1° generalized tonic-clonic seizures:** Phenytoin, fosphenytoin, or valproate constitutes first-line therapy. Lamotrigine or topiramate may be used as adjunctive therapy.
- **Secondarily generalized tonic-clonic seizures:** Same as for partial seizures.

Absence (Petit Mal) Seizures

- Begin in **childhood**; subside before adulthood. Often **familial.**
- **Hx/PE:** Present with brief **(5- to 10-second)**, often unnoticeable episodes of **impaired consciousness** occurring up to hundreds of times per day. Patients are **amnestic** during and immediately after seizures and may appear to be **daydreaming** or **staring.** Eye fluttering or lip smacking is common.
- **Dx:** EEG shows classic three-per-second spike-and-wave discharges.
- **Rx:** Ethosuximide is the first-line agent.

Status Epilepticus

- A **medical emergency** consisting of prolonged **(> 30-minute)** or repetitive seizures without a return to baseline consciousness.
- Common causes include anticonvulsant withdrawal/noncompliance, anoxic brain injury, EtOH/sedative withdrawal or other drug intoxication, metabolic disturbances (e.g., hyponatremia), trauma, and infection.
- **Dx:**
  - Determine the underlying cause with pulse oximetry, CBC, electrolytes, calcium, glucose, ABGs, LFTs, BUN/creatinine, ESR, and toxicology screen.
  - **Defer EEG and brain imaging until the patient is stabilized.**
  - Perform LP in the setting of fever or meningeal signs (only after having done a CT scan to ensure the safety of the LP).
- **Rx:**
  - Maintain **ABCs**; consider rapid intubation for airway protection.
  - Administer **IV benzodiazepine** (lorazepam or diazepam) plus a loading dose of **phenytoin.**
  - If seizures continue, intubate and load with **phenobarbital.** Consider an IV sedative (midazolam or pentobarbital) and initiate continuous EEG monitoring.
  - **Glucose, thiamine, and naloxone** may also be given to presumptively treat other potential etiologies.

Infantile Spasms (West Syndrome)

- Affects males more often than females; the initial event occurs between 3 and 12 months of age. Associated with a ⊕ family history.
- **Hx/PE:** Tonic, bilateral, symmetric **head jerks** that tend to occur in clusters of 5–10; **arrest of psychomotor development** at the age of seizure onset. The majority of patients have mental retardation.
- **Dx:** Abnormal interictal EEG (very high amplitude slow waves).
- **Rx:** Hormonal therapy with **ACTH**, prednisone, and clonazepam or valproic acid.

Benign Paroxysmal Positional Vertigo (BPPV)

- A common form of **peripheral vertigo** resulting from a **dislodged otolith** that causes disturbances in the semicircular canals.

- **Hx/PE:** Transient, episodic vertigo (lasting < 1 minute) and nystagmus triggered by changes in head position (classically while turning in bed or getting out of bed), together with nausea and vomiting.
- **Dx: Dix-Hallpike maneuver**—have the patient go from a sitting to a supine position while quickly turning the head to the side. If vertigo and/or nystagmus is reproduced, BPPV is the likely diagnosis.
- **Rx:** Usually subsides spontaneously in weeks to months. Repositioning exercises or the Epley maneuver (the reverse of Dix-Hallpike) may be beneficial.

DISORDERS OF THE NEUROMUSCULAR JUNCTION

Myasthenia Gravis

An **autoimmune disease** caused by antibodies that bind to **postsynaptic acetylcholine (ACh) receptors.** Occurs most often in young adult women and can be associated with **thyrotoxicosis, thymoma,** and other autoimmune disorders.

History/PE

- Fluctuating **fatigable ptosis or double vision,** bulbar symptoms, and **proximal muscle** weakness.
- **Symptoms typically worsen as the day progresses.**
- Patients may report difficulty with stairs, rising from a chair, brushing their hair, and swallowing.
- Respiratory compromise and aspiration are rare but potentially lethal complications and are termed **myasthenic crisis.**

Diagnosis

- **Edrophonium (Tensilon test):** Anticholinesterase → rapid amelioration of symptoms.
- **Ice test:** Place a pack of ice on one eye for five minutes; ptosis resolves transiently.
- An abnormal **single-fiber EMG** and/or a **decremental response to repetitive nerve stimulation** can yield additional confirmation.
- ACh antibodies are ⊕ in 80% of patients; anti–muscle-specific kinase (anti-MuSK) antibodies are ⊕ in 5%.
- Chest CT is used to evaluate for thymoma. Eighty-five percent of patients with thymoma have ⊕ antibodies against striated muscle.
- Follow serial FVCs to determine the need to intubate.

Treatment

- Anticholinesterase drugs (**neostigmine,** pyridostigmine) are used for symptomatic treatment.
- **Prednisone** and other immunosuppressants are mainstays of treatment.
- In severe cases, plasmapheresis or IVIG may provide temporary relief (days to weeks).
- **Resection of thymoma** can be curative.

Lambert-Eaton Myasthenic Syndrome

- Small cell lung carcinoma is a risk factor (90% of cases).
- **Hx/PE:** Weakness and fatigability of proximal muscles; depressed or absent DTRs. Extraocular and bulbar muscles are typically spared.

- **Dx:** Autoantibodies to presynaptic calcium channels; chest CT indicative of a lung neoplasm.
- **Rx:** Guanidine hydrochloride is the mainstay of treatment. Anticholinesterases may also improve symptoms. Tumor resection can reverse symptoms.

DEMENTIA

A chronic, progressive, global decline in multiple cognitive areas (see the mnemonic **The 5 A's of dementia**). Alzheimer's disease accounts for 70–80% of cases. The differential diagnosis is described in the mnemonic **DEMENTIAS**. Take care not to confuse delirium and dementia (see the Psychiatry section).

> **The 5 A's of dementia:**
>
> **A**phasia
> **A**mnesia
> **A**gnosia
> **A**praxia
> Disturbances in **A**bstract thought

Alzheimer's Disease (AD)

Risk factors include **age**, female gender, **family history, Down syndrome,** and low educational level. Pathology includes **neurofibrillary tangles, neuritic plaques** with **amyloid** deposition, amyloid angiopathy, and neuronal loss.

HISTORY/PE

Amnesia is usually the first presenting sign, followed by language deficits, acalculia, depression, agitation, and apraxia (inability to perform skilled movements). Mild cognitive impairment may precede AD by 10 years.

DIAGNOSIS

A **diagnosis of exclusion** that can be definitively **diagnosed only on autopsy.** MRI or CT may show atrophy and can rule out other causes. Neuropsychological testing helps distinguish dementia from depression. Also rule out hypothyroidism and subdural hematoma.

> **Differential diagnosis—**
>
> **DEMENTIAS**
>
> Neuro**D**egenerative diseases
> **E**ndocrine
> **M**etabolic
> **E**xogenous
> **N**eoplasm
> **T**rauma
> **I**nfection
> **A**ffective disorders
> **S**troke/**S**tructural

TREATMENT

- Supportive therapy for the patient and the family.
- **Cholinesterase inhibitors** (donepezil, rivastigmine, and galantamine, an NMDA receptor antagonist) are first-line therapy.
- Vitamin E (α-tocopherol) may also slow cognitive decline.
- **Survival is 5–10 years** from the onset of symptoms. Death is usually 2° to **aspiration pneumonia** or other infections.

MOVEMENT DISORDERS

Huntington's Disease

A rare, **hyperkinetic, autosomal-dominant** disease involving multiple **abnormal CAG triplet repeats** (< 29 is normal). The number of repeats expands in subsequent generations → earlier expression and more severe disease (**anticipation**). Life expectancy is 20 years from time of diagnosis.

HISTORY/PE

Presents at 30–50 years of age with gradual onset of **chorea, altered behavior,** and **dementia** (begins as irritability, moodiness, and antisocial behavior).

DIAGNOSIS

- A clinical diagnosis.
- **CT /MRI:** Cerebral atrophy (especially of the **caudate** and putamen).
- Molecular genetic testing to determine the number of CAG repeats.

TREATMENT

- There is no cure, and the disease cannot be halted. Symptomatic treatment only.
- Haloperidol for psychosis; reserpine to minimize unwanted movements.
- Genetic counseling should be offered to offspring.

Parkinson's Disease

An **idiopathic hypokinetic** disorder that usually begins at > 50–60 years of age. Due to **dopamine depletion** in the **substantia nigra.** Etiologies include **postencephalitic, toxic** (e.g., carbon disulfide, manganese, "designer drugs"), bihemispheric ischemic, traumatic, and iatrogenic (especially neuroleptic) insults.

HISTORY/PE

- The **"Parkinson's tetrad"** consists of the following:
    - **Resting tremor** (e.g., "pill rolling").
    - **Rigidity:** "Cogwheeling" is due to the combined effects of rigidity and tremor.
    - **Bradykinesia:** Slowed movements and difficulty initiating movements. Festinating gait (wide leg stance with short accelerating steps) without arm swing is also seen.
    - **Postural instability:** Stooped posture, impaired righting reflexes, freezing, falls.
- Other manifestations include masked facies, memory loss, and micrographia.

TREATMENT

- Dopamine agonists (**bromocriptine**) are first-line treatment for early disease.
- **Levodopa/carbidopa** are the mainstays of therapy.
- Selegiline (an MAO-B inhibitor) may be neuroprotective and may ↓ the need for levodopa.
- Catechol-O-methyltransferase (COMT) inhibitors (e.g., entacapone) ↑ the availability of levodopa to the brain and may ↓ motor fluctuations.
- If medical therapy fails, attempt **surgical pallidotomy** or chronic **deep brain stimulation.**

DEMYELINATING/DEGENERATIVE DISORDERS

Multiple Sclerosis (MS)

The pathogenesis is unclear, but there is evidence of an autoimmune or viral etiology. Both potential etiologies are thought to be **T-cell mediated.** The female-to-male ratio is 3:2; onset is typically at 20–40 years of age. More common as one moves farther away from the equator. Subtypes are **relapsing**/remitting, 2° progressive, and 1° progressive.

The classic triad in MS is scanning speech, intranuclear ophthalmoplegia, and nystagmus.

231

HISTORY/PE

- Multiple neurologic complaints separated in time and space that are not explained by a single lesion.
- Limb weakness, **optic neuritis**, paresthesias, diplopia, urinary retention, vertigo.
- Attacks are unpredictable but on average occur every 1.5 years, lasting for 6–8 weeks.
- Neurologic symptoms can wax and wane or be progressive. Prognosis is best with a relapsing and remitting history.
- Symptoms classically worsen with hot showers.
- Lhermitte's sign may be present (sharp pain traveling up or down the neck with flexion).

DIAGNOSIS

- **MRI: Multiple, asymmetric,** often **periventricular** white matter lesions (Dawson's fingers), especially in the **corpus callosum.** Active lesions enhance with gadolinium.
- **CSF:** Mononuclear pleocytosis (< 5 cells/μL), ↑ IgG index, or oligoclonal bands (nonspecific).
- Abnormal somatosensory or visual evoked potentials may also be present.

TREATMENT

- **Steroids** should be given during acute exacerbations.
- Immunomodulators alter relapse rates in relapsing/remitting MS and include interferon-α_{1a} (**A**vonex/Rebif), interferon-β_{1b} (**B**etaseron), and copolymer-1 (**C**opaxone).
- Mitoxantrone for worsening relapsing/remitting or progressive MS.

Guillain-Barré Syndrome (GBS)

- An **acute, rapidly progressive,** acquired demyelinating autoimmune disorder of the peripheral nerves → weakness.
- Associated with recent *Campylobacter jejuni* infection, viral infection, or influenza vaccination.
- Approximately 85% of patients make a complete or near-complete recovery (may take up to one year). The mortality rate is < 5%.

HISTORY/PE

- Rapidly progressive **ascending paralysis** (distal → proximal) involving the trunk, diaphragm, and cranial nerves.
- Autonomic symptoms, areflexia, and dysesthesias may be present.

DIAGNOSIS

- Evidence of diffuse demyelination on **EMG** and **nerve conduction studies.**
- Supported by a **CSF protein level > 55 mg/dL** with little or no pleocytosis (albuminocytologic dissociation).

TREATMENT

- Admit to the ICU in light of the risk of **respiratory failure.**
- **Plasmapheresis** and **IVIG** are first-line treatments. Steroids are **not indicated.**
- Aggressive physical rehabilitation is imperative.

Table 2.10-2. UMN vs. LMN Signs

CLINICAL FEATURES	UMN	LMN
Pattern of weakness	Pyramidal (arm extensors, leg flexors)	Variable
Tone	Spastic (↑; initially flaccid)	Flaccid (↓)
DTRs	↑ (initially ↓)	Normal, ↓, absent
Miscellaneous signs	Babinski's, other CNS signs	Atrophy, fasciculations

Amyotrophic Lateral Sclerosis (ALS)

- A **chronic, progressive degenerative disease** of unknown etiology characterized by loss of **upper and lower motor neurons** (UMNs/LMNs).
- Almost always progresses to respiratory failure and death. Also known as **Lou Gehrig's disease.**

HISTORY/PE

- Asymmetric, slowly progressive weakness affecting the arms, legs, and cranial nerves. Some patients initially present with fasciculations.
- Presents with **UMN signs** and/or **LMN signs** (see Table 2.10-2). Eye movements and sphincter tone are usually spared.

DIAGNOSIS

- The clinical presentation is usually diagnostic.
- **EMG/nerve conduction studies** reveal widespread denervation and fibrillation potentials.
- CT/MRI of the cervical spine to exclude structural lesions.
- Rule out systemic causes.

TREATMENT

Supportive measures and patient education.

NEOPLASMS

Intracranial neoplasms may be 1° (30%) or **metastatic (70%).**

- Of all 1° brain tumors, 40% are benign, and these rarely spread beyond the CNS.
- Metastatic tumors are most often from 1° **lung, breast, kidney, and GI tract neoplasms** and **melanoma.** Occur at the **gray-white junction** and **may be multiple discrete nodules;** characterized by rapid growth, invasiveness, necrosis, and neovascularization.

HISTORY/PE

- Symptoms depend on tumor type and location (see Table 2.10-3), local growth and **resulting mass effect,** cerebral edema, ↑ ICP, and ventricular obstruction.
- Symptoms develop gradually and include nausea and vomiting, headache, and focal neurologic deficits.

Most CNS tumors are metastatic. The most common 1° CNS tumors in adults are glioblastoma multiforme and meningioma. The most common 1° CNS tumors in children are medulloblastomas and astrocytomas.

Table 2.10-3. Most Common 1° Neoplasms

TUMOR	PRESENTATION	TREATMENT
Astrocytoma	Presents with headache and ↑ ICP. May cause unilateral paralysis in CN V–VII and CN X. Slow, **protracted course.** Prognosis much better than that of glioblastoma multiforme (GMB).	Resection if possible. Radiation.
GBM (grade IV astrocytoma)	Most common 1° brain tumor. Often presents with headache and ↑ ICP. Progresses rapidly. **Poor prognosis** (< 1 year from the time of prognosis).	Surgical removal/resection. Radiation and chemotherapy have variable results.
Meningioma	Originates from **dura mater or arachnoid.** Good prognosis. Incidence ↑ with age.	Surgical resection; radiation for unresectable tumors.
Acoustic neuroma (schwannoma)	Presents with ipsilateral hearing loss, tinnitus, vertigo, and signs of cerebellar dysfunction. Derived from **Schwann cells.**	Surgical removal.
Medulloblastoma	**Common in children.** Arises from fourth ventricle and leads to ↑ ICP. Highly malignant; may seed subarachnoid space.	Surgical resection coupled with radiation and chemotherapy.
Ependymoma	Common in children. May arise from ependyma of a ventricle (commonly the fourth) or the spinal cord; may → hydrocephalus.	Surgical resection. Radiation.

Two-thirds of 1° brain tumors in adults are supratentorial. One third of those in children are supratentorial.

- Personality changes, lethargy, intellectual decline, aphasias, seizures, and mood swings may also be seen.
- Metastases that tend to present with intracranial hemorrhage include renal cell carcinoma, thyroid cancer, choriocarcinoma, and melanoma.

DIAGNOSIS

- Contrast CT and MRI with gadolinium to localize and determine the extent of the lesion.
- Histologic diagnosis via CT-guided biopsy or surgical tumor debulking.

TREATMENT

- **Resection** (if possible), **radiation,** and **chemotherapy.**
- Therapy is highly dependent on tumor type, histology, progression, and site (see Table 2.10-3).
- **Corticosteroids** can be used to ↓ vasogenic edema. Management is often palliative.

Neurofibromatosis (NF)

The most common neurocutaneous disorder. There are two major types: neurofibromatosis 1 (NF1, or von Recklinghausen's syndrome) and neurofibromatosis 2 (NF2).

NF2 is associated with bilateral acoustic neuromas and a defective gene on chromosome 22.

HISTORY/PE

- Diagnostic criteria for **NF1** include two or more of the following:
    - Six **café-au-lait spots** (each ≥ 5 mm in children or ≥ 15 mm in adults).
    - Two neurofibromas of any type.
    - **Freckling in the axillary or inguinal area.**
    - **Optic glioma.**
    - **Two Lisch nodules (pigmented iris hamartomas).**
    - Bone abnormality.
    - A **first-degree relative** with NF1.
- Diagnostic criteria for **NF2** are as follows:
    - **Bilateral acoustic neuromas** or a first-degree relative with NF2 **and**
    - Unilateral acoustic neuromas **or** two of any of the following: neurofibromas, meningiomas, gliomas, or schwannoma.
    - Other features include seizures, skin nodules, and café-au-lait spots.

DIAGNOSIS

- **MRI of the brain, brain stem, and spine.**
- Complete dermatologic exam, ophthalmologic exams, and family history. Auditory testing is recommended.

TREATMENT

- There is no cure; treatment is symptomatic.
- Acoustic neuromas can be treated with surgery or radiosurgery.

Tuberous Sclerosis

HISTORY/PE

- Presents with **infantile spasms** and **"ash-leaf" hypopigmented lesions** on the trunk and extremities.
- Other skin manifestations include **sebaceous adenomas** (small red nodules on the nose and cheeks) and a **shagreen patch** (a rough papule in the lumbosacral region with an orange-peel consistency).
- Two retinal lesions are recognized: (1) mulberry tumors, which arise from the nerve head; and (2) phakomas, which are round, flat, gray lesions near the optic disk.
- Symptoms are 2° to small benign tumors that grow on the face, eyes, brain, kidney, and other organs.
- Mental retardation (↑ likelihood with early age of onset).
- CHF from cardiac rhabdomyoma.

DIAGNOSIS

- **Head CT:** Calcified tubers in the periventricular area. These lesions may on rare occasion transform into malignant astrocytomas.
- Skin lesions are enhanced by a Wood's UV lamp.

- **ECG:** Evaluate for rhabdomyoma of the heart, especially in the apex of the left ventricle (> 50% of patients).
- **Renal ultrasound:** May reveal renal hamartomas or polycystic disease.
- Angiomyolipomas (causing cystic or fibrous pulmonary changes).

TREATMENT

- Treatment should be based on symptoms.
- Maintain seizure control with clonazepam or valproic acid (as with infantile spasms).
- Surgical intervention may be indicated for ↑ ICP.

APHASIA

A general term for language disorders. Usually result from insults (e.g., strokes, tumors, abscesses) to the "dominant hemisphere" (usually the left).

Broca's Aphasia

- A **disorder of language production** with **intact comprehension.** Due to an insult to Broca's area in the **posterior inferior frontal gyrus.** Often 2° to a left superior **MCA stroke.**
- **Hx/PE: Impaired repetition,** frustration with awareness of deficits, arm and face **hemiparesis,** hemisensory loss, apraxia of oral muscles.
- **Rx: Speech therapy** (varying outcomes with intermediate prognosis).

Wernicke's Aphasia

- A **disorder of language comprehension** with **intact yet nonsensical production.**
- Due to an insult to Wernicke's area in the left posterior superior temporal lobe (perisylvian). Often 2° to left **inferior/posterior MCA** embolic stroke.
- **Hx/PE:** Frequent use of **neologisms** (made-up words) and paraphasic errors (word substitutions); **lack of awareness** of deficits.
- **Rx:** Treat the underlying etiology and institute speech therapy. Prognosis is poorer than that of Broca's aphasia.

> **B**roca's is **B**roken speech.
> **W**ernicke's is **W**ordy but makes no sense.

Broca's aphasia is also known as an expressive or nonfluent aphasia.

Wernicke's aphasia is also known as a fluent or receptive aphasia.

COMA

- A profound suppression of responses to external and internal stimuli. Due to either catastrophic structural CNS injury or diffuse metabolic dysfunction.
- Causes include **hemorrhage; infarction;** abscesses; tumors; endogenous electrolyte disturbances; endocrine or metabolic dysfunction; **exogenous toxins** (medications, EtOH, other drugs); infectious or inflammatory disease; and generalized seizure activity or postictal states.

HISTORY/PE

- Obtain a complete medical history, including current medications.
- Exam should include mental status, breathing pattern, papillary response, eye movements, cold-water calorics, and response to noxious stimuli.

DIAGNOSIS

- Typically made by H&P and exclusion of other etiologies.
- **EEG** can also be diagnostic and prognostic (alpha, spindle, and theta coma).

- MRI to exclude structural changes and ischemia.
- Rule out catatonic, hysterical, "locked-in," or persistent vegetative states, which can be confused with true coma.
- "Locked-in" patients are awake and alert but can move only their eyes and eyelids. Associated with central pontine myelinolysis, brain stem stroke, and advanced ALS.
- Persistent vegetative state is characterized by normal wake-sleep cycles but lack of awareness of self or the environment. The most common causes are trauma with diffuse cortical injury or hypoxic ischemic injury.

TREATMENT

Initial treatment consists of the following measures:

- **Stabilize the patient:** Attend to **ABCs.**
- **Reverse the reversible:** Administer **DONT**—Dextrose, Oxygen, Naloxone, and Thiamine.
- **Identify and treat the underlying cause** and associated complications.
- **Prevent further damage.**

NUTRITIONAL DEFICIENCIES

Table 2.10-4 describes the neurologic symptoms commonly associated with nutritional deficiencies.

Table 2.10-4. Neurologic Syndromes Associated with Nutritional Deficiencies

VITAMIN	SYNDROME	SIGNS/SYMPTOMS	CLASSIC PATIENTS	TREATMENT
Thiamine (vitamin B_1)	Wernicke's encephalopathy	Classic triad: **encephalopathy, ophthalmoplegia** (nystagmus, lateral rectus palsy, conjugate-gaze palsy), **ataxia** (polyneuropathy, cerebellar and vestibular dysfunction).	**Alcoholics, hyperemesis, starvation, renal dialysis,** AIDS. **Can be elicited by large-dose glucose administration.**	Reversible, almost immediately, with thiamine administration.
	Korsakoff's dementia	Above, plus amnesia, horizontal nystagmus.	Same as above.	Irreversible.
Cyanocobalamin (vitamin B_{12})[a]	Combined system disease (CSD) *or* subacute combined degeneration	Gradual, progressive onset. Symmetric paresthesias, leg stiffness, spasticity, paraplegia, bowel and bladder dysfunction. Dementia.	Patients with pernicious anemia.	B_{12} injections or large oral doses.
Folate[a]	Folate deficiency	Irritability, memory loss, personality changes without the neurologic systems of CSD.	**Alcoholics,** patients with pernicious anemia.	Reversible if corrected early.

[a] Associated with ↑ homocysteine and ↑ risk of vascular events.

Visual Field Defects

Figure 2.10-7 illustrates common visual field defects and the anatomic areas with which they are associated.

Closed-Angle Glaucoma

- Risk factors include older age, Asian ethnicity, **pupillary dilation** (prolonged time in a darkened area, stress, medications), anterior uveitis, and dislocation of the lens.
- **Hx/PE:** Extreme pain and blurred vision; nausea and vomiting may also be seen.
- **Dx:** Hard, red eye (from acute closure of a narrow anterior chamber angle); the pupil is dilated and nonreactive to light; ↑ intraocular pressure.
- **Rx:** This is a **medical emergency** that may lead to blindness; ↓ **intraocular pressure** with acetazolamide, then pilocarpine. **Laser iridotomy** is curative.

Open-Angle Glaucoma

- Risk factors include age > 40 years, **African-American ethnicity**, diabetes, and myopia.
- **Hx/PE:** Initially asymptomatic. Should be suspected in patients > 35 years of age who need **frequent lens changes** and have mild headaches, visual disturbances, and impaired adaptation to darkness. The earliest visual defect is seen in the peripheral nasal fields. **Cupping** of the optic disk is seen on funduscopic examination.
- **Dx:** Tonometry, ophthalmoscopic visualization of the optic nerve, and visual field testing are most important. A diseased trabecular meshwork that obstructs proper drainage of the eye → gradual ↑ pressure → progressive vision loss.

Open-angle glaucoma is much more common than closed-angle glaucoma and is almost always bilateral (closed angle is usually unilateral).

1. Right anopsia
2. Bitemporal hemianopsia
3. Left homonymous hemianopsia
4. Left upper quadrantic anopsia (right temporal lesion)
5. Left lower quadrantic anopsia (right parietal lesion)
6. Left hemianopsia with macular sparing

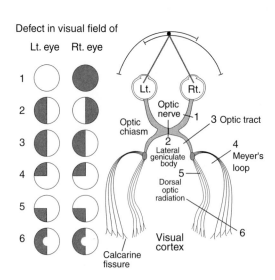

FIGURE 2.10-7.   Visual Field Defects.

- **Rx:** Prevention (ophthalmology exam every 3–5 years for all people > 40 years of age). Treat with topical β-blockers (timolol, betaxolol) to ↓ aqueous humor production or pilocarpine to ↑ aqueous outflow. Carbonic anhydrase inhibitors may also be used. If medication fails, laser trabeculoplasty can improve aqueous drainage.

Macular Degeneration

- More common among Caucasians, females, smokers, and those with a ⊕ family history.
- **Hx/PE: Painless loss of central vision.**
    - **Atrophic macular degeneration:** Causes gradual vision loss.
    - **Exudative macular degeneration:** Causes more rapid and severe vision damage.
- **Dx:** Funduscopy by an ophthalmologist reveals pigmentary or hemorrhagic disturbance in the macular region.
- **Rx:** Options are limited. Laser photocoagulation may delay loss of central vision in exudative macular disease.

In the United States, macular degeneration is the leading cause of permanent, bilateral visual loss in the elderly.

Retinal Occlusion

- Occurs in **elderly patients** and is often idiopathic.
- **Hx/PE:**
    - **Central retinal artery occlusion:** Sudden, painless, **unilateral blindness.** The pupil accommodates but is sluggishly reactive to direct light. Patients present with a **cherry-red spot** on the fovea, retinal swelling, and retinal arteries that may appear bloodless.
    - **Central retinal vein occlusion:** Rapid, painless vision loss. Retinal hemorrhage, cotton wool spots, and edema of the fundus may be seen on funduscopic exam.
- **Rx:**
    - **Central retinal artery occlusion: Thrombolysis** of the ophthalmic artery within **eight** hours of onset of symptoms. ↓ intraocular pressure through drainage of the anterior chamber. IV acetazolamide may improve retinal perfusion. If treatment is not instituted immediately, retinal infarction and permanent blindness may result.
    - **Central retinal vein occlusion:** Laser photocoagulation has variable results.

Obstetrics

Table 2.11-1 outlines normal physiologic changes associated with pregnancy.

TABLE 2.11-1. Normal Physiologic Changes During Pregnancy

ORGAN/SYSTEM	PHYSIOLOGIC CHANGE
Cervix	Softening and cyanosis at approximately four weeks. Thick mucus clot in the cervical os expelled at or near labor (**"bloody show"**). Mucus appears granular microscopically due to progesterone.
Uterus	Palpated above the pubic symphysis at **12 weeks.**
Vagina	Thick acidic secretions; violet colorations (Chadwick's sign) from ↑ blood flow.
Cardiovascular	↑ **cardiac output** (30–50%), **heart rate** (by 10–15 bpm), and **stroke volume.** ↓ systemic vascular resistance (progesterone → smooth muscle relaxation). ↓ **BP in the first trimester;** reaches a nadir at 24 weeks and normalizes by 40 weeks. Systolic murmur and audible S3 are normal; a **new diastolic murmur is not.** The heart is displaced by the uterus upward and to the left → cardiomegaly on CXR.
Endocrine	**Thyroid hormone:** ↑ estrogen levels → ↑ thyroid-binding globulin. Total and bound T_3/T_4 ↑, but active unbound hormone is unchanged. **Human placental lactogen (HPL):** Acts as an insulin antagonist to maintain fetal glucose levels → postprandial **hyperglycemia,** fasting **hyperinsulinemia/hypertriglyceridemia,** and exaggerated starvation **ketosis** response. Change can → or worsen gestational diabetes. **Cortisol:** ↑ total and free cortisol (produced by the fetal adrenal gland and the placenta).
GI	**Nausea and vomiting** (in up to 70%); resolves by 14–16 weeks when the hCG rise plateaus. ↑ **acid reflux** from ↓ gastroesophageal junction sphincter tone. **Constipation** from ↓ large bowel motility and ↑ water resorption. ↑ biliary cholesterol saturation predisposes to gallstone formation.
Hematologic	**Physiologic anemia:** Unequal ↑ in **plasma volume (50%)** and RBC mass (30%) → ↓ hemoglobin and hematocrit. However, a **hemoglobin < 11.0 mg/dL is never normal** and is likely due to iron deficiency. **WBC count:** ↑ throughout pregnancy to a mean of 10.5 million/mL, but can ↑ during labor to > 20 million/mL. **Hypercoagulable state:** DVT risk is highest in the puerperium. **The leading nonobstetric cause of postpartum death is thromboembolic disease (pulmonary embolism).**
Musculoskeletal	↑ motility of sacroiliac, sacrococcygeal, and pubic joints.
Pulmonary	↑ in **tidal volume (V_T)** of 40%; ↓ in total lung capacity, residual volume, and expiratory reserve volume. **Respiratory rate (RR) is unchanged.** ↑ minute ventilation ($V_T \times RR$) → ↑ alveolar and arterial Po_2 and ↓ alveolar and arterial Pco_2. **"Dyspnea of pregnancy"** is common and likely caused by ↑ V_T and ↓ Pco_2.

TABLE 2.11-1. Normal Physiologic Changes During Pregnancy (continued)

ORGAN/SYSTEM	PHYSIOLOGIC CHANGE
Renal	Kidneys dilate. **Dilation of the collecting system may be mistaken for hydronephrosis.** GFR ↑ **by 50%;** renal plasma flow ↑ by 30%. ↑ estrogen and progesterone stimulate the renin-angiotensin system. ↑ **aldosterone** contributes to water retention and ↑ plasma volume.
Skin	↑ estrogen may → changes that resemble cirrhotic disease, such as **striae** (on the abdomen, breast, and thighs), **spider angiomas,** and **palmar erythema.** **Hyperpigmentation** over the midline **(linea nigra),** face (chloasma), and perineum is due to ↑ α-melanocyte-stimulating hormone and steroids. **Diastasis recti:** Rectus muscles may separate in the midline, leaving part of the anterior uterus covered only by skin, fascia, and peritoneum.

PRENATAL CARE AND NUTRITION

The goal is to prevent, diagnose, and treat conditions that → adverse outcomes in pregnancy (see Table 2.11-2). In women with regular menstrual cycles, calculate the estimated date of delivery using **Nägele's rule.** Gestational

TABLE 2.11-2. Standard Prenatal Care

CATEGORY	RECOMMENDATIONS
Weight gain	Approximately 25–35 lbs for an average woman (15–25 lbs for obese women and more for thin women). An **additional 300 kcal/day** is needed during pregnancy and 500 kcal/day during breast-feeding.
Nutrition	Requirements for protein, iron, folate, calcium, and other vitamins/minerals in pregnancy are as follows: ▪ **Folate: 1 mg daily;** required to ↓ neural tube defects, especially three months prior to conception. ▪ **Iron:** Demand is ↑ by fetal needs and by expanding maternal blood supply. Supplement with **30–60 mg/day of elemental iron** in the latter half of pregnancy. ▪ Patients are advised to take prenatal vitamins, but most needs can be met through diet.
Prenatal labs Initial visit	**Heme:** CBC, blood type, Rh, and antibody screen. **Infectious disease:** UA and culture, rubella antibody titer, HBV surface antigen test, syphilis screen (RPR/VDRL), cervical gonorrhea and chlamydia PCR or culture, PPD, HIV (in high-risk groups). **Other:** Pap smear, glucose testing, sickle prep.
15–19 weeks	Maternal serum α-fetoprotein (MSAFP) or **triple screen (MSAFP, estriol, β-hCG).** Offer amniocentesis to patients > 35 years of age at the time of delivery.
18–20 weeks	Ultrasound to determine GA (if unknown or uncertain) and to survey fetal anatomy, amniotic fluid volume, and placental location.
26–28 weeks	Glucose challenge test; repeat hematocrit.
28 weeks	RhoGAM to Rh-antibody-⊖ women.
32–36 weeks	Cervical chlamydia and gonorrhea cultures in high-risk patients; repeat hematocrit. **Screen for group B streptococcus (GBS). If ⊕, give penicillin during labor** to prevent transmission to the infant.

age (GA) can be determined by fundal height, quickening (at 17–18 weeks), fetal heart tones (at 10 weeks via Doppler), or ultrasound (fetal crown–rump length at 5–12 weeks; biparietal diameter at 20–30 weeks).

PRENATAL DIAGNOSTIC TESTING

α-Fetoprotein (AFP)

- Produced by the fetus and found primarily in amniotic fluid. Small amounts cross the placenta and enter the maternal circulation.
- **MSAFP (15–20 weeks' gestation):** Results are reported as multiples of the median (MoMs) and depend on accurate gestational dating.
  - Causes of elevated MSAFP (> 2.5 MoMs) include open neural tube defects (anencephaly, spina bifida), abdominal wall defects (gastroschisis, omphalocele), multiple gestation, incorrect gestational dating, fetal death, and placental abnormalities (e.g., placental abruption).
  - Abnormally low MSAFP levels (< 0.5 MoM) warrant amniocentesis and karyotyping to rule out chromosomal abnormalities.
- **Triple screen:** Sensitivity for detecting chromosomal abnormalities is ↑ by adding estriol and β-hCG to MSAFP.
  - **Trisomy 18:** All three are ↓.
  - **Trisomy 21:** AFP and estriol are ↓ and β-hCG is ↑.

Amniocentesis

- Consists of transabdominal aspiration of amniotic fluid using an ultrasound-guided needle and evaluation of fetal cells for chromosomal abnormalities.
- There is ample fluid in **weeks 15–17** to perform the test. Risks are fetal-maternal hemorrhage (1–2%) and fetal loss (0.5%). Amniocentesis is indicated for the following:
  - In women who will be > **35 years of age at the time of delivery.**
  - In conjunction with an abnormal triple screen (together they detect 65% of fetuses with trisomy 21).
  - In Rh-sensitized pregnancy to obtain fetal blood type or to detect fetal hemolysis.
  - To evaluate fetal lung maturity via a lecithin-sphingomyelin ratio ≥ 2.5 or to detect the presence of phosphatidyl glycerol.

Chorionic Villus Sampling

- Transvaginal or transabdominal aspiration of chorionic villus tissue (the precursor to the placenta).
  - **Advantages:** Has a diagnostic accuracy comparable to that of amniocentesis; availability at **10–12 weeks' gestation.**
  - **Disadvantages:** A **1% risk of fetal loss and inability to diagnose neural tube defects.**
- Limb defects have been associated with chorionic villus sampling performed at ≤ 9 weeks.

Percutaneous Umbilical Blood Sampling

- Performed in the second and third trimesters, when umbilical cord vessels are large enough to puncture safely.
- Amniocentesis and chorionic villus sampling are now used preferentially because information can be obtained at an earlier date and because the techniques have a lower rate of fetal loss.

Nägele's rule—due date = last menstrual period (LMP) + nine months + seven days.

The triple screen is more sensitive than MSAFP alone for detecting trisomies.

Trisomy 18 = ↓ AFP, ↓ estriol, ↓ β-hCG.
Trisomy 21 = ↓ AFP, ↓ estriol, ↑ β-hCG.

HIGH-YIELD FACTS

OBSTETRICS

- Risks are fetal loss (1.8%), fetal-maternal hemorrhage, and infection. Percutaneous umbilical blood sampling is used for the following:
    - Assessment and treatment of Rh isoimmunization/erythroblastosis fetalis.
    - Fetal karyotyping.
    - Fetal infection (e.g., CMV, toxoplasmosis, rubella).
    - Evaluation of genetic diseases (e.g., sickle cell disease, thalassemia).
    - Evaluation of fetal acid-base status.

NORMAL LABOR AND DELIVERY

Stages of Labor

Table 2.11-3 and Figure 2.11-1 depict the normal stages of labor.

Tests of Fetal Well-Being

- **Nonstress test (NST):** Performed with the mother resting in the left lateral supine position (to prevent supine hypotension). Fetal heart rate is monitored externally by Doppler and correlated with spontaneous fetal movements as reported by the mother (see Table 2.11-4).
    - **Normal response:** Two accelerations of ≥ 15 bpm above baseline for at least 15 seconds over a 20-minute period.
    - **"Nonreactive":** Perform further tests (e.g., a biophysical profile). Lack of fetal heart rate accelerations may occur with any of the following: GA < 32 weeks, fetal sleeping, fetal CNS anomalies, maternal sedative or narcotic administration, and fetal hypoxia (rare).
- **Contraction stress test (CST):** Used in high-risk pregnancies to assess uteroplacental dysfunction. Fetal heart rate is monitored during spontaneous or induced (via nipple stimulation or oxytocin) contractions. Reactivity is determined as in the NST.
    - A "positive" CST is defined by late decelerations following 50% or more of contractions and raises concerns about fetal jeopardy. Must have at least three contractions in 10 minutes.

Factors affecting active phase—

3 P's:

Power
Passenger
Pelvis

TABLE 2.11-3. Stages of Labor

STAGE	STARTS/ENDS	DURATION		COMMENTS
First		**Primi**[a]	**Multi**[b]	
Latent	Onset of labor to 3–4 cm dilation	6–11 hrs	4–8 hrs	Prolongation seen with excessive sedation and hypertonic uterine contractions.
Active	4 cm to complete cervical dilation (10 cm)	4–6 hrs (1.2 cm/hr)	2–3 hrs (1.5 cm/hr)	Prolongation seen with **cephalopelvic disproportion.**
Second	Complete cervical dilation to delivery of infant	0.5–3.0 hrs	5–30 min	Baby goes through all cardinal movements of labor.
Third	Delivery of infant to delivery of placenta	0–0.5 hr	0–0.5 hr	Placenta separates and uterus contracts to establish hemostasis.

[a] Primiparous (first-time mother).

[b] Multiparous (prior pregnancy and delivery).

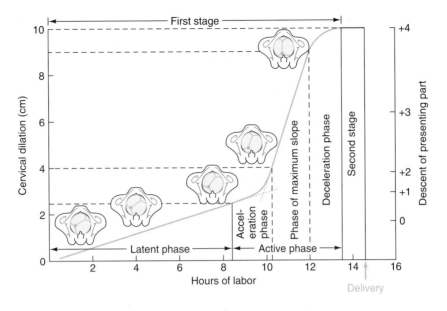

FIGURE 2.11-1. Stages of labor.

Cervical dilation, level of descent, and orientation of occipitoanterior presentation during various stages of labor. (Reproduced, with permission, from DeCherney AH. *Current Obstetric & Gynecologic Diagnosis & Treatment*, 8th ed. Stamford, CT: Appleton & Lange, 1994:211.)

- A "negative" CST (no late decelerations) is highly predictive of fetal well-being in conjunction with a normal NST (see Table 2.11-4 and Figure 2.11-2).
- **Biophysical profile (BPP):** Real-time ultrasound is used to assign a score of 2 (normal) or 0 (abnormal) to five parameters: fetal tone, breathing, movement, amniotic fluid volume, and NST.
  - A score of 8-10 is reassuring for fetal well-being.
  - A score of 0–2 is extremely worrisome for fetal asphyxia, and strong consideration should be given to immediate delivery if no nonhypoxic explanation is found.

> **When performing a BPP, remember to—**
>
> **Test the Baby, MAN!**
>
> Fetal **T**one
> Fetal **B**reathing
> Fetal **M**ovement
> **A**mniotic fluid volume
> **N**onstress test

TABLE 2.11-4. Fetal Heart Decelerations

TYPE	DESCRIPTION	MOST COMMON CAUSE
Early	Decelerations begin and end at approximately the same time as the maternal contraction.	Cephalic compression (**no fetal distress**).
Variable	Decelerations occur at any time during the maternal contraction.	Umbilical cord compression. Change mother's position (e.g., back to side).
Late	Decelerations begin at the peak of the contraction and persist until after the contraction has finished.	Uteroplacental insufficiency and fetal hypoxemia, possibly due to abruption or hypotension. Further testing for reassurance is necessary. If late decelerations are repetitive and severe, deliver the baby ASAP.

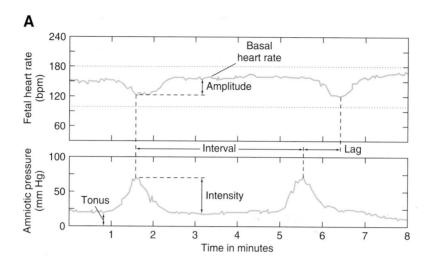

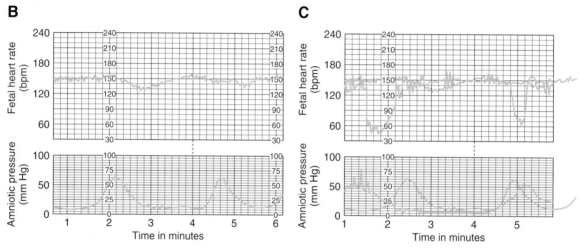

FIGURE 2.11-2. Fetal heart tracings.

(A) Schematic tracing. (B) Late deceleration. (C) Variable deceleration. (Reproduced, with permission, from DeCherney AH. *Current Obstetric & Gynecologic Diagnosis & Treatment*, 8th ed. Stamford, CT: Appleton & Lange, 1994:301.)

Hyperemesis Gravidarum

- **Intractable nausea and vomiting** that typically **persist beyond 14–16 weeks' gestation** → dehydration, electrolyte abnormalities, and **poor weight gain or weight loss.**
- More common in nulliparous and **molar pregnancies** (with ↑ β-hCG).
- **Hx/PE:** Differentiate from "morning sickness," acid reflux, and gastroenteritis.
- **Dx:** Evaluate for ketonemia, ketonuria, hyponatremia, and hypokalemic-hypochloremic metabolic alkalosis.
- **Rx:** Frequent small meals; antiemetics and IV hydration.

Gestational Diabetes Mellitus

Occurs in **3–5% of all pregnancies, usually in late pregnancy.** Hyperglycemia in the first trimester usually suggests preexisting diabetes. May result from insulin antagonist hormones from the placenta (e.g., HPL, cortisol). Risk factors include obesity, a family or personal history of diabetes, recurrent abortions, stillbirths, maternal age > 25 years, a prior macrosomic (> 4000 g) or congenitally deformed infant, and prior polyhydramnios.

HISTORY/PE

Typically asymptomatic. Edema, polyhydramnios, or a **large-for-GA infant (> 90th percentile) may be warning signs.**

DIAGNOSIS

- UA reveals glycosuria.
- Diagnosis requires two abnormal glucose tests from any of the following:
  - **Fasting serum glucose > 126 mg/dL.**
  - Random glucose > 200 mg/dL.
  - **Abnormal glucose challenge test,** routinely performed at 24–28 weeks' gestation. If > 140, a three-hour glucose tolerance test is required.
  - Confirm with a three-hour (100-g) glucose tolerance test showing any two of the following: fasting > 95 mg/dL; one hour > 180; two hours > 155; three hours > 140.

Hyperglycemia in the first trimester suggests preexisting diabetes.

TREATMENT

- **Mother:**
  - Tight maternal glucose control improves outcomes.
  - Start with the **ADA diet** and regular exercise.
  - **Add insulin** if dietary control is insufficient.
  - Give intrapartum insulin and dextrose to maintain tight control during delivery.
- **Fetus:**
  - Obtain periodic ultrasound and NSTs to assess fetal growth and well-being.
  - May need to induce labor at 39–40 weeks.

A fetus that is large for GA may indicate occult diabetes.

COMPLICATIONS

More than 50% of patients go on to **develop glucose intolerance and/or type 2 DM** later in life.

Pregestational Diabetes and Pregnancy

Poorly controlled DM (HbA$_{1C}$ > 8%) is associated with an ↑ **risk of congenital malformations** and ↑ maternal/fetal morbidity during labor and delivery.

TREATMENT

- **Mother:**
  - Routine prenatal screening/care and nutritional counseling.
  - Renal, ophthalmologic, and cardiac evaluation to assess for end-organ damage.
  - Strict glucose control (with insulin for type 1 DM) to minimize fetal defects.
    - **Fasting morning:** ≤ 90 mg/dL.
    - **Two-hour postprandial:** < 120 mg/dL.

TABLE 2.11-5. Complications of Pregestational Diabetes Mellitus

MATERNAL COMPLICATIONS	FETAL COMPLICATIONS
DKA (type 1) or HHNK (type 2)	Macrosomia
Preeclampsia/eclampsia	Cardiac and renal defects
Cephalopelvic disproportion (from macrosomia) and need for C-section	Neural tube defects (e.g., sacral agenesis)
	Hypocalcemia
Preterm labor	Polycythemia
Infection	Hyperbilirubinemia
Polyhydramnios	Intrauterine growth restriction (IUGR)
Postpartum hemorrhage	Hypoglycemia from hyperinsulinemia
Maternal mortality	Respiratory distress syndrome (RDS)
	Birth injury (e.g., shoulder dystocia)
	Perinatal mortality

- Fetus:
    - **16–20 weeks:** Ultrasound to determine fetal age and growth and to detect growth disturbances and polyhydramnios; triple screen to screen for developmental anomalies.
    - **20–22 weeks:** Ultrasound to evaluate for fetal cardiac anomalies.
    - **Third trimester:** Close fetal surveillance (e.g., NST, CST, BPP). Admit at 32–36 weeks if maternal DM has been poorly controlled or fetal parameters are a concern.
- Delivery and postpartum:
    - Maintain normoglycemia (80–100 mg/dL) during labor.
    - Consider early delivery if there is poor maternal glucose control, preeclampsia, macrosomia, or evidence of fetal lung maturity.
    - Cesarean delivery is indicated for fetal macrosomia.
- Continue glucose monitoring postpartum. Insulin needs rapidly ↓ after delivery.

COMPLICATIONS

See Table 2.11-5.

Gestational and Chronic Hypertension

- **Gestational hypertension** (formerly known as pregnancy-induced hypertension) is idiopathic hypertension without significant proteinuria (< 300 mg/L) that begins in the second half of pregnancy, during labor, or within 48 hours of delivery. Some patients may go on to develop preeclampsia. Retrospective diagnosis is made 1–12 weeks after delivery.
- **Chronic hypertension** is present before conception and at < 20 weeks' gestation or may persist for > 12 weeks postpartum. Treatment is as follows:
    - Monitor BP closely and treat with appropriate antihypertensives (e.g., methyldopa, β-blockers, hydralazine, calcium channel blockers).
    - **Do not give ACEIs or diuretics,** as ACEIs are known to → uterine ischemia and diuretics can aggravate low plasma volume to the point of uterine ischemia. Complications are similar to those of preeclampsia.

Preeclampsia and Eclampsia

- **Preeclampsia** is defined as **new-onset hypertension and proteinuria** occurring at > 20 weeks' gestation.
- **Eclampsia** is defined as preeclampsia plus **seizures**.
- **HELLP syndrome** is a variant of preeclampsia with a poor prognosis (see the mnemonic).
  - The etiology is unknown, but clinical manifestations are explained by vasospasm → hemorrhage and organ necrosis.
  - Risk factors include nulliparity, black ethnicity, extremes of age (< 20 or > 35), multiple gestation, molar pregnancy, renal disease (due to SLE or type 1 DM), a family history of preeclampsia, and chronic hypertension.
- **Hx/PE:** See Table 2.11-6 for the signs and symptoms of preeclampsia and eclampsia.
- **Dx:** Modalities include UA, 24-hour urine protein, CBC, electrolytes, BUN/creatinine, uric acid, precise measurement of fetal age, **amniocentesis** (to assess **fetal lung maturity**), LFTs, PT/PTT, fibrinogen and fibrin split products (for DIC), urine toxicology screen, ultrasound, and NST/CST/BPP (as indicated).
- **Rx:** The only cure for preeclampsia/eclampsia is **delivery of the fetus.** See Table 2.11-6 for management.

Teratogenic Drugs

Table 2.11-7 summarizes the effects of common teratogens.

Signs of severe preeclampsia are persistent headache or other cerebral or visual disturbances, persistent epigastric pain, and hyperreactive reflexes.

OBSTETRIC COMPLICATIONS OF PREGNANCY

Intrauterine Growth Restriction (IUGR)

Defined as fetal weight < 10th percentile for GA. Suspect IUGR if there is a discrepancy of > 4 between fundal height (in centimeters) and GA (in weeks) on exam. Occurs in 3–7% of pregnancies. See Table 2.11-8 for differences between symmetric and asymmetric IUGR.

DIAGNOSIS

- **Serial** ultrasound evaluation every 3–4 weeks.
- Fetal monitoring with NST, CST, and BPP; Doppler flow studies to evaluate umbilical artery flow.

TREATMENT

- **Steroids** (e.g., betamethasone) to accelerate fetal lung maturity.
- Consider early delivery, particularly with asymmetric IUGR, since uterine environment later in pregnancy is critical.

Oligohydramnios

- A deficiency of amniotic fluid volume defined as an **amniotic fluid index (AFI) < 5** on ultrasound. Without rupture of membranes (ROM), it is associated with a 40-fold ↑ in perinatal mortality.
- Etiologies include **fetal urinary tract abnormalities** (e.g., renal agenesis, polycystic kidney disease, GU obstruction), **chronic uteroplacental insufficiency** (associated with a small-for-GA fetus), or **ROM.**

Oligohydramnios almost always indicates the need to assess fetal well-being.

	SIGNS AND SYMPTOMS	MANAGEMENT	COMPLICATIONS
Mild preeclampsia	BP > **140/90** on two occasions > 6 hours apart. Rapid weight gain and nondependent edema. Proteinuria (> 300 mg/24 hrs or 1–2 ⊕ urine dipsticks).	If the patient is close to term or preeclampsia worsens, induce delivery with IV oxytocin, prostaglandins, or amniotomy. If the patient is far from term, treat with modified bed rest and **expectant management.**	Prematurity, fetal distress, stillbirth, placental abruption, seizure, DIC, cerebral hemorrhage, serous retinal detachment, fetal/maternal death.
Severe preeclampsia	BP > **160/110** on two occasions > 6 hours apart. **Renal:** Proteinuria (> 5 g/24 hrs or 3–4 ⊕ urine dipsticks) or oliguria (< 500 mL/24 hrs). **Cerebral changes:** Headache, somnolence. **Visual changes:** Blurred vision, scotomata. **Hyperactive reflexes/clonus.** **HELLP syndrome:** RUQ/epigastric pain. Oligohydramnios or IUGR.	**Control BP** with labetalol and/or hydralazine (goal < 160/110 with a diastolic BP of 90–100 to maintain fetal blood flow). Deliver by C-section if the mother is stable. **Prevent seizures with continuous magnesium sulfate (MgSO$_4$) drip.** Watch for signs of Mg^{2+} toxicity (loss DTRs, respiratory paralysis, coma). **Continue seizure prophylaxis for 24 hours postpartum.** Treat Mg^{2+} toxicity with IV Ca^{2+} gluconate.	Same as above.
Eclampsia	The most common signs preceding an eclamptic attack are **headache, visual changes,** and **RUQ/epigastric pain.** **Seizures** are severe if not controlled with anticonvulsant therapy.	ABCs with supplemental O$_2$. Seizure control/prophylaxis with **MgSO$_4$.** If seizures recur, give IV diazepam. Control BP (labetalol and/or hydralazine). Limit fluids; Foley for strict I/Os. Monitor Mg^{2+} blood levels and Mg^{2+} toxicity; monitor fetal status. Initiate delivery if the patient is stable and convulsions are controlled. Postpartum management is the same as that for preeclampsia. Seizures may occur antepartum (25%), intrapartum (50%), and postpartum (25%); most occur within 48 hours after delivery.	Cerebral hemorrhage, aspiration pneumonia, hypoxic encephalopathy, thromboembolic events, fetal/maternal death.

- **Hx/PE:** Usually asymptomatic, but IUGR or fetal distress may be present.
- **Dx:** Rule out inaccurate gestational dates.
- **Rx:** Treat the underlying cause if possible. Patients with ROM may benefit from amnio infusion.

TABLE 2.11-7. Common Teratogenic Drugs

Teratogen[a]	Effect
Alcohol	Fetal alcohol syndrome (microcephaly, midfacial hypoplasia, mental retardation, IUGR, cardiac defects).
Cocaine	Bowel atresias, IUGR, microcephaly.
Streptomycin	CN VIII damage/ototoxicity.
Tetracycline	Tooth discoloration, inhibition of bone growth, small limbs, syndactyly.
Sulfonamides	Kernicterus.
Quinolones	Cartilage damage.
Isotretinoin	Heart and great vessel defects, craniofacial dysmorphism, deafness.
Iodide	Congenital goiter, hypothyroidism, mental retardation.
Methotrexate	CNS malformations, craniofacial dysmorphism, IUGR.
DES	Clear cell adenocarcinoma of the vagina/cervix, genital tract abnormalities (cervical hood, T-shaped uterus, hypoplastic uterus), cervical incompetence.
Thalidomide	Limb reduction (phocomelia), ear and nasal anomalies, cardiac and lung defects, pyloric or duodenal stenosis, GI atresia.
Coumadin	Stippling of bone epiphyses, IUGR, nasal hypoplasia, mental retardation.
ACEIs	Oligohydramnios, fetal renal damage.
Lithium	Ebstein's anomaly, other cardiac diseases.
Carbamazepine	Fingernail hypoplasia, IUGR, microcephaly, neural tube defects.
Phenytoin	Nail hypoplasia, IUGR, mental retardation, craniofacial dysmorphism, microcephaly.
Valproic acid	Neural tube defects, craniofacial and skeletal defects.

[a] The fetus is most susceptible during gestational weeks 3–8 (organogenesis).

- **Complications:** Musculoskeletal abnormalities (e.g., clubfoot, facial distortion); **pulmonary hypoplasia;** fetal hypoxia due to umbilical cord compression and IUGR.

Polyhydramnios

- An excess of amniotic fluid volume, defined by an **AFI > 20** on ultrasound. May be present in normal pregnancies, but fetal chromosomal or developmental abnormalities are common.
- Etiologies include **maternal DM, multiple gestation,** isoimmunization, pulmonary abnormalities (e.g., cystic lung malformations), fetal anomalies

TABLE 2.11-8. Types of Intrauterine Growth Restriction

	SYMMETRIC	ASYMMETRIC
Prevalence	20% of cases	80% of cases
Ultrasonic parameters		
Biparietal diameter	↓	Normal
Head circumference	↓	Normal
Abdominal circumference	↓	↓
Femur length	↓	Normal
Time of insult	Early in pregnancy	Late in pregnancy
Etiology	Fetal problem:	Placenta mediated:
	Cytogenetic	Hypertension
	Infection	Poor nutrition
	Anomalies	Maternal smoking

(e.g., duodenal atresia, tracheoesophageal fistula, **anencephaly**), and twin-twin transfusion syndrome.

- **Hx/PE:** Usually asymptomatic, or exam may reveal fundal height greater than expected.
- **Dx:** Evaluation includes ultrasound for fetal anomalies, glucose testing for DM, and Rh screen.
- **Rx:** Etiology specific.
- **Complications:** Preterm labor, fetal malpresentation, cord prolapse.

Rhesus Isoimmunization

Rhesus (Rh) factor is an antigenic protein located on RBCs in Rh-⊕ individuals. Transmission is autosomal dominant. When fetal RBCs leak into maternal circulation, maternal anti-Rh IgG antibodies can form. These antibodies can cross the placenta → hemolysis of fetal Rh-⊕ RBCs (**erythroblastosis fetalis;** see Figure 2.11-3). Hemolytic disease usually occurs during the second

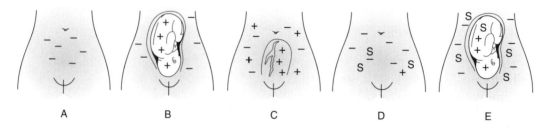

FIGURE 2.11-3. Rh disease.

(A) Rh-⊖ woman before pregnancy. (B) Pregnancy occurs. The fetus is Rh-⊕. (C) Separation of the placenta. (D) Following delivery, Rh isoimmunization occurs in the mother, and she develops antibodies (S = antibodies). (E) The next pregnancy with an Rh-⊕ fetus. Maternal antibodies cross the placenta, enter the bloodstream, and attach to Rh-⊕ cells, causing hemolysis. RhoGAM is given to the Rh-⊖ mother to prevent sensitization. (Adapted, with permission, from DeCherney AH. *Current Obstetric & Gynecologic Diagnosis & Treatment*, 8th ed. Stamford, CT: Appleton & Lange, 1994:339.)

pregnancy owing to rapid production of anti-Rh IgG antibodies by memory plasma cells.

HISTORY/PE

Inquire about prior events that may have exposed the mother to Rh-⊕ blood, including ectopic pregnancy, **abortion**, blood transfusions, **prior delivery of an Rh-⊕ child**, amniocentesis, or other traumatic procedures during pregnancy.

DIAGNOSIS

- **Maternal:** On initial visit, test for ABO and Rh blood groups and perform antibody screening (indirect Coombs' test). If ⊖, repeat Coombs' test at 26–28 weeks. If ⊕, test serially for high titers of maternal anti-Rh IgG (> 1:16).
- **Fetal:** Assess during pregnancy using amniocentesis or ultrasound-guided umbilical blood sampling for fetal blood type, Coombs' titer, bilirubin levels, hematocrit, and reticulocytes—or determine Rh status and hematocrit postnatally using fetal cord blood.

TREATMENT

- **Prevention:**
    - If the mother is Rh ⊖ at 28 weeks and (1) the father is Rh ⊕, (2) the father's Rh status is unknown, or (3) paternity is uncertain, **give RhoGAM (Rh immune globulin)**.
    - If the baby is Rh ⊕, give RhoGAM postpartum as well.
    - Give RhoGAM to Rh-⊖ mothers who undergo abortion (therapeutic or spontaneous) or who have had an ectopic pregnancy, amniocentesis, vaginal bleeding, or placenta previa/placental abruption.
- Sensitized Rh-⊖ mothers with titers > 1:16 should be closely monitored with serial ultrasound and amniocentesis for evidence of fetal hemolysis.
- In severe cases, initiate preterm delivery when fetal lungs are mature.
- Prior to delivery, intrauterine blood transfusions may be given to correct a low fetal hematocrit.

RhoGAM (Rh immune globulin) destroys Rh-⊕ cells in maternal circulation and prevents Rh sensitization.

COMPLICATIONS

- Fetal hypoxia and acidosis, kernicterus, prematurity, death.
- **Hydrops fetalis** (↓ protein and oncotic pressure, edema, jaundice, high-output cardiac failure) occurs when hemoglobin drops to < 7 g/dL.

Gestational Trophoblastic Disease (GTD)

A range of proliferative trophoblastic abnormalities that can be benign (e.g., hydatidiform mole) or malignant (e.g., choriocarcinoma). Risk factors for GTD include extremes of age (< 20 or > 40), a diet deficient in folate or β-carotene, and blood group (e.g., a type A woman impregnated by a type O man). Molar pregnancy may progress to malignant GTD, including invasive moles (10–15%) and choriocarcinoma (2–5%). **Hydatidiform mole** (or molar pregnancy) accounts for approximately **80% of cases of GTD**. Subtypes are as follows:

Preeclampsia in the first trimester is pathognomonic for hydatidiform mole.

- **Complete moles:** Usually result from sperm fertilization of an empty ovum; have a chromosomal pattern of 46,**XX** and are paternally derived.
- **Incomplete (partial) moles:** Result when a normal ovum is fertilized by two sperm (or a haploid sperm that duplicates its chromosomes). Usually have a chromosomal pattern of 69,**XXY** and **contain fetal tissue.**

History/PE

- Presents with first-trimester **uterine bleeding** (most common), **hyperemesis gravidarum, preeclampsia/eclampsia** at < 24 weeks, **uterine size greater than dates**, and hyperthyroidism (hypertension, tachycardia, tachypnea). No fetal heartbeat is detected.
- Pelvic exam may reveal enlarged ovaries with bilateral theca-lutein cysts that will resolve after treatment. It may also reveal possible **expulsion of grapelike molar clusters** into the vagina or blood in the cervical os.

Partial moles can contain fetal parts.

Diagnosis

- Look for **markedly ↑ serum β-hCG** (usually > 100,000 mIU/mL) and a **"snowstorm" appearance on pelvic ultrasound** with no gestational sac or fetus present.
- CXR may show lung metastases.

Treatment

- D&C reveals "cluster-of-grapes" tissue (see Figure 2.11-4).
- **Type and screen is critical; follow β-hCG** closely and **prevent pregnancy for one year** to ensure accurate monitoring.
- Treat malignant disease with **chemotherapy** (methotrexate or dactinomycin) and **residual uterine disease with hysterectomy.**
- Chemotherapy and irradiation are highly successful for metastases (90%).

Complete hydatidiform mole has a "snowstorm" appearance on pelvic ultrasound.

Complications

Malignant GTD, pulmonary or CNS metastases, trophoblastic pulmonary emboli, acute respiratory insufficiency.

Third-Trimester Bleeding

- Any bleeding **after 20 weeks' gestation.** Prior to 20 weeks, bleeding is referred to as threatened abortion.
- Complicates 3–5% of pregnancies.
- The **most common causes are placental abruption and placenta previa** (see Table 2.11-9 and Figure 2.11-5).

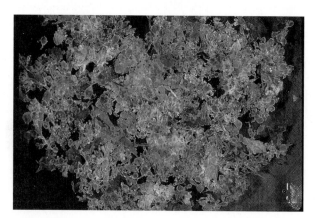

FIGURE 2.11-4.   Hydatidiform mole.

Note the characteristic "bunch-of-grapes" appearance on this gross specimen. (Reproduced courtesy of Dr. Raoul Fresco, Loyola University.)

TABLE 2.11-9. Placental Abruption vs. Placenta Previa

	PLACENTAL ABRUPTION	PLACENTA PREVIA
Pathophysiology	**Premature** (before onset of labor) **separation** of normally implanted placenta.	**Abnormal placental implantation:** ▪ **Total:** Placenta covers cervical os. ▪ **Marginal:** Placenta extends to margin of os. ▪ **Low-lying:** Placenta in close proximity to os.
Incidence	1 in 100.	1 in 200.
Risk factors	Hypertension, abdominal/pelvic trauma, tobacco or cocaine use, previous abruption, rapid decompression of overdistended uterus.	Prior C-sections, grand multiparous, advanced maternal age, multiple gestation, prior placenta previa.
Symptoms	**Painful, dark** vaginal bleeding that does not spontaneously cease. Abdominal pain, uterine hypertonicity. Fetal distress.	**Painless, bright red** bleeding that often ceases in 1–2 hours with or without uterine contractions. First bleeding episode at 29–30 weeks. Usually no fetal distress.
Diagnosis	**Primarily clinical.** Transabdominal/transvaginal ultrasound sensitivity is only 50%; look for retroplacental clot; most useful for ruling out previa.	**Transabdominal/transvaginal ultrasound sensitivity is > 95%;** look for abnormally positioned placenta.
Management	Stabilize patient with mild abruption and premature fetus; **manage expectantly** (hospitalize, start IV and fetal monitoring; type and cross blood, bed rest). **Moderate to severe abruption:** Immediate delivery (vaginal delivery with amniotomy if mother and fetus are stable; C-section for maternal or fetal distress).	**NO vaginal exam!** **Stabilize patient with premature fetus;** manage expectantly. Give tocolytics ($MgSO_4$). Serial ultrasound to assess fetal growth; resolution of partial previa. Assess fetal lung maturity with amniocentesis and augment with betamethasone. **Deliver by C-section. Indications for delivery include persistent labor, life-threatening bleeding, fetal distress, documented fetal lung maturity, and 36 weeks' GA.**
Complications	Hemorrhagic shock. Coagulopathy: **DIC** in 10%. Recurrence risk is 5–16%; rises to 25% after two previous abruptions. Fetal hypoxia.	↑ risk of placenta accreta. Vasa previa (fetal vessels crossing the internal os). Preterm delivery, premature rupture of membranes (PROM), IUGR, congenital anomalies. Recurrence risk is 4–8%.

▪ Other causes include bloody show, ruptured vasa previa, early labor, ruptured uterus, marginal placental separation, genital tract lesions and trauma, and placenta accreta (placental adherence to myometrium).

HIGH-YIELD FACTS

OBSTETRICS

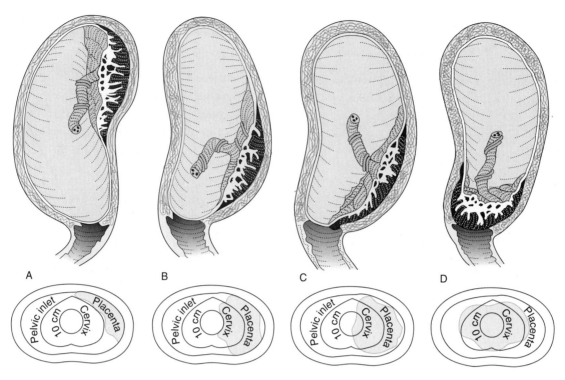

FIGURE 2.11-5. **Placental implantation.**

(A) Normal placenta. (B) Low implantation. (C) Partial placenta previa. (D) Complete placenta previa. (Adapted, with permission, from DeCherney AH. *Current Obstetric & Gynecologic Diagnosis & Treatment*, 8th ed. Stamford, CT: Appleton & Lange, 1994:404.)

ABNORMAL LABOR AND DELIVERY

Failure to Progress

- Risk factors include chorioamnionitis, postdated pregnancy, occiput posterior position, nulliparity, epidural anesthesia, macrosomia, pregnancy complications, nonreassuring fetal heart rate, older maternal age, high station at full dilatation, and pelvic contraction.
- Table 2.11-10 outlines the stages of failure to progress and delineates its treatment.

Premature Rupture of Membranes (PROM)

Defined as **spontaneous ROM** before onset of labor. May be precipitated by vaginal or cervical infections, abnormal membrane physiology, and cervical incompetence. Preterm PROM occurs at < 37 weeks' gestation. Prolonged ROM is defined as rupture > 18 hours prior to delivery. Risk factors include low socioeconomic status (SES), young maternal age, smoking, and STDs.

HISTORY/PE

Patients often report a **"gush"** of clear or blood-tinged amniotic fluid. Uterine contractions may be present.

TABLE 2.11-10.   Failure to Progress

STAGE	DEFINITION	TREATMENT
First		
Latent	Failure to have progressive cervical change: ■ **Prima:** > 20 hours ■ **Multi:** > 14 hours	Therapeutic rest via parenteral analgesia; oxytocin; amniotomy; cervical ripening.
Active	Failure to have progressive cervical change after reaching 3–4 cm.	Amniotomy; oxytocin; C-section if the previous interventions are ineffective.
Second	Arrest of fetal descent: ■ **Prima:** > 3 hours ■ **Multi:** > 2 hours	Close observation with a ↓ in epidural rate and continued oxytocin. Assisted vaginal delivery (forceps or vacuum). C-section.

DIAGNOSIS

- Sterile speculum exam reveals **pooling** of amniotic fluid in the vaginal vault, a ⊕ **Nitrazine paper test** (paper turns blue in alkaline amniotic fluid), and a ⊕ **fern test** (a ferning pattern is seen under a microscope after amniotic fluid dries on a glass slide).
- Ultrasound to assess amniotic fluid volume.
- Cultures or smears to rule out infections. Minimize infection risk; **do not** perform digital vaginal exams if gestational age is less than 34 weeks.
- Check fetal heart tracing, maternal temperature, WBC count, and uterine tenderness for evidence of chorioamnionitis.

TREATMENT

- **Depends on GA and fetal lung maturity.** In general, if there is no sign of infection, delivery is delayed with **tocolytics** in the form of β-agonists (e.g., ritodrine, terbutaline), magnesium, NSAIDs (e.g., indomethacin), or calcium channel blockers (e.g., nifedipine).
- **Prophylactic antibiotics** are given to prevent infection.
- **Corticosteroids** (e.g., betamethasone or dexamethasone × 48 hours) can be given to promote fetal lung maturity.
- If signs of infection or fetal distress develop, give antibiotics (ampicillin and gentamicin) and induce labor. If the patient is penicillin allergic, gentamicin and clindamycin are appropriate.

COMPLICATIONS

Preterm labor and delivery, chorioamnionitis, placental abruption, cord prolapse.

Preterm Labor

Defined as onset of labor between **20 and 37 weeks' gestation.** Occurs in approximately 10% of all U.S. pregnancies and is the 1° cause of neonatal morbidity and mortality. Risk factors include multiple gestation, infection, PROM, uterine anomalies, previous preterm labor or delivery, polyhydramnios, placental abruption, poor maternal nutrition, and low SES. **Most patients have no identifiable risk factors.**

To minimize the risk of infection, do not perform digital vaginal exams on women with PROM at < 34 weeks' GA.

HISTORY/PE

Patients may have menstrual-like cramps, onset of low back pain, pelvic pressure, and new vaginal discharge or bleeding.

DIAGNOSIS

- Requires **regular uterine contractions** ($\geq$ 3 contractions of 30 seconds each over a 30-minute period) and **concurrent cervical change** at < 37 weeks' gestation.
- **Assess for contraindications to tocolysis** (e.g., infection, nonreassuring fetal testing, placental abruption).
- Perform a **sterile speculum exam** to rule out PROM.
- Obtain an **ultrasound** to rule out fetal or uterine anomalies, verify GA, and assess fetal presentation and amniotic fluid volume.
- Obtain cultures for chlamydia, gonorrhea, and group B strep. Obtain a UA and urine culture.

Preterm labor = regular uterine contractions + concurrent cervical change at < 37 weeks' gestation.

TREATMENT

- Hydration and bed rest.
- Unless contraindicated, begin **tocolytic therapy** and give **steroids** to accelerate fetal lung maturation. Give **penicillin or ampicillin for group B strep prophylaxis** if preterm delivery is likely.

COMPLICATIONS

RDS, intraventricular hemorrhage, PDA, necrotizing enterocolitis, retinopathy of prematurity, bronchopulmonary dysplasia, death.

Fetal Malpresentation

Breech presentation is the most common fetal malpresentation.

Defined as any presentation other than vertex (i.e., head closest to birth canal, chin to chest, occiput anterior). Risk factors include **prematurity**, prior breech delivery, uterine anomalies, poly- or oligohydramnios, multiple gestations, preterm PROM, hydrocephalus, anencephaly, and placenta previa. **Breech presentations** are the most common (3% of all deliveries) and involve presentation of the fetal lower extremities or buttocks into the maternal pelvis (see Figure 2.11-6). Subtypes include the following:

- **Frank breech (50–75%):** Thighs are flexed and knees are extended.
- **Footling breech (20%):** One or both legs are extended below the buttocks.
- **Complete breech (5–10%):** Thighs and knees are flexed.

DIAGNOSIS

Use Leopold maneuvers (a series of uterine palpations) to identify fetal lie (transverse or vertical) and presentation (vertex or breech).

TREATMENT

- **Follow:** Up to 75% spontaneously change to vertex by week 38.
- **External version:** If the fetus has not reverted spontaneously, apply pressure to the maternal abdomen to turn the infant to vertex. The success rate is roughly 75%. Risks are placental abruption and cord compression, so be prepared for an emergency C-section if needed.
- **Trial of breech vaginal delivery:** Attempt **only if delivery is imminent;** otherwise contraindicated. Complications include cord prolapse and/or head entrapment.

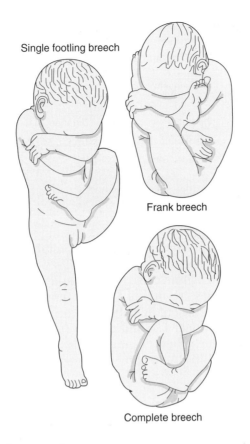

Single footling breech

Frank breech

Complete breech

FIGURE 2.11-6. Types of breech presentations.

(Reproduced, with permission, from DeCherney AH. *Current Obstetric & Gynecologic Diagnosis & Treatment*, 8th ed. Stamford, CT: Appleton & Lange, 1994:411.)

- **Elective C-section:** The standard of care in many hospitals, but it has not been shown to improve outcome.

Indications for Cesarean Section

See Table 2.11-11 for indications.

PUERPERIUM

Postpartum Hemorrhage

- Defined as a loss of **> 500 mL of blood for vaginal delivery** or **> 1000 mL for C-section** occurring before, during, or after delivery of the placenta. Table 2.11-12 summarizes common causes.
- Complications include acute blood loss (potentially fatal), anemia due to chronic blood loss (predisposes to puerperal infection), and **Sheehan's syndrome** (see below).

Postpartum Infections

- Genital tract infection with a temperature ≥ **38°C** for **at least two of the first ten postpartum days (not including the first 24 hours).**

TABLE 2.11-11. **Indications for Cesarean Section**

Maternal Factors	Fetal and Maternal Factors	Fetal Factors
Prior classical C-section (vertical incision predisposes to uterine rupture with vaginal delivery)	Cephalopelvic disproportion (most common cause of 1° C-section)	Fetal malposition (e.g., posterior chin, transverse lie, shoulder presentation)
Active genital herpes infection	Placenta previa/placental abruption	Fetal distress
Cervical carcinoma	Failed operative vaginal delivery	Cord compression
Maternal trauma/demise	Post-term pregnancy (relative indication)	Erythroblastosis fetalis (Rh incompatibility)

- Endometrial infection is most common. Incidence is ↑ after C-section.
- Risk factors include emergent C-section, PROM, prolonged labor, multiple intrapartum vaginal exams, and intrauterine manipulations.
- Etiologies are outlined in the mnemonic **the 7 W's.** Perform a pelvic exam to rule out hematoma or lochial block.
- **Dx:** Consider UA and culture (for UTI) and blood cultures (for sepsis). Consider other diagnoses (e.g., pelvic abscess, **septic pelvic thrombophlebitis**) if the three-drug regimen is not effective after 48 hours.

TABLE 2.11-12. **Common Causes of Postpartum Hemorrhage**

	Uterine Atony	Genital Tract Trauma	Retained Placental Tissue
Risk factors	Uterine overdistention (multiple gestation, macrosomia, polyhydramnios). Exhausted myometrium (rapid or prolonged labor, oxytocin stimulation). Uterine infection. Conditions interfering with contractions (anesthesia, myomas, $MgSO_4$).	Precipitous labor. Operative vaginal delivery (forceps, vacuum extraction). Large infant. Inadequate episiotomy repair.	Placenta accreta/increta/percreta. Placenta previa. Uterine leiomyomas. Preterm delivery. Previous C-section/curettage.
Diagnosis	Palpation of soft, enlarged, "boggy" uterus. **Most common cause of postpartum hemorrhage (90%).**	Manual and visual inspection of lower genital tract for any laceration > 2 cm long.	Manual and visual inspection of placenta and uterine cavity for missing cotyledons. Ultrasound may also be used to inspect uterus.
Treatment[a]	Bimanual **uterine massage** (usually successful). **Oxytocin** infusion. **Methergine** (methylergonovine) if not hypertensive. **Prostin** ($PGF_{2\alpha}$) if not asthmatic.	Surgical repair of the physical defect.	Manual removal of remaining placental tissue. Curettage with suctioning (take care not to perforate the uterine fundus).

[a] For all uterine causes, when bleeding persists after conventional therapy, uterine/internal iliac artery ligation or hysterectomy can be lifesaving.

- **Rx:** Hospitalize and give **broad-spectrum IV antibiotics** (e.g., clindamycin and gentamicin) **until patients have been afebrile for 48 hours.** Add ampicillin for complicated cases.

Sheehan's Syndrome (Postpartum Pituitary Necrosis)

- Defined as pituitary ischemia and necrosis → anterior pituitary insufficiency 2° to massive obstetric hemorrhage and shock.
- The 1° cause of anterior pituitary insufficiency in adult females. The **most common presenting syndrome is failure to lactate** (due to ↓ prolactin levels).
- Other symptoms include weakness, lethargy, cold insensitivity, genital atrophy, and menstrual disorders.

Lactation and Breast-Feeding

- **Physiology:** During pregnancy, ↑ estrogen and progesterone → breast hypertrophy and inhibition of prolactin release. After delivery of the placenta, hormone levels ↓ markedly and prolactin is released, stimulating milk production. Periodic infant suckling → further release of **prolactin** and **oxytocin,** which stimulate myoepithelial cell contraction and milk ejection ("let-down reflex").
- **Breast-feeding:** Colostrum ("early breast milk") contains protein, fat, **secretory IgA,** and minerals. Within one week postpartum, mature milk with protein, fat, lactose, and water is produced.
    - High IgA levels in colostrum provide passive immunity for the infant and protect against enteric bacteria.
    - Other benefits include ↓ incidence of allergies, facilitation of mother-child bonding, and maternal weight loss.
    - Contraindications to breast-feeding include HIV infection, active HBV and HCV, and use of certain medications (e.g., tetracycline, chloramphenicol, warfarin).

Mastitis

- Cellulitis of the periglandular tissue caused by nipple trauma from breast-feeding coupled with introduction of **S. aureus** from the infant's nostrils into the nipple ducts.
- **Hx/PE:** Symptoms often begin 2–4 weeks postpartum; are **usually unilateral;** and include focal breast tenderness, erythema, edema, warmth, and possible purulent nipple drainage.
- **Dx:** Differentiate from simple breast engorgement. Infection is suggested by focal symptoms, a ⊕ breast milk culture, ↑ WBC count, and fever.
- **Rx: Continued breast-feeding** and PO antibiotics (e.g., penicillin, dicloxacillin, erythromycin). Incision and drainage of breast abscess if present.

SPONTANEOUS ABORTION (SAB)

Loss of the fetus prior to the 20th week of pregnancy. Some 75% of cases occur before the 16th week, with 75% of these occurring before the eighth week. Approximately 20% of clinically recognized pregnancies terminate in SAB. ↑ risk is associated with a history of incompetent cervix, cervical coniza-

The 7 W's of post-partum fever:

Womb (endomyometritis)
Wind (atelectasis, pneumonia)
Water (UTI)
Walk (DVT, pulmonary embolism)
Wound (incision, episiotomy)
Weaning (breast engorgement, abscess, mastitis)
Wonder drugs (drug fever)

Breast-feeding is contraindicated in maternal HIV infection, active hepatitis, and use of certain medications.

The treatment of mastitis includes antibiotics and continued breast-feeding.

TABLE 2.11-13. **Types of Spontaneous Abortion**

TYPE	DESCRIPTION	DIAGNOSIS	TREATMENT
Complete	All products of conception (POC) expelled; pain ceases, but spotting may persist.	Os is closed; ultrasound shows empty uterus. POC is submitted to pathology to confirm fetal tissue.	D&C if ↑ likelihood that abortion was incomplete.
Incomplete	Mild cramping and bleeding; some POC expelled. Visible tissue in the vagina or endocervical canal.	Os is open; ultrasound reveals retained fetal tissue.	D&C to remove remaining POC and to control bleeding. Hemodynamic stabilization for heavy bleeding.
Threatened	No POC expelled; membranes remain intact. Uterine bleeding is present; abdominal pain may be present. The fetus is still viable.	Os is closed; ultrasound is normal.	Avoid heavy activity. Pelvic rest for 24–48 hours with gradual resumption of activities, but abstinence from coitus and douching.
Inevitable	No POC expelled, but considered inevitable. Uterine bleeding and cramps.	Os is open +/– ROM.	D&C or expectant management. Surgical evacuation of uterine contents. Prostaglandin suppositories are an alternative.
Missed	Pregnancy has ceased to develop. No POC is expelled; fetal tissue is retained. No uterine bleeding; symptoms of pregnancy disappear. Brownish vaginal discharge.	Os is closed; ultrasound reveals **no fetal cardiac activity. Fetal tissue is retained.**	D&C; prostaglandin suppositories are an alternative. DIC is a serious but rare complication whose risk ↑ with ↑ GA.
Septic	Infection with abortion. Endometritis → septicemia. Maternal mortality is 10–15%.	Hypotension, hypothermia, oliguria, respiratory distress if in shock; ↑ WBC.	Complete uterine evacuation, D&C; IV antibiotics.
Recurrent	≥ 2 consecutive SABs or a total of three SABs. If early, often due to chromosomal abnormalities → karyotyping of both parents. Incompetent cervix should be suspected with a history of painless dilation of the cervix and delivery of a normal fetus between 18 and 32 weeks.	**Evaluate for uterine abnormalities.** Cervical cultures for gonococcus, chlamydia, and group B streptococcus should be obtained before the procedure.	Surgical cerclage procedures to suture the cervix closed until labor or ROM occurs with subsequent removal prior to delivery. Restriction of activities.
Intrauterine fetal demise	Absence of fetal cardiac activity.	Uterus small for GA; no fetal heart tones or movement on ultrasound.	Induce labor and evacuate the uterus to avoid DIC at GA > 16 weeks.

tion or loop electrosurgical excision procedure (LEEP), cervical injury, DES exposure, and anatomical abnormalities of the cervix. Additional risk factors are as follows:

- **First trimester: Fetal factors (chromosomal abnormalities).**
- **Second trimester:** Maternal factors (cervical incompetence, infection, hypercoagulable states); maternal trauma, infection, dietary deficiency, DM, hypothyroidism, or anatomic malformation.

HISTORY/PE

See Table 2.11-13 for types of SAB.

DIAGNOSIS

- ↓ levels of hCG.
- **Ultrasound:**
    - Can identify the gestational sac 5–6 weeks from the LMP, a fetal pole at six weeks, and fetal cardiac activity at 6–7 weeks.
    - With accurate dating, a small, irregular intrauterine sac without a fetal pole on transvaginal ultrasound is diagnostic of an abnormal pregnancy.
- CBC is warranted in the presence of heavy bleeding.
- **Maternal Rh type should be determined and RhoGAM given if the type is Rh ⊖.**
- All recovered tissue should be preserved and assessed by a pathologist and sent for chromosomal analysis.

COMPLICATIONS

Retained tissue and prolonged bleeding can occur with prostaglandin use.

Gynecology

The differential diagnosis of a breast mass includes fibrocystic disease, fibroadenoma, mastitis/abscess, fat necrosis, and breast cancer.

Intraductal papilloma is a common cause of bloody nipple discharge.

Fibrocystic Breast Disease

Exaggerated stromal tissue response to hormones and growth factors. Microscopic findings include cysts (gross and microscopic), papillomatosis, adenosis, fibrosis, and ductal epithelial hyperplasia. Primarily affects women 30–50 years of age; rarely found in postmenopausal woman. Associated with trauma and caffeine use.

HISTORY/PE

- Presents with **painful, often multiple masses in both breasts.**
- Nipple discharge may also be present.
- Rapid **fluctuation** in the size of the masses is common.
- During the premenstrual phase, pain and mass size ↑.

DIAGNOSIS

- See Figure 2.12-1 for an algorithm of a breast mass workup.
- Mammography is of limited use. Ultrasound can help differentiate a cystic from a solid mass.
- Aspiration of a discrete mass that is suggestive of a cyst is indicated to alleviate pain as well as to confirm the cystic nature of the mass.
    - Fine-needle aspiration (FNA) cytology or needle biopsy of suspicious lesions may be used.

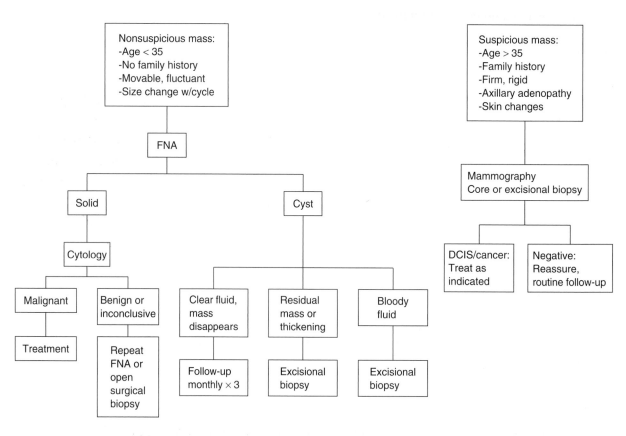

FIGURE 2.12-1. Workup of a breast mass.

- Perform an excisional biopsy if no fluid is obtained or if the fluid is bloody on aspiration.
- There is an ↑ risk of **breast cancer** if ductal epithelial hyperplasia or cellular atypia is present.

TREATMENT

- Danazol may be given for severe pain but is rarely used owing to its side effects (acne, hirsutism, edema).
- Simple mastectomy or extensive removal of breast tissue is rarely indicated.

Fibroadenoma

A benign, slow-growing breast tumor with epithelial and stromal components. **The most common breast lesion in women < 30 years of age.** Cystosarcoma phyllodes is a large fibroadenoma.

HISTORY/PE

- Presents as a round or ovoid, rubbery, discrete, relatively mobile, nontender mass 1–5 cm in diameter.
- Does not occur after menopause unless the patient is on HRT.

DIAGNOSIS

- **Breast ultrasound** can differentiate cystic from solid masses.
- **Needle biopsy or FNA.**
- Excision with pathologic exam if the diagnosis remains uncertain.

TREATMENT

Excision is curative, but recurrence is common.

Breast Cancer

The most common cancer (affects one in nine women) and the second most common cause of cancer death in women (after lung cancer). The distribution by quadrant is as follows: **45% occur in the upper outer quadrant**, 15% in the upper inner quadrant, 5% in the lower inner quadrant, 10% in the lower outer quadrant, and 25% in the subareolar area. Risk factors include the following:

- Female gender, older age.
- Breast cancer in a first-degree relative.
- BRCA1 and BRCA2 mutations (associated with early onset).
- A personal history of breast cancer.
- A **high-fat and low-fiber diet.**
- A history of fibrocystic change with cellular atypia.
- ↑ **exposure to estrogen (nulliparity, early menarche, late menopause).**
- First full-term pregnancy after age 35.
- Late menarche is associated with ↓ risk.

HISTORY/PE

- **Early findings:** May present as a single, nontender, firm-to-hard mass with ill-defined margins or as mammographic abnormalities with no palpable mass.

↑ exposure to estrogen (early menarche, late menopause, nulliparity) ↑ the risk of breast cancer.

- **Later findings:** Skin or nipple retraction, axillary lymphadenopathy, breast enlargement, redness, edema, pain, fixation of mass to the skin or chest wall.
- **Late findings:**
  - Ulceration; supraclavicular lymphadenopathy; edema of the arm; metastases to the bone, lung, and liver.
  - Prolonged unilateral scaling erosion of the nipple with or without discharge (may be Paget's disease of the nipple).
- **Metastatic disease:**
  - Back or bone pain, jaundice, weight loss.
  - A firm or hard axillary node > 1 cm.
  - Axillary nodes that are matted or fixed to the skin (stage III); ipsilateral supraclavicular or infraclavicular nodes (stage IV).

DIAGNOSIS

Diagnostic measures are as follows (see also Figure 2.12-1):

- **Mammography:** Look for ↑ density with microcalcifications and irregular borders.
- **Ultrasound:** To distinguish a solid mass from a benign cyst.
- **Tumor markers for recurrent breast cancer: CEA and CA 15-3 or CA 27-29.**
- **Receptor status of tumor:** Determine estrogen receptor (ER), progesterone receptor (PR), and HER2/neu status.
- **Metastatic disease:**
  - **Labs:** ↑ ESR, ↑ alkaline phosphatase (liver and bone metastases), ↑ calcium.
  - **CXR:** To evaluate for pulmonary metastases.
  - **CT of the chest, abdomen, pelvis, and brain:** To look for metastases.
  - **Bone scan:** ↑ uptake indicates metastases to bone.

TREATMENT

- **Pharmacologic:**
  - All hormone receptor–⊕ patients should receive tamoxifen.
  - ER-⊖ patients should receive chemotherapy.
  - **Trastuzumab,** a monoclonal antibody that binds to HER2/neu receptors on the cancer cell, is highly effective in HER2/neu-expressive cancers.
- **Surgical options** include the following:
  - Partial mastectomy plus axillary dissection followed by radiation therapy.
  - Modified radical mastectomy (total mastectomy plus axillary dissection).
  - **Contraindications to breast-conserving therapy** include large tumor size, subareolar location, multifocal tumors, fixation to the chest wall, or involvement of the nipple or overlying skin.
  - Invasive cancer requires axillary dissection.
- **Stage IV:** Treat with radiotherapy and hormonal therapy; mastectomy may be required for local symptom control.
- **TNM staging (I–IV) is the most reliable indicator of prognosis.**
  - ER- and PR-⊕ status is associated with a favorable course.
  - Cancer localized to the breast has a 75–90% cure rate. With spread to the axilla, the five-year survival is 40–50%.
  - Aneuploidy is associated with a poor prognosis.

COMPLICATIONS

Pleural effusion occurs in 50% of patients with metastatic breast cancer; edema of the arm is common.

CONTRACEPTION

- The relative advantages and disadvantages of common contraceptive methods are outlined in Table 2.12-1.

TABLE 2.12-1. Contraceptive Methods

METHOD	DESCRIPTION/ADVANTAGES	DISADVANTAGES
Behavioral methods		
Rhythm	Uses body temperature and cervical mucus consistency to predict time of fertility.	Unreliable compared to other methods.
Coitus interruptus	Withdrawal of the penis before ejaculation.	High failure rate.
Barrier methods		
Diaphragm/cervical cap	A dome-shaped sheet of rubber or latex placed over the cervix. Must be fitted by a physician and remain in the vagina 6–8 hours after intercourse.	Possible allergy to latex or spermicides; risk of UTI and toxic shock syndrome (TSS).
Condoms	A latex sheath covers the penis during intercourse.	Possible allergy to latex or spermicides.
IUD	A plastic/metal device placed in the uterus; → a local sterile inflammatory reaction within the uterine wall such that sperm are engulfed and destroyed.	↑ vaginal bleeding, uterine perforation, IUD migration, infection, ↑ risk of PID and ectopic pregnancy.
Hormonal methods		
OCPs (combination estrogen and progestin)	Suppress ovulation by inhibiting FSH/LH; change the consistency of cervical mucus, making the endometrium unsuitable for implantation. Highly reliable, with a failure rate < 1%. Protect against endometrial and ovarian cancer; associated with an ↓ incidence of pelvic infections and ectopic pregnancy. Menses are more predictable, lighter, and less painful.	Require daily compliance; no STD protection; 10–30% have breakthrough bleeding; ↑ risk of thromboembolism (pulmonary embolism, DVT). Side effects of estrogen include bloating, weight gain, breast tenderness, nausea, and headache. Side effects of progestin include depression, acne, and hypertensive crisis.
Progestin-only "minipills"	**Lactating women can use;** can start immediately postpartum. No effect on milk production or on the baby.	Higher failure rate than OCPs (ovulation continues in 40%); requires strict compliance (taking pill at the same time each day).
Depo-Provera (medroxyprogesterone)	Provides contraception for > 1 year; eliminates noncompliance with daily OCPs; can be used by lactating women. IM injection every three months for a maximum of two years.	Irregular vaginal bleeding; 50% of patients are infertile for 10 months after last injection.

TABLE 2.12-1. Contraceptive Methods (continued)

METHOD	DESCRIPTION/ADVANTAGES	DISADVANTAGES
Hormonal methods (continued)		
Levonorgestrel (Norplant)	Progestin-only subdermal implant. Suppresses ovulation, thickens cervical mucus, and makes the endometrium unsuitable for implantation. Subcutaneous implants provide contraception for five years. Prompt fertility when discontinued.	Some 30% of breakthrough pregnancies are ectopic. Also associated with irregular vaginal bleeding, weight gain, galactorrhea, acne, breast tenderness, and headache. Can be difficult to remove.
Postcoital "morning-after pill"	Progesterone +/− estrogen taken within 72 hours of unprotected sex to suppress ovulation or inhibit implantation	Nausea, vomiting, fatigue, headache, dizziness, breast tenderness.
Surgical sterilization		
Tubal litigation, vasectomy	Tubes are ligated, cauterized, or mechanically occluded.	Essentially irreversible; associated with bleeding, infection, failure, and ectopic pregnancy.

- **Absolute contraindications to OCPs** are as follows:
  - Pregnancy.
  - A history of thromboembolic disorders (past or present).
  - A history of stroke or CAD (past or present).
  - Breast cancer (known or suspected).
  - Undiagnosed abnormal vaginal bleeding.
  - Estrogen-dependent cancer (known or suspected).
  - A benign or malignant tumor of the liver (past or present).
  - Cigarette smoking in women > 35 years of age.
- **Absolute contraindications to IUD use** include the following:
  - Pregnancy.
  - A history of PID.
  - Acute cervical, uterine, or salpingeal infection.
  - Suspected gynecologic malignancy.
  - Undiagnosed abnormal vaginal bleeding.

DYSMENORRHEA

1° Dysmenorrhea

Menstrual pain associated with ovulatory cycles in the **absence of pathologic findings.** Caused by uterine vasoconstriction, anoxia, and sustained contractions mediated by prostaglandin. Onset is within 1–2 years of menarche; may become more severe with time. The frequency of cases ↑ up to age 20 and then ↓ with age.

- Hx/PE:
  - Presents with low, midline, wavelike, crampy pelvic pain that often radiates to the back or inner thighs.
  - Cramps may last for one or more days and may be associated with nausea, diarrhea, headache, and flushing.
  - No pathologic findings on pelvic exam.

- **Dx:** Diagnosis is by clinical impression.
- **Rx:** NSAIDs; OCPs may be given to suppress ovulation.

2° Dysmenorrhea

Menstrual pain for which an organic cause exists (e.g., endometriosis). Onset is after menarche, sometimes in the 30–40s.

- **Hx/PE:** Look for findings that point to organic causes such as endometriosis or PID.
- **Dx: Laparoscopy** to differentiate endometriosis from PID; **MRI** to detect submucous myomas.
- **Rx:** Etiology specific.

Endometriosis

An aberrant growth of endometrium outside the uterus, particularly in the dependent parts of the pelvis and ovaries. Has a 2% prevalence among fertile women. **Adenomyosis is endometrial tissue in the myometrium that makes the uterus symmetrically enlarged and globular.**

HISTORY/PE

- Pain does not correlate with the extent of disease.
- Cyclic pain begins 2–7 days before the onset of menses and becomes increasingly severe until flow slackens.
- 2° dysmenorrhea occurs twice as often in women with endometriosis.
- May present with **dyspareunia** (painful intercourse), infertility, and rectal pain with bleeding.
- Pelvic exam:
  - Tenderness is best detected at the time of menses.
  - Nodularity of the uterosacral ligaments and cul-de-sac may be found.
  - The uterus may be fixed in retroversion due to adhesions.

DIAGNOSIS

- **Clinical impression.**
- **Laparoscopy** is the 1° diagnostic modality. Classic lesions have a **blue-black ("raspberry") or dark brown ("powder-burned") appearance.** Ovaries may show a characteristic "chocolate cyst."
- **Ultrasound:** Reveals complex fluid-filled masses that cannot be distinguished from neoplasms.
- **MRI:** More sensitive and specific than ultrasound, especially for adnexal masses.

TREATMENT

- **Depends on the extent and location of disease** as well as on **symptom severity and the desire for future fertility.**
- **Pharmacologic: Inhibit ovulation** for 4–9 months to prevent cyclic stimulation of endometrial implants. Options are as follows:
  - **GnRH analogs:** Nafarelin or leuprolide.
  - **Danazol:** Suppresses menstruation by inhibiting midcycle FSH and LH surges.
  - Combination OCPs.

- **Surgery** is indicated for moderate to extensive endometriosis.
  - For patients < **35 years of age,** resect the lesions and free adhesions. Some 20% of patients can become pregnant.
  - For patients > **35 years of age,** those disabled by pain, and/or those with involvement of both ovaries, TAH/BSO may be necessary.

ENDOCRINOLOGY

Amenorrhea

Menarche typically occurs between 11 and 15 years of age and may be 1° or 2°. Etiologies are outlined in Table 2.12-2.

HISTORY/PE

- **1° amenorrhea:** No menses by age 16; no sexual characteristics by age 14.
- **2° amenorrhea:** Absence of menses for three consecutive months in women who have passed menarche.

DIAGNOSIS

Workup is as follows (see also Figures 2.12-2 and 2.12-3):

- Ultrasound to determine the presence of the uterus. If the uterus is absent, consider karyotyping.
- **Pregnancy test: Pregnancy is the most common cause of 2° amenorrhea.**

TABLE 2.12-2.   Causes of Amenorrhea

CAUSE/LABS	1° AMENORRHEA	2° AMENORRHEA
Anatomic abnormalities		
Normal FSH	Müllerian anomalies, vaginal agenesis, imperforate hymen.	Asherman's syndrome,[a] cervical stenosis.
↑ LH	Testicular feminization.	
Ovarian or uterine dysfunction		
↑ FSH	Ovarian failure, gonadal dysgenesis (Turner's).	Premature ovarian failure; 1° hypogonadism before age 40; menopause.
↓ or normal FSH	Steroidogenic enzyme defects, constitutional developmental delay.	PCOS.
↑ β-hCG		Pregnancy.
Central regulatory disorders		
↓ or normal FSH	Hypothalamic dysfunction (Kallmann's syndrome, anorexia, excess exercise, weight loss, stress, tumor, infection); 1° pituitary dysfunction (rate).	Hypothalamic dysfunction (anorexia, excess exercise, weight loss, stress); pituitary dysfunction (Sheehan's syndrome, panhypopituitarism); hyperprolactinemia.

[a] Asherman's syndrome is associated with endometritis, scarring after delivery, or D&C. It is the most common anatomic cause of amenorrhea.

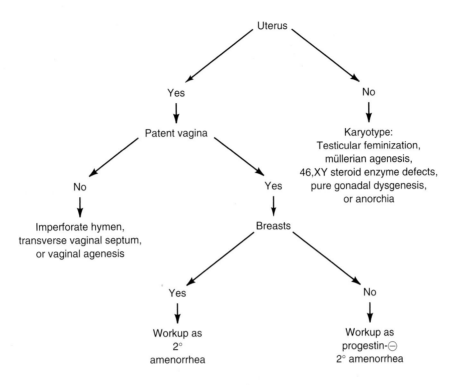

FIGURE 2.12-2. **Workup for patients with primary amenorrhea.**

(Reproduced, with permission, from DeCherney AH. *Current Obstetric & Gynecologic Diagnosis & Treatment*, 8th ed. Stamford, CT: Appleton & Lange, 1994:1010.)

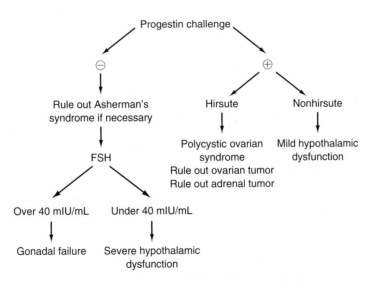

FIGURE 2.12-3. **Workup for patients with 2° amenorrhea without hyperprolactinemia.**

(Reproduced, with permission, from DeCherney AH. *Current Obstetric & Gynecologic Diagnosis & Treatment*, 8th ed. Stamford, CT: Appleton & Lange, 1994:1012.)

- If β-hCG is ⊖:
  - Obtain FSH, LH, prolactin, TSH, and free T_4.
    - ↑ FSH indicates ovarian failure.
    - ↑ prolactin (which inhibits the release of LH and FSH) points to thyroid pathology. Order an MRI of the pituitary to rule out tumor.
    - ↑↑ prolactin points to a prolactin-secreting pituitary adenoma.
  - Obtain potassium, creatinine, and liver enzymes.
  - Assess testosterone levels (in hirsute or virilized women). If testosterone is ↑, rule out hyperandrogenism and adrenal hyperplasia, PCOS, and ovarian tumor.
  - Conduct a 1-mg overnight dexamethasone suppression test to look for signs of hypercortisolism.
  - Obtain a Pap smear and vaginal smear to assess estrogen effect.
- **Progestin withdrawal test:** In nonpregnant women with a normal pelvic exam and normal labs, give a 10-day course of progestin.
  - Absence of withdrawal menses points to a possible pregnancy, uterine abnormality, or estrogen deficiency.
  - Occurrence of withdrawal bleeding indicates anovulation that is likely due to noncyclic gonadotropin secretion, pointing to PCOS or idiopathic anovulation.

TREATMENT

- **Hypothalamic:** Reverse the underlying cause and induce ovulation with gonadotropins.
- **Tumors:** Excision.
- **Premature ovarian failure (age < 40 years):**
  - **Uterus present:** Estrogen + progestin.
  - **Uterus absent:** Estrogen.

Abnormal Uterine Bleeding

Normal menstrual bleeding lasts an average of four days (range is 2–7 days) and → a mean blood loss of 40 mL.

PREMENOPAUSAL UTERINE BLEEDING

HISTORY/PE

- Assess the duration and amount of flow, related pain, and relationship to last menstrual period (LMP).
- Look for clots and assess the degree of inconvenience caused by the bleeding.
- Assess the extent of the bleeding:
  - **Menorrhagia:** ↑ amount of flow (> 80 mL of blood loss per cycle) or prolonged bleeding (flow lasting > 8 days); may → anemia.
  - **Oligomenorrhea:** ↑ length of time between menses (35–90 days between cycles).
  - **Polymenorrhea:** Frequent menstruation (< 21-day cycle); anovular.
  - **Metrorrhagia:** Bleeding between periods.
  - **Menometrorrhagia:** Excessive and irregular bleeding.
- Assess the nature of the bleeding:
  - **Anovulatory bleeding:** Dysfunctional uterine bleeding; overgrowth of endometrium due to estrogen stimulation without adequate progesterone to stabilize growth.
  - **Ovulation bleeding:** A single episode of spotting between regular menses (common).

- **Pelvic exam:** Look for pregnancy, uterine myomas, adnexal masses, or infections.

DIAGNOSIS

- **Labs:** β-hCG, CBC, ESR.
- If bleeding is **ovulatory** (associated with regular menses), further workup is indicated to rule out pathology.
    - Obtain platelet count, bleeding time, and PT/PTT.
    - Check for cervical masses and polyps.
    - Perform a D&C or hysteroscopy and obtain a biopsy if necessary.
- If bleeding is **anovulatory** (irregular, excessive bleeding with no organic causes):
    - Obtain cervical smears as needed for cytologic and culture studies.
    - Order TFTs.
    - **Ultrasound:** Evaluate endometrial thickness; look for intrauterine or ectopic pregnancy or adnexal masses.
    - **MRI:** Diagnose myomas and adenomyosis.
    - Endometrial biopsy (> 35 years) to rule out hyperplasia.

TREATMENT

- **Dysfunctional uterine bleeding:**
    - Give progestins to stabilize endometrial growth.
    - Medroxyprogesterone acetate or norethindrone × 14 days, medical curettage, withdrawal bleeding.
    - For active bleeding, use any combination OCP.
- **Heavy bleeding:**
    - Danazol for intractable bleeding.
    - Estrogen 25 mg IV q 6 h × 4 doses stabilizes the endometrial lining and stops bleeding within one hour.
    - GnRH agonists (leuprolide or nafarelin).
    - OCPs to thicken the endometrium and control the bleeding.
- **Menorrhagia:**
    - NSAIDs to ↓ blood loss.
    - Prolonged use of progestin can → intermittent bleeding.

Pregnancy is the most common cause of abnormal uterine bleeding and amenorrhea. Always check a pregnancy test!

POSTMENOPAUSAL UTERINE BLEEDING

Vaginal bleeding that occurs ≥ 6 months following the cessation of menstrual function is cancer until proven otherwise. Etiologies include atrophic endometrium, endometrial proliferation or hyperplasia, endometrial or cervical cancer, and administration of estrogens without progestins.

HISTORY/PE

- Generally presents with **painless uterine bleeding.**
- May present with pain if the cervix is stenotic, bleeding is severe and rapid, or infection or torsion is present.
- Look for vulvar and vaginal bleeding, ulcers, or **neoplasms.**

DIAGNOSIS

- A cytologic smear of the cervix and vaginal pool should be taken.
- Perform **transvaginal ultrasound to measure endometrial thickness:**
    - **< 4 mm:** Points to a very low likelihood of hyperplasia or endometrial cancer.

- **> 4 mm:** Endocervical curettage and endometrial aspiration are warranted.

TREATMENT

- **Simple or complex endometrial hyperplasia:**
  - Cyclic progestin therapy (medroxyprogesterone acetate or norethindrone acetate) for 21 days each month × 3 months.
  - A repeat D&C or endometrial biopsy should be performed. If tissue is normal and estrogen replacement therapy is to be reinstituted, a progestin should be prescribed.
  - **Surgery:** Aspiration curettage.
- **Endometrial hyperplasia with atypical cells or carcinoma** warrants a **hysterectomy.**

COMPLICATIONS

Endometrial cancer. Complex hyperplasia with atypia has a high risk of becoming adenocarcinoma.

Hirsutism and Virilization

Hirsutism is excessive sexual hair. **Virilization** is excessive androgenic influence.

HISTORY/PE

- Presents with excessive hair on the chin, upper lip, abdomen, and chest.
- Acne, balding, deep voice, ↑ strength, clitoromegaly, and amenorrhea are seen in severe cases.

Hypertrichosis is excessive nonsexual hair; the etiology may be drug related or hereditary.

DIAGNOSIS

- ↑ androgens (testosterone > 2 ng; DHEAS > 7 μg/mL): Rule out adrenal or ovarian neoplasm.
  - ↑ **serum testosterone:** Suspect an ovarian tumor.
  - ↑ **DHEAS:** Suspect an adrenal source (adrenal tumor, Cushing's syndrome, congenital adrenal hyperplasia).
- See Table 2.12-3 for further diagnostic measures.

TREATMENT

Treat the underlying cause of hyperandrogenism.

Polycystic Ovarian Syndrome (PCOS)

One of the most common endocrine disorders in reproductive women. Also known as Stein-Leventhal syndrome.

HISTORY/PE

- Presents with **hirsutism** (70%), obesity (40%), and virilization (20%).
- Amenorrhea and/or abnormal uterine bleeding is frequently seen.
- **Infertility** is common.

TABLE 2.12-3. Workup of Hirsutism and Virilization

TESTOSTERONE	DHEAS	DISEASE	WORKUP
> 200 ng/dL	Normal	Ovarian neoplasm.	Adrenal CT, pelvic ultrasound.
Variable	> 7 μg/mL	Adrenal tumor, Cushing's syndrome.	Adrenal CT, dexamethasone suppression test.
> 70 ng/dL	↑ but < 7 μg/mL	PCOS, adrenal hyperplasia, Cushing's syndrome.	No further workup; rule out congenital adrenal hyperplasia and Cushing's syndrome.
Normal	Normal	↓ end-organ sensitivity.	Free testosterone, androstenediol glucuronide.

- Acanthosis nigricans +/− bilateral ovarian enlargement may be present.
- **HAIR-AN syndrome** is a variant of PCOS that → hyperandrogenism, insulin resistance, and acanthosis nigricans.

DIAGNOSIS

- **Labs:**
  - ↑ LH/FSH ratio (> 2:1).
  - ↑ testosterone (total +/− free).
  - ↑ androstenedione, ↑ DHEAS, ↓ glucose/insulin ratio.
- **Ultrasound:** Polycystic ovaries typically show multiple, 2- to 8-mm, subcapsular preantral follicles forming a black **"pearl necklace" sign** (see Figure 2.12-4).

TREATMENT

- **Infertility:**
  - Clomiphene or other drugs for ovulatory stimulation.
  - If clomiphene fails, metformin, gonadotropin therapy, and ovarian drilling may be tried.

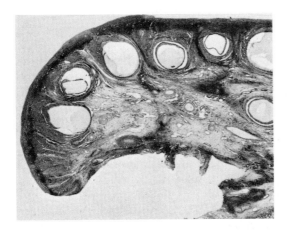

FIGURE 2.12-4. Polycystic ovary with prominent multiple cysts.

(Reproduced, with permission, from DeCherney AH. *Current Obstetric & Gynecologic Diagnosis & Treatment*, 8th ed. Stamford, CT: Appleton & Lange, 1994:747.)

- If the above treatment fails, IVF may be tried.
- OCP or progestin to ↓ the risk of endometrial hyperplasia/carcinoma.
- Address cardiovascular risk factors and lipid levels.
- Diet, weight loss, and exercise.

COMPLICATIONS

↑ risk of early-onset type 2 DM; ↑ long-term risk of breast and endometrial cancer owing to unopposed estrogen secretion.

Menopause

Cessation of menses for a minimum of 12 months due to cessation of follicular development. Average age of onset is 51. Premature menopause is ovarian failure and menstrual cessation before age 40.

HISTORY/PE

- See the mnemonic HAVOC.
- Other symptoms include insomnia, anxiety/irritability, vaginal bleeding, poor concentration, mood changes, dyspareunia, and loss of libido.

DIAGNOSIS

- ↑ FSH and ↑ LH.
- Vaginal cytologic exam shows low estrogen effect with parabasal cells.
- DEXA scan for osteoporosis.
- Lipid profile.

TREATMENT

- **Vasomotor symptoms:**
  - HRT; combination estrogen and progestin.
  - Posthysterectomy patients do not need progestin.
  - Clinicians should review the risks and benefits of HRT with their patients. Long-term HRT for symptom prevention is no longer indicated.
  - Contraindications to HRT include vaginal bleeding, suspected or known breast cancer, endometrial cancer, a history of thromboembolism, chronic liver disease, and hypertriglyceridemia.
  - Clonidine to ↓ the frequency of hot flashes.
- **Vaginal atrophy:**
  - **Long term: Estradiol vaginal ring.**
  - **Short term:** Estrogen vaginal cream will relieve symptoms.
- **Osteoporosis:** Daily calcium supplementation and exercise.

COMPLICATIONS

- Dyspareunia from vaginal atrophy and ↓ vaginal lubrication.
- Overall health risks exceed the benefits derived from the use of combined estrogen plus progestin for an average of five years (↑ the risk of coronary heart disease, cardiovascular accidents, pulmonary embolism, invasive breast cancer, and gallbladder disease).

> **Menopause wreaks HAVOC:**
>
> **H**ot flashes (vasomotor instability)
> **A**trophy of the
> **V**agina
> **O**steoporosis
> **C**oronary artery disease

TABLE 2.12-4. Infertility Workup

	MALE	FEMALE
History/PE	Testicular injury or infection. Medications (steroids, cimetidine, spironolactone). Thyroid or liver disease → abnormalities of spermatogenesis Signs of hypogonadism, ⊕ varicocele on physical exam.	Age (incidence ↑ with age). Previous STDs. Abortions, pregnancies, and menstrual cycle characteristics (length, duration, premenstrual symptoms).
Diagnosis	Semen analysis: ↓ sperm count and motility (accounts for **40% of infertility cases**). ↑ FSH, ↑ LH, ↓ testosterone = 1° testicular failure (hypergonadotropic hypogonadism). ↓ FSH, ↓ LH, ↓ testosterone = 2° testicular failure (hypogonadotropic hypogonadism). Check prolactin.	**Basal body temperature** to evaluate ovulation (↓ temperature at time of menses, then an ↑ two days after LH surge at the time of progesterone rise). Hysterosalpingogram, endometrial biopsy, postcoital test, antisperm antibodies, luteal progesterone levels.
Treatment	Intrauterine insemination, donor insemination, IVF.	Induction of ovulation with **clomiphene;** tubal or uterine surgery; GnRH analogs (for fibroids and endometriosis); IVF.

Infertility

- Etiologies include abnormal spermatogenesis (40%), anovulation (30%), and female anatomic defects (20%). Ten percent of cases are of unknown etiology.
- Hx/PE: Pregnancy does not result after 12 months of normal, unprotected sexual activity (see Table 2.12-4).
- Dx:
  - **Pathology in the male partner is the most frequent cause.**
  - Consider laparoscopy if male and female workup is ⊖.
- Rx: Etiology specific. If unexplained, consider IVF.

ECTOPIC PREGNANCY

A condition in which a fertilized ovum implants in an area other than the endometrial lining of the uterus. Occurs in 1 in 100 pregnancies. The most common location is the **ampulla** of the oviduct (95%). Risk factors include a **history of PID,** prior ectopic pregnancy, tubal/pelvic surgery, DES exposure in utero, and IUD use.

The ampulla of the oviduct is the most common location for an ectopic pregnancy.

HISTORY/PE

- Suspect in any pregnant woman in the first trimester who presents with the **classic triad of amenorrhea, light vaginal bleeding, and lower abdominal/pelvic pain.** Specific manifestations include the following:
  - **Pain:** May be pelvic or abdominal, localized or generalized.
  - **Bleeding:** Abnormal uterine bleeding (75% of patients).
  - **2° amenorrhea:** Affects 50% of patients.
  - **Syncope (33% of patients):** Presents with dizziness and light-headedness.

- Examination reveals diffuse or localized abdominal tenderness as well as adnexal and/or cervical motion tenderness. A tender pelvic or adnexal mass may be palpable.
- **Ruptured ectopic pregnancy** (a surgical emergency) may present with sudden sharp abdominal pain accompanied by orthostatic hypotension, tachycardia, generalized abdominal and adnexal tenderness with rebound tenderness, shoulder pain, and shock.

↑ β-hCG in the absence of an intrauterine pregnancy on ultrasound is worrisome for ectopic pregnancy.

DIAGNOSIS

- ↑ β-hCG in the absence of intrauterine pregnancy on ultrasound is highly suspicious. β-hCG levels are lower compared with normal pregnancies of the same duration. Follow the rate of ↑. **Failure of serum level to double every 48 hours is suggestive of ectopic pregnancy.**
- **Serum progesterone** is often less than normal but is nonspecific.
- **Transabdominal ultrasound** (β-hCG of 5000 mIU/mL) or transvaginal ultrasound (β-hCG of 1500 mIU/mL), **which is more sensitive,** is used to look for intrauterine pregnancy and to rule out ectopic pregnancy (see Table 2.12-5). **An empty uterine cavity demonstrated by abdominal ultrasound with a β-hCG of 6500 mIU/mL is virtually diagnostic.**
- **Culdocentesis:** Withdrawal of ≥ 5 mL of nonclotting blood from the cul-de-sac through the vagina. Can be done to check for blood in the pouch of Douglas, but has a high false-⊖ rate. Rarely done anymore.

TREATMENT

- **Expectant management:** For asymptomatic, compliant patients with low or ↓ β-hCG titers (< 200 mIU/mL) and a low risk of rupture.
- **Medical management: Methotrexate** is effective for small (< 3-cm) unruptured ectopic pregnancies in asymptomatic, compliant women. Follow β-hCG levels, CBC, creatinine, and AST.
- **Surgical treatment:**
  - **Salpingostomy:** The tube is incised and only the product of conception is removed.
  - **Salpingectomy:** The entire tube is removed.
  - **Salpingo-oophorectomy:** Both the tube and ovary are removed.
- RhoGAM should be given to any Rh-⊖ mother.

COMPLICATIONS

Inevitable loss of fetus, hemorrhagic shock, future ectopic pregnancy, infertility, maternal death, Rh sensitization.

TABLE 2.12-5. Diagnosis of Ectopic Pregnancy

TRANSVAGINAL ULTRASOUND	β-hCG	DAYS SINCE LMP
Gestational sac	1500	35
Fetal pole	5000	40
Fetal heart motion	11,000	45

Vaginitis

The most common gynecologic condition encountered by physicians. *Lactobacillus*, the predominant organism in the vagina, keeps the vagina slightly acidic to inhibit the growth of harmful organisms. When these bacteria are replaced with anaerobic bacteria and other organisms, vaginitis occurs. Feminine hygiene products, medications (OCPs, antibiotics), STDs, intercourse, and stress can all alter the normal vaginal pH (normal is 3.8–4.2) → overgrowth of pathogens.

HISTORY/PE

- Determine the LMP and ask about recent sexual activity and use of OCPs, tampons, or douches.
- Note the presence or absence of vaginal burning, pain, pruritus, and profuse or malodorous discharge.
- Normal secretions are as follows:
  - **Midcycle estrogen surge:** Clear, elastic, mucoid secretions.
  - **Luteal phase/pregnancy:** Thick and white; adhere to the vaginal wall.
- Examine the vulva, vaginal walls, and cervix.

DIAGNOSIS

- See Table 2.12-6 for common findings.
- Check the pH of the discharge.
- Obtain a wet smear with saline and a KOH smear ("whiff test").
- Obtain a Gram stain of vaginal discharge to rule out STDs and a clean-catch urine culture and UA to rule out UTI.

The diagnosis of vaginitis is made with a wet prep (for Trichomonas and bacterial vaginitis) or KOH prep (for yeast).

Cervicitis

- **Inflammation of the uterine cervix.** Because the female genital tract is contiguous from the vulva to the fallopian tubes, there is some overlap between vulvovaginitis and cervicitis. Etiologies are as follows:
  - **Infectious (most common):** *Chlamydia*, gonococcus, *Trichomonas*, HSV, HPV.
  - **Noninfectious:** Trauma, radiation exposure, malignancy.
- Hx/PE: Yellow-green mucopurulent discharge; ⊕ **cervical motion tenderness; absence of other signs of PID.**
- Dx/Rx: See the discussion of STDs.

Pelvic Inflammatory Disease (PID)

A polymicrobial infection of the **upper genital tract** associated with *Neisseria gonorrhoeae* (one-third of cases), *Chlamydia trachomatis* (one-third of cases), and endogenous aerobes/anaerobes. The lifetime risk is 1–3%. Risk factors include non-Caucasian ethnicity, douching, smoking, prior PID, and IUD use. A ↓ risk is associated with the use of OCPs or barrier methods. Occurs most often in young, nulliparous, sexually active women with multiple sex partners.

HISTORY/PE

- Presents with lower abdominal pain, **fever** and chills, menstrual disturbances, and a purulent cervical discharge.
- **Cervical motion (chandelier sign) and adnexal tenderness** are also seen.
- RUQ pain may indicate perihepatitis (Fitz-Hugh–Curtis syndrome).

Chandelier sign is defined as severe cervical motion tenderness that makes the patient "jump for the chandelier" on exam.

TABLE 2.12-6. **Causes of Vaginitis**

	BACTERIAL VAGINOSIS	TRICHOMONAS	YEAST
Incidence	50% (most common).	25%.	25%.
Etiology	**Not an STD.** Caused by overgrowth of *Gardnerella* and other anaerobes.	Protozoal flagellates affect the vagina, Skene's duct, and lower urinary tract as well as the lower GU tract in men.	Usually *Candida*.
Risk factors	Pregnancy, IUD use, frequent douching.	Tobacco use, unprotected sex with multiple partners, IUD.	**DM, antibiotic use, pregnancy, steroids,** HIV, OCP use, IUD use, young age at first intercourse, ↑ frequency of intercourse.
History	Odor.	Discharge.	Pruritus.
Exam	Mild vulvar irritation.	Strawberry petechiae in the upper vagina/cervix.	Erythematous, excoriated vulva/vagina.
Discharge	Homogenous, **grayish-white, fishy**/stale odor.	Profuse, malodorous, **yellow-green, frothy.**	Thick, white, **cottage-cheese texture.**
Vaginal pH	> 4.5 (5.0–6.0).	> 4.5 (5.0–7.0).	Normal.
Saline smear[a]	**"Clue cells"** (epithelial cells coated with bacteria; see Figure 2.12-5).	**Motile trichomonads** (flagellated organisms that are slightly larger than WBCs).	Nothing.
KOH prep	⊕ whiff test (fishy smell).	Nothing.	Pseudohyphae (see Figure 2.12-5).
Treatment	PO metronidazole or clindamycin × 7 days.	PO metronidazole. Treat partners and test for other STDs.	**Uncomplicated:** Topical azole × 1–3 days. **Complicated** (≥ 4 episodes in one year, noncandidal, HIV, DM, steroids, pregnancy): Two weeks of topical antifungals or fluconazole × 2 doses.
Complications	PID, endometritis, vaginal cuff cellulitis when invasive procedures are done (e.g., biopsy, C-section, IUD placement).		**No topical azole for pregnant women.**

[a] If there are many WBCs and no organism on saline smear, suspect *Chlamydia.*

HIGH-YIELD FACTS

GYNECOLOGY

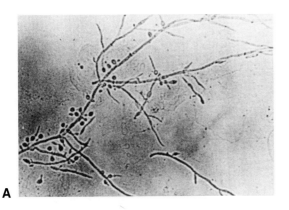 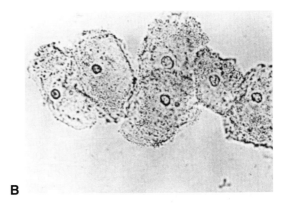

A **B**

FIGURE 2.12-5. Causes of vaginitis.

(A) Candidal vaginitis. Branched and budding *Candida albicans* organisms are evident on KOH preparation of vaginal discharge. (B) *Gardnerella vaginalis*. Saline wet mount of vaginal fluid reveals granulations on vaginal epithelial cells ("clue cells") due to adherence of *G. vaginalis* organisms to the cell surface. (Reproduced, with permission from DeCherney AH. *Current Obstetric & Gynecologic Diagnosis & Treatment*, 8th ed. Stamford, CT: Appleton & Lange, 1994:692.)

DIAGNOSIS

- Diagnosis is complicated by the fact that many women have mild symptoms that are not readily recognized as PID.
- **Labs:** WBC > 10,000, ↑ ESR (> 15 mm/hr), ↑ CRP.
- Cervical or vaginal discharge with WBCs on saline microscopy.
- Obtain an endocervical culture for *N. gonorrhoeae* and *C. trachomatis*.
- Order a β-hCG and ultrasound to rule out pregnancy and to evaluate the possibility of tubo-ovarian abscess.

TREATMENT

- **Antibiotic treatment should not be delayed** while awaiting culture results. All sexual partners should be examined and treated appropriately.
- **Outpatient antibiotic regimens** are as follows:
  - **Regimen A:** Cefoxitin with probenecid × 1 dose.
  - **Regimen B:** Ceftriaxone IM × 1 dose + doxycycline × 14 days.
  - **Regimen C:** Ofloxacin × 14 days + metronidazole × 14 days.
- **Admit the following for IV antibiotics:**
  - Patients in whom surgical emergencies such as appendicitis cannot be ruled out.
  - Tubo-ovarian abscess (admit for at least 24 hours before switching to outpatient).
  - Pregnant patients.
  - Patients who are unable to follow or tolerate an outpatient regimen.
  - Those who have failed to respond clinically to outpatient therapy.
  - Those with severe illness, nausea/vomiting, or high fever.
  - Immunodeficient patients (HIV-⊕ patients with low CD4 counts or those who are taking immunosuppressant drugs).
- **Inpatient antibiotic regimens:**
  - Cefoxitin or cefotetan + doxycycline × 14 days.

■ Clindamycin + gentamicin × 14 days.
■ **Surgery:**
  ■ Tubo-ovarian abscess may require surgical excision (30% of cases) or transcutaneous/transvaginal aspiration. Unilateral salpingo-oophorectomy is acceptable for unilateral abscess.
  ■ Hysterectomy and BSO may be necessary for overwhelming infection or in cases of chronic disease with intractable pelvic pain.

COMPLICATIONS

■ Some 25% of women with acute disease develop repeated episodes of infection, chronic pelvic pain, dyspareunia, **ectopic pregnancy,** or **infertility.**
■ RUQ pain (Fitz-Hugh–Curtis syndrome) may indicate an associated perihepatitis (abnormal liver function, shoulder pain).
■ The risk of infertility ↑ with repeated episodes of salpingitis and is estimated to approach 10% after the first episode, 25% after the second episode, and 50% after a third episode.

Toxic Shock Syndrome (TSS)

An acute illness caused by preformed *S. aureus* toxin (TSST-1) that can → scalded skin syndrome, bullous impetigo, necrotizing pneumonitis, and enterotoxin food poisoning. **More than 90% of patients are women of childbearing age;** often occurs within five days of the onset of a menstrual period in women who have used **tampons.** Nonmenstrual cases are nearly as common as menstrual cases; organisms from the nasopharynx, bones, vagina, rectum, and wounds have all been associated with the illness.

HISTORY/PE

■ Presents with **abrupt onset of fever, vomiting,** and watery diarrhea.
■ A **diffuse macular erythematous rash** is also seen.
■ Nonpurulent conjunctivitis is common.
■ **Desquamation, especially of the palms and soles,** generally occurs during recovery within 1–2 weeks of illness.

DIAGNOSIS

Blood cultures are ⊖ because symptoms result from preformed toxin and are not due to the invasive properties of the organism.

TREATMENT

■ Rapid rehydration; removal of sources of toxin (e.g., removal of tampons, drainage of abscess).
■ Antistaphylococcal drugs (nafcillin, oxacillin); management of renal or cardiac failure.

GYNECOLOGIC NEOPLASMS

The 1° cancers affecting women, in order of frequency, are lung, breast, colon, and endometrial. The most common gynecologic cancers are endometrial, ovarian (carries the highest mortality), cervical, and vulvar. Table 2.12-7 outlines common findings associated with endometrial, cervical, vulvar, and ovarian cancers.

TABLE 2.12-7. **Gynecologic Neoplasms**

	ENDOMETRIAL	CERVICAL	VULVAR	OVARIAN
Patients affected	Postmenopausal, 50–70 years of age.	Premenopausal, > 40 years of age.	Postmenopausal, > 50 years of age.	Postmenopausal, > 50 years of age.
History	Vaginal bleeding (80% of patients), pain (late finding).	Metrorrhagia, postcoital spotting, discharge (bloody or purulent, odorous, nonpruritic). May be asymptomatic.	Prolonged vulvar irritation; **pruritus;** history of genital warts.	Often asymptomatic, but may present with ↑ abdominal girth from ascites, GI and GU complaints, thrombophlebitis, and lower abdominal pain/pressure.
Exam	Palpable abdominal and pelvic masses.	Cervical ulceration; bladder/rectal dysfunction.	**Early:** Resembles chronic vulvar dermatitis. **Late:** Presents with a large, cauliflower-like or hard ulcerated area in the vulva.	**Early:** Pelvic exam may be normal, or may present with a palpable adnexal mass and pedal edema. **Late:** Palpable mass, ascites.
Risk factors	**Excess estrogen:** Well-differentiated tumor with high survival rates.[a] Thin, multiparous African-American women have more aggressive tumors with a poorer prognosis.	HPV infection, venereal warts, early sexual activity, multiple sex partners, smoking, family history.	**HPV (types 16,18, 31),** infrequent medical exams, diabetes, obesity, hypertension, evidence of cardiovascular disease.	Nulliparity, breast cancer, family history. OCP use is protective.
Screening tests	None (Pap smear is only 50% effective).	Annual Pap smear for sexually active women.		None (routine ultrasound and, CA-125 are not cost-efficient).
Precursor lesion	Endometrial hyperplasia (treatment is progesterone).	Cervical intraepithelial neoplasia (CIN) is a common diagnosis; most often seen in women 25–40 years of age. Associated with HPV.	Vulvar intraepithelial neoplasia (VIN).	None.

HIGH-YIELD FACTS

GYNECOLOGY

TABLE 2.12-7. Gynecologic Neoplasms (continued)

	ENDOMETRIAL	CERVICAL	VULVAR	OVARIAN
Diagnostic tests	**Endometrial/ endocervical biopsy;** Pap smear is not reliable. Vaginal ultrasound shows thickened endometrium → hypertrophy and neoplastic change.	⊕ **Pap smear;** punch +/– cone biopsy.	VIN I and II are associated with mild and moderate dysplasia with ↑ risk → advanced stages and carcinoma. VIN III = carcinoma in situ.	Ultrasound, abdominal CT, CA-125 for epithelial cancers; α-fetoprotein (AFP) and β-hCG for germ cell cancers.
Treatment	TAH/BSO with lymph node dissection; progesterone; radiotherapy. Treat advanced cases with chemotherapy.	**Early:** Radiotherapy, radical hysterectomy and lymph-adenectomy. **Advanced:** Irradiation/ chemotherapy (surgery would harm the bladder and rectum without being effective).	**Surgical:** ▪ **In situ:** Excise with wide margin. ▪ **Invasive:** (1) Radical vulvectomy and regional lymphadenectomy or (2) wide local excision of the 1° tumor with inguinal lymph node dissection. **Radiation:** To ↓ tumor burden and for metastatic or recurrent disease.	TAH/BSO and peritoneal washing for cytology with or without pelvic and aortic node sampling; tumor debulking; chemotherapy.
Prevention	Progesterone to oppose estrogen; low-fat diet; weight control.	Safe sex (condoms) to ↓ the risk of HPV infection; smoking cessation; routine Pap smears.	None.	OCPs; prophylactic BSO in patients with a strong family history.
Notes	Adenocarcinomas.	Some 5% are squamous cell carcinomas and 15% adenocarcinomas. **Uremia** is the most common cause of death in end-stage cervical cancer.	Approximately 87% are squamous cell carcinomas and 6% malignant melanomas; the remainder include basal cell carcinoma and Paget's disease. obstruction.	Complications include ovarian rupture, torsion, hemorrhage, infections, and infarction. The most common cause of death is bowel

[a] **Excess estrogen exposure** is associated with a history of unopposed estrogen use, late menopause, obesity, nulliparity, and tamoxifen use for breast cancer.

Uterine Leiomyoma (Fibroids)

The most common **benign** neoplasm of the female genital tract. The tumor is discrete, round, firm, and often multiple. It is composed of smooth muscle and connective tissue that is hormonally responsive; its size often ↑ in pregnancy and ↓ after menopause. Malignant transformation to **leiomyosarcoma is rare (0.1–0.5%).**

History/PE

- The majority of patients are asymptomatic.
- Symptomatic patients may present with the following:
    - **Bleeding:** Longer, heavier periods; anemia.
    - **Pressure:** Pelvic pressure and bloating; constipation and rectal pressure; urinary frequency or retention.
    - **Pain:** 2° dysmenorrhea, dyspareunia.
    - **Pelvic symptoms:** A firm, nontender, irregular enlarged ("lumpy-bumpy"), or cobblestone uterus may be seen.

Diagnosis

- **CBC:** To look for anemia.
- **Ultrasound:** To look for **uterine myomas;** can also exclude ovarian masses.
- **MRI:** Can delineate intramural and submucous myomas.

Treatment

- **Pharmacologic:**
    - Medroxyprogesterone acetate or danazol to slow or stop bleeding.
    - GnRH analogs (leuprolide or nafarelin) to **↓ the size of myomas, suppress further growth, and ↓ surrounding vascularity.**
- **Surgery:** Emergent surgery is indicated for torsion of a pedunculated myoma.
- **Women of childbearing years:** Myomectomy.
- **Women who have completed childbearing:** Total or subtotal abdominal or vaginal hysterectomy.

Complications

Infertility may be due to a myoma that distorts the uterine cavity and plays a role similar to that of an IUD.

Cervical Intraepithelial Neoplasia (CIN)

- An abnormal Pap smear in an asymptomatic woman with no grossly visible cervical changes.
- Hx/PE: No specific symptoms or signs; the cervix appears grossly normal
- Dx:
    - **Pap smear:** Reveals dysplasia or carcinoma in situ (see Table 2.12-8).
    - **Colposcopy:** Reveals an atypical transformation zone with white patches and vascular atypia that indicates areas of greatest cellular activity.
    - Colposcopically directed **punch biopsy** and endocervical curettage.

If a uterine mass continues to grow after menopause, pathologic evaluation is crucial to rule out malignancy.

HIGH-YIELD FACTS

GYNECOLOGY

TABLE 2.12-8. Pap Smear Findings

DYSPLASIA	CIN	BETHESDA SYSTEM
Benign	Benign	Normal
Benign with inflammation	Benign with inflammation	Normal, ASCUS[a]
Mild dysplasia	CIN I	Low-grade SIL[b]
Moderate dysplasia	CIN II	High-grade SIL
Severe dysplasia	CIN III	High-grade SIL
Carcinoma in situ	CIN III	High-grade SIL
Invasive cancer	Invasive cancer	Invasive cancer

[a] ASCUS = atypical squamous cells of undetermined significance.

[b] SIL = squamous intraepithelial lesion.

TREATMENT

- **CIN I:** Pap smear or colposcopy every 3–4 months for one year. With resolution, patients can return to an annual Pap smear.
- **CIN II and CIN III:**
    - **Exocervix:** Laser or cryotherapy.
    - **Endocervix:** Conization with the loop electrosurgical excision procedure (LEEP) or cold knife biopsy.

Cervical Cancer

Risk factors for cervical cancer include the following:

- Multiparity, smoking, early initiation of intercourse, ↑ number of sexual partners, HIV infection.
- **HPV:** Types 6 and 11 → mild dysplasia; types 16,18, and 31 → higher-grade cellular changes.

HISTORY/PE

- Often asymptomatic.
- May present with **postcoital bleeding,** menorrhagia, pelvic pain, or vaginal discharge.
- Look for **cervical discharge/ulceration** or pelvic mass (see Table 2.12-9).

DIAGNOSIS

- ⊕ **Pap smear.** However, treatment is never justified until a definitive diagnosis has been established through biopsy.
- Cervical biopsy and endocervical curettage or conization to determine the extent and depth of invasion of the cancer.
- Clinical staging (under anesthesia) to estimate gross spread.
- The depth of penetration of malignant cells beyond the basement membrane serves as a reliable clinical guide to the extent of cancer within the cervix as well as a predictor of the likelihood of metastases.
- **Imaging:** Abdominal and pelvic CT or MRI.

Infection with HPV types 16, 18, and 31 → the risk of cervical cancer.

- Carcinoma in situ (stage 0):
  - **Women who have completed childbearing:** TAH.
  - **Women who wish to retain the uterus:** Cervical conization or ablation of the lesion with cryotherapy or laser.
- Invasive carcinoma:
  - **Microinvasive carcinoma (stage IA):** Simple extrafascial hysterectomy.
  - **Stage I (limited to cervix):** Hysterectomy.
  - **Radiation therapy:**
    - **Stage II:** Upper two-thirds of the vagina or parametria.
    - **Stage III:** Lower third of the vagina or pelvic side wall; all cases of hydronephrosis.
    - **Stage IV:** Bladder or rectal involvement or distant metastases.
  - Radical surgery → fewer long-term complication than irradiation and may allow preservation of ovarian function; it is therefore the preferred mode of therapy in younger women.
- Close follow-up with Pap smears every three months for one year and every six months for another year is necessary after cryotherapy.

COMPLICATIONS

- Metastases to regional lymph nodes occur with ↑ frequency from stage I to IV.
- GU complications include the following:
  - Ureters are often obstructed lateral to the cervix → hydroureter, hydronephrosis, and renal insufficiency.
  - Almost **two-thirds** of untreated patients die of uremia when ureteral obstruction is bilateral.

Ovarian Tumors

Most ovarian tumors are benign, but malignant tumors are the leading cause of death from reproductive tract cancer. Death most commonly results from **bowel obstruction**. The lifetime risk is 1.6%. Risk factors include the following:

TABLE 2.12-9. Benign vs. Malignant Pelvic Masses

FINDING	BENIGN	MALIGNANT
Exam: pelvic mass		
Mobility	Mobile	Fixed
Consistency	Cystic	Solid or firm
Location	Unilateral	Bilateral
Cul-de-sac	Smooth	Nodular
Transvaginal ultrasound: adnexal mass		
Size	< 8 cm	> 8 cm
Consistency	Cystic	Solid or cystic and solid
Septations	Unilocular	Multilocular
Location	Unilateral	Bilateral
Other	Calcifications	Ascites

- Age, low parity, ↓ fertility, delayed childbearing.
- A ⊕ family history. Patients with one affected first-degree relative have a 5% lifetime risk. With two or more affected first-degree relatives, the risk is 75%.
- The BRCA1 mutation carries a 45% lifetime risk of ovarian cancer. The BRCA2 mutation is associated with a 25% lifetime risk.
- **Lynch II syndrome,** or hereditary nonpolyposis colorectal cancer (HNPCC), is associated with an ↑ risk of colon, ovarian, endometrial, and breast cancer.
- OCPs ↓ risk.

Any palpable ovary or adnexal mass in a premenarchal or postmenopausal patient is suggestive of ovarian neoplasm.

HISTORY/PE

- Both benign and malignant ovarian neoplasms are generally asymptomatic.
- Mild, nonspecific GI symptoms or pelvic pressure/pain may be seen.
- Early disease is typically not detected on routine pelvic exam.
- Some 75% of woman present with **advanced malignant disease,** as evidenced by abdominal pain and bloating, a palpable abdominal mass, and ascites.
- Table 2.12-9 differentiates the benign and malignant characteristics of pelvic mass.

DIAGNOSIS

- **Tumor markers (see Table 2.12-10):** ↑ CA-125 is associated with epithelial cell cancer (90% of ovarian cancers).
  - **Premenopausal women:** ↑ CA-125 may point to benign disease such as endometriosis.
  - **Postmenopausal women:** ↑ CA-125 (> 35 units) indicates an ↑ likelihood that the ovarian tumor is malignant.
- **Transvaginal ultrasound:**
  - **Screen high-risk women.**
  - See Table 2.12-9 to differentiate benign and malignant ovarian/adnexal masses.

TREATMENT

Treatment of **ovarian masses** is as follows:

- **Premenarchal women:** Masses > 2 cm require exploratory laparotomy.

TABLE 2.12-10. Ovarian Tumor Markers

OVARIAN TUMOR	MARKER
Epithelial	CA-125
Endodermal sinus	AFP
Embryonal carcinoma	AFP, hCG
Choriocarcinoma	hCG
Dysgerminoma	LDH

- **Premenopausal women:**
  - Observation for 4–6 weeks for asymptomatic, mobile, unilateral simple cystic masses < 8–10 cm. Most will resolve spontaneously.
  - Surgical evaluation is warranted for masses > 8–10 cm as well as for those that are unchanged on repeat pelvic exam and ultrasound.
  - If malignancy is suspected, preoperative workup includes CXR, LFTs and TFTs, and basic hematology studies.
- **Postmenopausal women:**
  - Asymptomatic, unilateral simple cysts < 5 cm in diameter with a **normal CA-125** should be **closely followed with ultrasound.**
  - Palpable masses warrant surgical evaluation by exploratory laparotomy.

Treatment of **ovarian cancer** is as follows:

- **Surgery:**
  - Surgical staging followed by TAH/BSO with omentectomy, peritoneal washings and biopsies, and pelvic and para-aortic lymphadenectomy.
  - Benign neoplasms warrant tumor removal or unilateral oophorectomy.
  - **Postoperative chemotherapy** is routine except for women with early-stage or low-grade ovarian cancer.
- Radiation therapy is effective for dysgerminomas.

PREVENTION

- Women with the BRCA1 gene mutation should be screened annually with ultrasound and CA-125 testing. Prophylactic oophorectomy is recommended by age 35 or whenever childbearing is completed.
- OCP use ↓ risk.

URINARY INCONTINENCE

Defined as the involuntary loss of urine due to either bladder or sphincteric dysfunction.

HISTORY/PE

- Table 2.12-11 outlines the types of incontinence along with their distinguishing features and treatment.
- Exclude fistula in cases of total incontinence. Look for neurologic abnormalities in cases of urge incontinence (spasticity, flaccidity, rectal sphincter tone) or distended bladder in overflow incontinence.

DIAGNOSIS

- UA and urine culture to exclude UTI.
- Serum creatinine to exclude renal dysfunction.
- Cystogram to demonstrate fistula sites and descensus of the bladder neck.

Causes of urinary incontinence without specific urogenital pathology—

DIAPPERS

Delirium/confusional state
Infection
Atrophic urethritis/vaginitis
Pharmaceutical
Psychiatric causes (esp. depression)
Excessive urinary output (hyperglycemia, hypercalcemia, CHF)
Restricted mobility
Stool impaction

TABLE 2.12-11. **Types of Incontinence**

TYPE	HISTORY OF URINE LOSS	ETIOLOGY	TREATMENT
Total	Uncontrolled loss at all times and in all positions.	Sphincteric efficiency is lost (previous surgery, nerve damage, cancer infiltration). Abnormal connection between the urinary tract and the skin (fistula).	Surgery.
Stress	Activities that ↑ intra-abdominal pressure (coughing, sneezing, lifting); not common in the supine position.	Urethral sphincteric insufficiency due to laxity of pelvic floor musculature; common in multiparous women or after pelvic surgery.	Surgery centers on placing the bladder neck into the appropriate anatomical location.
Urge[a]	Preceded by a strong, unexpected urge to void that is unrelated to position or activity.	Detrusor hyperreflexia or sphincter dysfunction due to inflammatory conditions or neurogenic disorders of the bladder.	Anticholinergic medications or TCAs.
Overflow[b]	Patients with chronic urinary retention.	Chronically distended bladder with ↑ intravesical pressure that just exceeds the outlet resistance, allowing a small amount of urine to dribble out.	Placement of urethral catheter in acute settings. Treat underlying diseases. Timed voiding.

[a]Etiologies include inhibited contractions, local irritation (cystitis, stone, tumor), and CNS causes.
[b]Etiologies include physical agents (tumor, stricture), neurologic factors (lesions), and medications.

Pediatrics

Neurology   318

    CEREBRAL PALSY   318

    FEBRILE SEIZURES   319

    NEUROBLASTOMA   320

    WILMS' TUMOR   320

Includes neglect as well as physical, sexual, and emotional abuse. Suspect abuse if (1) the history is **discordant with physical findings,** and/or (2) there is a **delay** in obtaining appropriate medical care.

HISTORY/PE

- Infants may have apnea, seizures, or failure to thrive (FTT).
- Neglect may → poor hygiene and behavioral abnormalities.
- Exam findings include the following:
    - Oddly situated (e.g., face, thighs) **ecchymoses of varying ages or patterned injuries** (e.g., immersion burns, cigarette burns, belt marks).
    - **Spiral fractures** of the humerus and femur in children < 3 years of age suggest abuse until proven otherwise.
    - **Epiphyseal/metaphyseal injuries** can occur in infants from pulling or twisting of the limbs.
    - **Rib injuries** in children < 2 years of age.
    - Findings of **STDs or genital trauma** point to sexual abuse.

DIAGNOSIS

- Rule out conditions that mimic abuse—e.g., bleeding disorders, mongolian spots (bruises), osteogenesis imperfecta (fractures), bullous impetigo (blisters may mimic cigarette burns), and "coining" (an alternative treatment in certain cultures).
- **Skeletal survey and bone scan can show fractures in various stages of healing.**
- Test for gonorrhea, chlamydia, and HIV if sexual abuse is suspected.
- Rule out shaken baby syndrome by performing an ophthalmologic exam for **retinal hemorrhages** (see Clinical Images), CT for **subdural hemorrhages,** and MRI for white matter changes.

TREATMENT

- **Document injuries.**
- **Notify child protective services** for evaluation and possible removal of the child from the home.
- Hospitalize if necessary to stabilize injuries or to protect the child.

Consider abuse if the caretaker's story does not match the child's injury.

Spiral fractures suggest child abuse.

Intrauterine risk factors include maternal alcohol and drug use, exogenous hormones (e.g., OCPs), lithium, and congenital infection. Classified by the presence or absence of cyanosis:

- **Noncyanotic conditions** have left-to-right shunts, in which oxygenated blood from the lungs is shunted back into the pulmonary circulation.
- **Cyanotic conditions** have a right-to-left shunt, in which deoxygenated blood is shunted into the systemic circulation.

Ventricular Septal Defect (VSD)

An opening in the ventricular septum allows blood to flow between ventricles. VSD is the **most common congenital heart defect.** More common in patients with Apert's syndrome (cranial deformities; fusion of fingers and toes), Down syndrome, cri-du-chat syndrome, and trisomies 13 and 18.

Left-to-right shunts— the 3 D's:

VS**D**
AS**D**
P**D**A

HIGH-YIELD FACTS

PEDIATRICS

297

HISTORY/PE

- Symptoms depend on the degree of **left-to-right** shunting. Small defects are usually **asymptomatic** at birth, whereas large defects can present with frequent respiratory infections, FTT, and CHF.
- Examination reveals a **pansystolic murmur at the lower left sternal border** and a **loud pulmonic S2.** In severe defects, systolic thrill, cardiomegaly, and crackles may be present.

DIAGNOSIS

Echocardiogram is diagnostic. ECG may show RVH or LVH but is normal with small VSDs.

TREATMENT

- Most small VSDs close spontaneously.
- Large VSDs (or those in Down syndrome patients) require early surgical repair to prevent complications (e.g., Eisenmenger's syndrome).
- Treat existing CHF with diuretics, inotropes, and ACEIs; treat respiratory infections.
- Endocarditis and septic emboli prophylaxis (e.g., amoxicillin) before dental or pulmonary procedures.

VSD is the most common congenital heart defect.

Atrial Septal Defect (ASD)

A condition in which an opening in the atrial septum allows blood to flow between the atria. **Left-to-right shunting** occurs as a result of lower right-sided pressures. Consequently, **blood flow to the lungs is ↑.**

HISTORY/PE

- Usually presents in late childhood or early adulthood. Symptom onset and severity depend on the size of the defect.
- Large defects → CHF.
- Characterized by easy fatigability, frequent respiratory infections, and FTT.
- Examination reveals a right ventricular heave; a wide and **fixed, split S2;** and a systolic ejection murmur at the upper left sternal border (from ↑ flow across the pulmonary valve).

ASD has a fixed, split S2.

DIAGNOSIS

- **Echocardiogram with color flow Doppler** reveals blood flow between the atria (diagnostic), paradoxic ventricular wall motion, and a dilated right ventricle.
- ECG shows **right-axis deviation** with ostium secundum defects (most common).
- CXR reveals cardiomegaly and ↑ **pulmonary vascular markings.**

In Eisenmenger's syndrome, left-to-right shunt → pulmonary hypertension and shunt reversal.

TREATMENT

- Small defects may close spontaneously and do not require treatment.
- **Antibiotic prophylaxis** before dental procedures is required for ostium primum defects to prevent bacterial endocarditis.
- Surgical closure in infants with CHF and patients with > 2:1 ratio of pulmonary-to-systemic blood flow. Early correction prevents complications such as **arrhythmias**, right ventricular dysfunction, and **Eisenmenger's syndrome.**

Patent Ductus Arteriosus (PDA)

Failure of the ductus arteriosus to close in the first few days of life → a **left-to-right shunt** from the aorta to the pulmonary artery. Risk factors include high altitude (low O_2 tension) and maternal first-trimester **rubella** infection.

HISTORY/PE

- More common in **premature infants** and **females.**
- **Typically asymptomatic,** but may present with FTT, recurrent lower respiratory tract infections, lower extremity clubbing, and CHF symptoms.
- Examination reveals a **wide pulse pressure;** a **continuous "machinery murmur"** at the second left intercostal space at the sternal border; a **loud S2;** and **bounding peripheral pulses.**

DIAGNOSIS

- A color flow Doppler demonstrating blood flow from the aorta into the pulmonary artery is diagnostic.
- With larger PDAs, echocardiography shows left atrial and left ventricular enlargement.
- ECG may show LVH, and CXR may show cardiomegaly.
- Small PDAs often have no signs of cardiomegaly.

TREATMENT

- Give **indomethacin** unless the PDA is needed for survival (e.g., transposition of the great vessels, tetralogy of Fallot, hypoplastic left heart).
- If indomethacin fails or if the child is > 6–8 months of age, surgical closure is preferred.

Coarctation of the Aorta

Constriction of a portion of the aorta → ↑ flow proximal to and ↓ flow distal to the coarctation. Risk factors include **Turner's syndrome** and male sex. One-fourth of patients have a bicuspid aortic valve.

HISTORY/PE

- Often presents in childhood with **asymptomatic hypertension.**
- Dyspnea on exertion, syncope, claudication, epistaxis, and headache may be present.
- On examination, **systolic BP is higher in the upper extremities** and may be **greater in the right arm than in the left.** Femoral pulses are weak or delayed; a late systolic murmur is heard in the left axilla; and apical impulse is forceful.
- Advanced cases may have **lower extremity wasting** from ↓ blood flow.

DIAGNOSIS

- Obtain an ECG (showing LVH), echocardiography, and color flow Doppler.
- Cardiac catheterization (aortography) is diagnostic.
- CXR may reveal a **"3" sign** due to pre- and postdilatation of the coarctation segment with aortic wall indentation and **"rib notching"** due to collateral circulation through intercostal arteries.

Coarctation is a cause of 2° hypertension in children.

In advanced cases of coarctation, patients may have a well-developed upper body and lower extremity wasting.

TREATMENT

- **Surgical correction** or **balloon angioplasty** (controversial).
- Continue **endocarditis prophylaxis** even after treatment.

Transposition of the Great Vessels

A condition in which pulmonary and systemic circulations exist in **parallel.** The aorta is connected to the right ventricle and the pulmonary artery to the left ventricle. **Without a septal defect or a PDA, it is incompatible with life.** Risk factors include Apert's syndrome, Down syndrome, cri-du-chat syndrome, and trisomies 13 and 18.

HISTORY/PE

- **Critical illness and cyanosis typically occur immediately after birth.**
- Examination reveals tachypnea and progressive respiratory failure. Some patients have signs of CHF.

DIAGNOSIS

- Echocardiography.
- CXR may show a narrow heart base and absence of the main pulmonary artery segment (**"egg-shaped silhouette"**).

TREATMENT

- If present, keep the PDA open with **prostaglandin E$_1$ (PGE$_1$).**
- **Balloon atrial septostomy** if immediate surgery is not feasible.
- **Surgical correction** (arterial or atrial switch).

Tetralogy of Fallot

Consists of (1) VSD, (2) right ventricular outflow obstruction (pulmonary stenosis), (3) RVH, and (4) overriding aorta. Early cyanosis results from right-to-left shunting across the VSD. Risk factors include Down syndrome, cri-du-chat syndrome, and trisomies 13 and 18.

HISTORY/PE

- Presents during infancy with **cyanosis, dyspnea,** and fatigability. Children often **squat for relief** (↑ systemic vascular resistance) during hypoxemic episodes (**"tet" spells**).
- Hypoxemia may → FTT or mental status changes.
- Examination reveals a **systolic ejection murmur** at the left sternal border (due to right ventricular outflow obstruction) as well as **right ventricular lift,** a single S2, and possibly signs of CHF.

DIAGNOSIS

- **Echocardiography** and catheterization.
- CXR shows a **"boot-shaped"** heart with ↓ pulmonary vascular markings.
- ECG shows right-axis deviation and RVH.

TREATMENT

- Administer **PGE$_1$** to keep the PDA open.
- Treat cyanotic spells with O$_2$, propranolol, knee-chest position, fluids, and morphine.

In transposition of the great vessels, a PDA or septal defect is life sustaining, allowing the mixing of pulmonary and systemic blood flow.

Right-to-left shunts—

the 5 T's:

Tetralogy
Transposition
Truncus arteriosus
Tricuspid atresia
Total anomalous pulmonary venous return

Tetralogy of Fallot—

PROVe

Pulmonary stenosis
RVH
Overriding aorta
VSD

*Transposition—the most common cyanotic heart disease of **infancy.***

*Tetralogy—the most common cyanotic heart disease of **childhood.***

*Both are treated with **PGE$_1$.***

- Temporary palliation can be achieved through creation of an artificial shunt (e.g., balloon atrial septostomy) before definitive surgical correction.

Childhood Vaccinations

Table 2.13-1 summarizes recommended childhood immunizations. Contraindications and precautions are as follows:

- **Contraindications:**
  - Current moderate to severe illness (with or without fever).
  - Severe allergy to a vaccine component or a prior dose of vaccine.
  - Encephalopathy within seven days of prior pertussis vaccination.
  - Anaphylactic egg allergy for influenza vaccine (do prior skin testing).
  - Recent administration of antibody-containing blood products (for live injected vaccines).
  - Avoid live vaccines (oral polio vaccine, varicella, MMR) in immunocompromised and pregnant patients (exception: HIV patients without immunocompromise may receive MMR and varicella).
- **Precautions:**
  - Progressive neurologic disorders.
  - Prior reactions to pertussis vaccine (fever > 40.5°C, shocklike state, persistent crying for > 3 hours within 48 hours of vaccination, or seizure within three days of vaccination).
- The following are **not contraindications** to vaccination:
  - Mild illness and/or low-grade fever.
  - Current antibiotic therapy.
  - Prematurity.

TABLE 2.13-1. Immunization Schedule

Vaccine[a-c]	Birth	2 Months	4 Months	6 Months	12–15 Months	15–18 Months	2 Years	4–6 Years
HBV	x	x		x				
DTaP		x	x	x		x		x
Hib		x	x	x	x			
IPV		x	x	x				x
PPV		x	x	x	x			
MMR					x			x
Varicella					x			
HAV							x	

[a] Influenza vaccine is indicated in patients > 6 months old.

[b] HAV vaccine is recommended at age two in certain regions and high-risk groups.

[c] PPV is recommended for all children aged 2–23 months and certain children > 24 months, but fewer doses are needed.

Note: DTaP = diphtheria, tetanus, and pertussis; Hib = *Haemophilus influenzae* type B; IPV = inactivated polio vaccine; PPV = pneumococcal polysaccharide vaccine; MMR = measles, mumps, and rubella.

Developmental Milestones

Table 2.13-2 highlights major developmental milestones.

Failure to Thrive (FTT)

Defined as persistent weight below the third to fifth percentile for age or "falling off the growth curve" (i.e., crossing two major percentile lines on a growth chart). Risk factors include chronic illness, poverty, low maternal age, chaotic environments, genetic disease (e.g., CF), inborn errors of metabolism, and HIV. Classified as follows:

- **Organic:** When an underlying medical condition is present (e.g., mechanical GI dysfunction; structural abnormalities; infection; endocrine, cardiac, pulmonary, or neurologic diseases).
- **Nonorganic (most cases):** When psychosocial factors are thought to be the cause. Examples include inadequate or improper feeding.

TABLE 2.13-2. Developmental Milestones

AGE	GROSS MOTOR	FINE MOTOR	LANGUAGE	SOCIAL/COGNITIVE
2 months	Lifts head/chest when prone.	Tracks past midline.	Alerts to sound, coos.	Recognizes parent, social smile.
4–5 months	Rolls front to back, back to front (5 months).	Grasps rattle.	Orients to voice, "ah-goo," razzes.	Enjoys looking around, laughs.
6 months	Sits unassisted.	Transfers objects, raking grasp.	Babbles.	Stranger anxiety.
9–10 months	Crawls, pulls to stand.	Uses three-finger pincer grasp.	Says mama/dada (nonspecific).	Waves bye-bye, plays pat-a-cake.
12 months	Cruises (11 months), walks alone.	Uses two-finger pincer grasp.	Says mama/dada (specific).	Imitates actions.
15 months	Walks backward.	Uses cup.	Uses 4–6 words.	Temper tantrums.
18 months	Runs, kicks a ball.	Builds tower of 2–4 cubes.	Names common objects.	Copies parent in tasks (e.g., sweeping).
2 years	Walks up/down steps with help, jumps.	Builds tower of six cubes.	Uses two-word phrases.	Follows two-step commands, removes clothes.
3 years	Rides tricycle, climbs stairs with alternating feet (3–4 years).	Copies a circle, uses utensils.	Uses three-word sentences.	Brushes teeth with help, washes/dries hands.
4 years	Hops.	Copies a cross.	Counts to ten.	Cooperative play.

HISTORY/PE

- Patients are of **low weight for age and height** and experience minimal weight gain or weight loss.
- Plot height, weight, and head circumference on a growth chart and compare to population norms.
- Look for signs of systemic disease.
- Take a diet history and observe caregiver-child interaction.

DIAGNOSIS/TREATMENT

- Start a calorie count. **Supplement nutrition** if breast-feeding is inadequate.
- Tests include CBC, electrolytes, creatinine, albumin, and total protein.
- Consider a sweat chloride test (for CF), UA and culture, stool culture/O&P, and assessment of bone age.
- **Hospitalize** if there is evidence of neglect or severe malnourishment.

Hospitilize children if there is evidence of neglect or severe malnourishment.

GENETIC DISEASE

Tables 2.13-3 and 2.13-4 outline common genetic diseases and their associated abnormalities.

Cystic Fibrosis (CF)

An **autosomal-recessive** disorder caused by mutations in the CFTR gene (chloride channel) on **chromosome 7** and characterized by widespread **exocrine gland dysfunction.** CF is the most common severe genetic disease in the United States and is most frequently found in **Caucasians.**

HISTORY/PE

- Some 50% of cases present with FTT or respiratory compromise.
- Characterized by **recurrent pulmonary infections** (especially with *Pseudomonas* and *S. aureus*) with subsequent cyanosis, digital clubbing, cough, dyspnea, **bronchiectasis,** hemoptysis, chronic sinusitis, rhonchi, rales, hyperresonance to percussion, and nasal polyposis.
- Some 15% of infants present with **meconium ileus.** Patients usually have greasy stools and flatulence.
- **Malabsorption syndromes,** pancreatitis, rectal prolapse, esophageal varices, biliary cirrhosis, **abnormal glucose tolerance,** type 2 DM, "salty taste," and unexplained hyponatremia may be present.
- Most males are infertile.

DIAGNOSIS

Sweat chloride test > 60 mEq/L for those < 20 years of age and > 80 mEq/L in adults; genetic testing.

TREATMENT

- Pulmonary manifestations are managed with **chest physical therapy, bronchodilators, anti-inflammatory agents, antibiotics,** and DNase.
- Administer **pancreatic enzymes** and **fat-soluble vitamins A, D, E, and K** for malabsorption.

TABLE 2.13-3. **Genetic Diseases**

DISEASE	GENETIC ABNORMALITY	COMMON CHARACTERISTICS
Down syndrome	Trisomy 21	The most common chromosomal disorder and the cause of mental retardation. Associated with advanced maternal age. Presents with mental retardation, flat facial profile, prominent epicanthal folds, and simian crease. Associated with duodenal atresia and congenital heart disease (the most common malformation is septum primum–type ASD due to endocardial cushion defects). Associated with an ↑ risk of acute lymphocytic leukemia (ALL).
Edwards' syndrome	Trisomy 18	Presents with severe mental retardation, rocker-bottom feet, low-set ears, micrognathia, clenched hands, and prominent occiput. Associated with congenital heart disease. Death usually occurs within one year of birth.
Patau's syndrome	Trisomy 13	Presents with severe mental retardation, microphthalmia, microcephaly, cleft lip/palate, abnormal forebrain structures, and polydactyly. Associated with congenital heart disease. Death usually occurs within one year of birth.
Klinefelter's syndrome (male)	XXY	Presence of inactivated X chromosome (Barr body). One of the most common causes of hypogonadism in males. Presents with testicular atrophy; eunuchoid body shape; tall, long extremities; gynecomastia; and female hair distribution.
Turner's syndrome (female)	XO	The most common cause of 1° amenorrhea. No Barr body. Presents with short stature, ovarian dysgenesis, webbing of the neck, and coarctation of the aorta.
Double Y males	XYY	Observed with ↑ frequency among inmates of penal institutions. Phenotypically normal, very tall, severe acne, antisocial behavior (seen in 1–2% of XYY males).
Phenylketonuria	↓ phenylalanine hydroxylase or ↓ tetrahydrobiopterin cofactor	Screened for at birth. Tyrosine becomes essential and phenylalanine builds up → excess phenyl ketones. Mental retardation, fair skin, eczema, musty body odor. Treat with ↓ phenylalanine and ↑ tyrosine in diet.
Fragile X syndrome	An X-linked defect affecting the methylation and expression of FMR1 gene	The second most common cause of genetic mental retardation. Presents with macro-orchidism; long face with a large jaw; large, everted ears; and autism. Triplet repeat disorder that may show genetic anticipation.

HIGH-YIELD FACTS

PEDIATRICS

TABLE 2.13-4. Lysosomal Storage Diseases[a]

DISEASE	ETIOLOGY	MODE OF INHERITANCE
Fabry's disease	Caused by deficiency of α-galactosidase A → accumulation of ceramide trihexoside. Finding: renal failure.	X-linked recessive.
Krabbe's disease	Absence of galactosylceramide β-galactoside → accumulation of galactocerebroside in the brain. Optic atrophy, spasticity, early death.	Autosomal recessive.
Gaucher's disease	Caused by deficiency of β-glucocerebrosidase → glucocerebroside accumulation in brain, liver, spleen, and bone marrow (Gaucher's cells with characteristic "crinkled paper" enlarged cytoplasm). Type I, the more common form, is compatible with a normal life span.	Autosomal recessive.
Niemann-Pick disease	Deficiency of sphingomyelinase → buildup of sphingomyelin and cholesterol in reticuloendothelial and parenchymal cells and tissues. Patients die by age 3.	Autosomal recessive. No man **PICKs (Niemann-PICK)** his nose with his **sphinger.**
Tay-Sachs disease	Absence of hexosaminidase A → GM$_2$ ganglioside accumulation. Death occurs by age 3. Cherry-red spot visible on macula. Carrier rate is 1 in 30 in Jews of European descent (1 in 300 for others).	**Tay-saX lacks heXosaminidase.**
Metachromatic leukodystrophy	Deficiency of arylsulfatase A → accumulation of sulfatide in the brain, kidney, liver, and peripheral nerves.	Autosomal recessive.
Hurler's syndrome	Deficiency of α-L-iduronidase → corneal clouding and mental retardation.	Autosomal recessive.
Hunter's syndrome	Deficiency of iduronate sulfatase. Mild form of Hurler's with no corneal clouding and mild mental retardation.	X-linked recesive. **Hunters** aim for the **X.**

[a] Each of these syndromes is caused by a deficiency in a lysosomal enzyme.

- Nutritional counseling and support are essential for health maintenance.
- Patients who have severe disease (but who can tolerate surgery) may be candidates for lung or pancreas transplants.

GASTROENTEROLOGY

Intussusception

A condition in which one portion of the bowel telescopes into an adjacent segment, usually proximal to the ileocecal valve (see Figure 2.13-1). The **most common cause of bowel obstruction in the first two years of life** (males > females). The cause is often unknown. Risk factors include Meckel's diverticulum, intestinal lymphoma (> 6 years of age), Henoch-Schönlein pur-

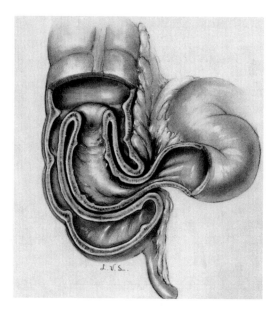

FIGURE 2.13-1.   Intussusception.

A segment of bowel telescopes into an adjacent segment, causing obstruction. (Reproduced, with permission, from Way L. *Current Surgical Diagnosis & Treatment*, 10th ed. Stamford, CT: Appleton & Lange, 1994:1222.)

pura, parasites, polyps, adenovirus or rotavirus infection, celiac disease, and CF.

HISTORY/PE

Intussusception is the most common cause of bowel obstruction in the first two years of life.

- Presents with **abrupt-onset colicky abdominal pain** in apparently healthy children, often with drawing up of the legs and vomiting.
- The classic triad is **abdominal pain, vomiting,** and **blood per rectum** (only 1 in 3 patients).
- Young infants may have pallor and sweating.
- Advanced signs include bloody mucus in stools (**red "currant jelly" stool**), lethargy, and fever.
- On exam, look for abdominal tenderness, ⊕ stool guaiac, and a palpable "sausage-shaped" RUQ abdominal mass.

DIAGNOSIS/TREATMENT

- Correct any volume or electrolyte abnormalities and check CBC (for leukocytosis).
- Abdominal plain films (showing small bowel obstruction) and ultrasound may be helpful.
- **Air-contrast barium enema** is diagnostic and often curative. If the child is unstable or enema reduction is unsuccessful, perform **surgical reduction** and resection of gangrenous bowel.

Pyloric Stenosis

Hypertrophy of the pyloric sphincter → gastric outlet obstruction. **Firstborn males** are more often affected.

HISTORY/PE

- Nonbilious emesis → projectile emesis after every feeding in the first **two weeks to four months** of life. Babies feed well initially but eventually suffer from malnutrition and dehydration.
- Examination may reveal a palpable **olive-shaped, mobile, nontender epigastric mass** and visible gastric peristaltic waves.

DIAGNOSIS

- **Abdominal ultrasound** showing a hypertrophic pylorus is diagnostic.
- Barium studies reveal a narrow pyloric channel ("**string sign**") or a **pyloric beak**.
- Check for **hypochloremic, hypokalemic metabolic alkalosis** due to persistent emesis.

TREATMENT

- Correct existing dehydration and acid-base/electrolyte abnormalities. NG tube placement may be necessary.
- **Surgical correction** with **pyloromyotomy**.

> *For pyloric stenosis, first correct metabolic abnormalities and then perform pyloromyotomy.*

IMMUNOLOGY

Immunodeficiency Disorders

Congenital immunodeficiencies are rare and often present with **chronic or recurrent infections** (e.g., chronic thrush), unusual or opportunistic organisms, incomplete treatment response, or FTT. Categorization is based on the 1° immune system component that is abnormal (see Table 2.13-5):

- **B-cell deficiencies: Most common** (50%). Typically present **after six months of age** with recurrent sinopulmonary, GI, and urinary tract infections with **encapsulated organisms** (*H. influenzae, Streptococcus pneumoniae, Neisseria meningitidis*).

> *DiGeorge syndrome is a —*
>
> **CATCH-22**
>
> **C**ongenital heart disease
> **A**bnormal facies
> **T**hymic aplasia
> **C**left palate
> **H**ypocalcemia
> **22**q deletion

TABLE 2.13-5. Pediatric Immunodeficiency Disorders

DISORDER	DESCRIPTION	INFECTION/RISK TYPE	DIAGNOSIS/TREATMENT
B cell			
X-linked agammaglobulinemia (**Bruton's**)	A **B**-cell deficiency in **boys** only.	Life threatening; *Pseudomonas* infections.	Quantitative immunoglobulin levels; treat with prophylactic antibiotics and IVIG.
Common variable immunodeficiency	Immunoglobulin level drops in the **20s** and **30s**.	↑ pyogenic upper and lower respiratory infections; ↑ risk of lymphoma and autoimmune disease.	Quantitative Ig levels; treat with IVIG.
IgA deficiency	Mild; the most common immunodeficiency.	Usually asymptomatic; patients may develop recurrent infections. Anaphylactic transfusion reaction due to anti-IgA antibodies is a common presentation.	Quantitative IgA levels; treat . infections

TABLE 2.13-5. **Pediatric Immunodeficiency Disorders (continued)**

DISORDER	DESCRIPTION	INFECTION/RISK TYPE	DIAGNOSIS/TREATMENT
T cell			
Thymic aplasia (DiGeorge syndrome)	See mnemonic. Presents with tetany (2° to hypocalcemia) in the first days of life.	Variable risk of infection. ↑↑ infections with fungi and *Pneumocystis carinii* pneumonia (PCP).	Absolute lymphocyte count; mitogen stimulation response; delayed hypersensitivity skin testing. Treat with bone marrow transplantation and IVIG for antibody deficiency; PCP prophylaxis. Alternative—thymus transplant.
Combined			
Ataxia-telangiectasia	**Oculocutaneous telangiectasias** and progressive **cerebellar ataxia.** Caused by a **DNA repair defect.**	↑↑ incidence of non-Hodgkin's lymphoma and gastric carcinoma.	No treatment.
Severe combined immunodeficiency (SCID)	Severe lack of B and T cells.	Severe, frequent bacterial infections; chronic candidiasis; and opportunistic organisms. **Needs PCP prophylaxis.**	Treat with bone marrow transplant or stem cell transplant and IVIG for antibody deficiency.
Wiskott-Aldrich syndrome	An **X-linked** disorder with less severe B- and T-cell dysfunction. Patients have **eczema,** ↑↑ IgE/IgA, ↓↓ IgM, and **thrombocytopenia.** Classic presentation: bleeding, eczema, recurrent otitis media.	↑ risk of atopic disorders, lymphoma/ leukemia, and infection from *S. pneumoniae, S. aureus,* and *H. influenzae* type B.	Treatment is supportive (IVIG and antibiotics). Patients rarely survive to adulthood.
Phagocytic			
Chronic granulomatous disease	An X-linked or autosomal-recessive disease with deficient superoxide production by PMNs and macrophages. Anemia, lymphadenopathy, and hypergamma-globulinemia may be present.	Chronic pulmonary, GI, and urinary tract infections; osteomyelitis and hepatitis. Infecting organisms are catalase ⊕.	Absolute neutrophil count with neutrophil assays. **Nitroblue tetrazolium test is diagnostic for chronic granulomatous disease.** Treat with **daily TMP-SMX;** judicious use of antibiotics during infections. IFN-α can reduce the incidence of serious infection.

TABLE 2.13-5.   Pediatric Immunodeficiency Disorders (continued)

Disorder	Description	Infection/Risk Type	Diagnosis/Treatment
Phagocytic (continued)			
Chédiak-Higashi syndrome	An autosomal-recessive disorder → a defect in neutrophil chemotaxis. Syndrome includes oculocutaneous albinism, neuropathy, and neutropenia.	↑ incidence of overwhelming infections with *S. pyogenes, S. aureus,* and *Pseudomonas* spp.	Bone marrow transplant is the treatment of choice.
Complement			
C1 esterase deficiency (hereditary angioneurotic edema)	An autosomal-dominant disorder with recurrent episodes of angioedema lasting 2–72 hours and provoked by stress or trauma.	Can → life-threatening airway edema.	**Total hemolytic complement (CH50)** to assess the quantity and function of complement. Treat with daily prophylactic **danazol.** Purified C1 esterase and FFP can be used prior to surgery.
Terminal complement deficiency (C5–C9)	Inability to form membrane attack complex (MAC).	Recurrent meningococcal or gonococcal infections. Rarely, lupus or glomerulonephritis.	**Meningococcal vaccine** and **appropriate antibiotics.**

- **T-cell deficiencies:** Tend to present earlier (1–3 months) with **opportunistic and low-grade fungal, viral, and intracellular bacterial infections** (e.g., mycobacteria). 2° B-cell dysfunction may also be seen.
- **Phagocyte deficiencies:** Characterized by mucous membrane infections, **abscesses,** and poor wound healing. **Catalase-⊕ (e.g., *S. aureus*) and gram-⊖ enteric organisms** are common. Delayed umbilical cord separation may be an early sign.
- **Complement deficiencies:** Characterized by recurrent **bacterial** infections with **encapsulated organisms.**

Kawasaki Disease

A multisystem acute vasculitis that primarily affects young children (80% are < 5 years of age), particularly those of Asian ancestry.

Diagnosis

- **Subacute-phase** manifestations are **thrombocytosis and ↑ ESR.**
- **Acute-phase** manifestations are as follows (fever plus ≥ 4 of the criteria below are required for diagnosis):
    - Fever (usually > 40°C) for at least five days.
    - Bilateral, nonexudative, painless conjunctivitis.

309

- Polymorphous rash (primarily truncal).
- Cervical lymphadenopathy (often unilateral, with at least one node > 1 cm).
- Diffuse mucous membrane erythema (e.g., strawberry tongue).
- Erythema of the palms and soles; indurative edema of the hands and feet; late desquamation of fingertips.

TREATMENT

- **High-dose aspirin** (for inflammation and fever) and **IVIG** (to prevent aneurysms).
- **Corticosteroids** may ↑ aneurysm formation and are currently **contraindicated.**

COMPLICATIONS

Untreated patients are at risk for **coronary artery aneurysms** (40%) and MI. Prognosis is tied to the severity of cardiac involvement.

INFECTIOUS DISEASE

Bronchiolitis

An acute inflammatory illness of the small airways that primarily affects **infants** and **children < 2 years of age. RSV** is the **most common cause.** Progression to respiratory failure is a potentially fatal complication. For severe RSV, risk factors include age < 6 months, prematurity, heart or lung disease, and immunodeficiency.

HISTORY/PE

- Low-grade **fever, rhinorrhea, cough, apnea** (in young infants).
- Examination reveals **tachypnea, wheezing,** crackles, prolonged expiration, and **hyperresonance to percussion.**

DIAGNOSIS

- CXR reveals hyperinflation of the lungs, interstitial infiltrates, and atelectasis.
- ELISA of nasal washings for RSV is highly sensitive and specific.

The most common cause of bronchiolitis is RSV.

TREATMENT

- Treat mild disease with outpatient management using fluids, nebulizers, and O_2 if needed.
- Hospitalize in the presence of marked respiratory distress, O_2 saturation of < 92%, toxic appearance, dehydration/poor oral feeding, a history of **prematurity** (< 34 weeks), **age < 3 months,** underlying **cardiopulmonary disease,** or unreliable parents.
- Treat inpatients with contact isolation, hydration, and O_2. A trial of aerosolized albuterol may be attempted with continuation of albuterol therapy if effective.
- **RSV prophylaxis** with injectable poly- or monoclonal antibodies **(RespiGam or Synagis)** is recommended in winter for high-risk patients.

Croup (Laryngotracheobronchitis)

An acute inflammatory disease of the larynx, primarily within the **subglottic** space. Pathogens include parainfluenza virus type 1 (PIV-1; the **most com-**

mon), PIV-2 and -3, RSV, influenza, rubeola, adenovirus, and *Mycoplasma pneumoniae.*

HISTORY/PE

Prodromal URI symptoms are typically followed by low-grade fever, mild dyspnea, inspiratory stridor that worsens with agitation, a hoarse voice, and a characteristic **barking cough** (usually at night).

DIAGNOSIS

- **Clinical** impression.
- AP neck film may show subglottic narrowing (see Figure 2.13-2).
- Table 2.13-6 differentiates croup from epiglottitis and tracheitis.

TREATMENT

- **Mild cases:** Outpatient management with **cool mist therapy** and fluids.
- **Moderate cases:** May require oral **corticosteroids.**
- **Severe cases** (e.g., respiratory distress at rest, inspiratory stridor): Hospitalize and give **nebulized racemic epinephrine.**

Epiglottitis

A serious and rapidly progressive infection of **supraglottic structures** (e.g., epiglottis, arytenoids). Prior to immunization, **H. influenzae type B** was the 1° pathogen. Common causes now include *Streptococcus* spp, nontypable *H. influenzae*, and viral agents.

Epiglottitis may → life-threatening airway obstruction.

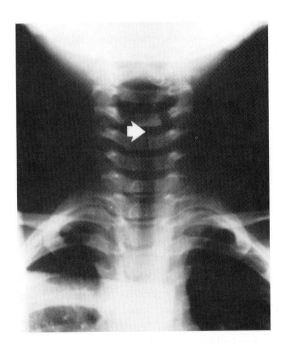

FIGURE 2.13-2. Croup.

The x-ray shows marked subglottic narrowing of the airway ("steeple sign"). (Reproduced, with permission, from Saunders C. *Current Emergency Diagnosis & Treatment,* 4th ed. Stamford, CT: Appleton & Lange, 1992:448.)

TABLE 2.13-6.   Characteristics of Croup, Epiglottitis, and Tracheitis

	CROUP	EPIGLOTTITIS	TRACHEITIS
Age group	3 months to 3 years	3–7 years	3 months to 2 years
Incidence in children presenting with stridor	88%	8%	2%
Pathogen	PIV	*H. influenzae*	Often *S. aureus*
Onset	Prodrome (1–7 days)	Rapid (4–12 hours)	Prodrome (3 days) → acute decompensation (10 hours)
Fever severity	Low grade	High grade	Intermediate grade
Associated symptoms	Barking cough, hoarseness	Muffled voice, drooling	Variable respiratory distress
Position preference	None	Seated, neck extended	None
Response to racemic epinephrine	Stridor improves	None	None
CXR findings	"Steeple sign" on AP film	"Thumbprint sign" on lateral film	Subglottic narrowing

Throat examination may precipitate laryngospasm and airway obstruction.

HISTORY/PE

- Acute-onset high **fever** (39–40°C), **dysphagia, drooling, muffled voice,** inspiratory retractions, cyanosis, **soft stridor.**
- Patients sit with the neck hyperextended and chin protruding ("**sniffing dog**" position) and lean forward in a "**tripod**" position to maximize air entry.
- Untreated infection can → life-threatening airway obstruction and respiratory arrest.

DIAGNOSIS

- Clinical impression.
- In light of potential laryngospasm and airway compromise, **do not examine the throat** unless an anesthesiologist is present.
- Definitive diagnosis is made via direct fiberoptic visualization of cherry-red, swollen epiglottis and arytenoids.
- Lateral x-ray shows a swollen epiglottis obliterating the valleculae ("**thumbprint sign**"; see Figure 2.13-3).

TREATMENT

- This disease is a true emergency. Keep the patient (and parents) calm, call anesthesia, and **transfer the patient to the OR.**
- Treat with **endotracheal intubation or tracheostomy** and **IV antibiotics** (ceftriaxone or cefuroxime).

Otitis Media

A middle ear infection commonly caused by **S. pneumoniae, H. influenzae,** or **Moraxella catarrhalis.** Children are predisposed owing to a shorter, more

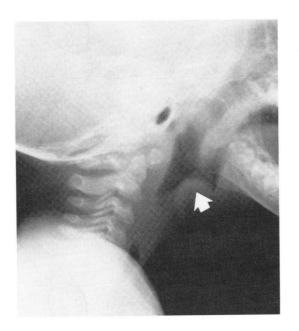

FIGURE 2.13-3. **Epiglottitis.**

The classic swollen epiglottis ("thumbprint sign"; arrow) and obstructed airway are seen on lateral neck x-ray. (Reproduced, with permission, from Saunders C. *Current Emergency Diagnosis & Treatment*, 4th ed. Stamford, CT: Appleton & Lange, 1992:447.)

horizontal eustachian tube. Risk factors include viral URIs, trisomy 21, CF, immunodeficiencies, smoke exposure, day-care attendance, bottle feeding, cleft palate, and prior otitis media.

HISTORY/PE

- Parents may report **fever, ear tugging, hearing loss, irritability,** crying, feeding difficulties, and vomiting.
- Classic exam findings are **erythema**, opacity, **bulging,** and ↓ **mobility** (with insufflation) of the **tympanic membrane** with **loss of the light reflex and bony landmarks.**
- The tympanic membrane may be perforated (see Figure 2.13-4).

DIAGNOSIS

Diagnosis is clinical. Erythema alone is insufficient (can be caused by vigorous crying).

TREATMENT

- Treat with **amoxicillin × 10 days.**
- Patients with treatment failure (persistent ear pain, fever, or bulging tympanic membrane) after three days can be switched to amoxicillin–clavulanic acid, ceftriaxone, or cefuroxime.

Viral Exanthems

Table 2.13-7 outlines the clinical presentation of common viral exanthems.

The clinical diagnosis of otitis media must include erythema, bulging, and ↓ mobility of the tympanic membrane.

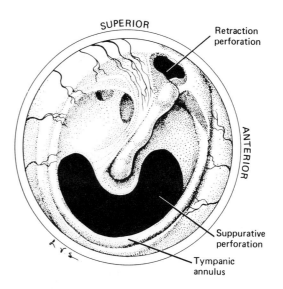

FIGURE 2.13-4. Perforated tympanic membrane.

Common sites of tympanic membrane perforation. (Reproduced, with permission, from Saunders C. *Current Emergency Diagnosis & Treatment*, 4th ed. Stamford, CT: Appleton & Lange, 1992:433.)

NEONATOLOGY

Apgar Scoring

APGAR:

Appearance (color)
Pulse (heart rate)
Grimace (reflex irritability)
Activity (muscle tone)
Respiratory effort

A rapid scoring system that helps evaluate the need for neonatal resuscitation. Each of five parameters (see the mnemonic **APGAR**) is assigned a score of 0–2 at one and five minutes after birth.

- Scores of **8–10** typically reflect good cardiopulmonary adaptation.
- Scores of **4–7** indicate the possible need for resuscitation. Infants should be observed, stimulated, and possibly given ventilatory support.
- Scores of **0–3** indicate the need for immediate resuscitation.

Congenital Malformations

Table 2.13-8 describes selected congenital malformations.

Direct hyperbilirubinemia is always pathologic.

Neonatal Jaundice

Elevated serum bilirubin concentration (> 5 mg/dL) due to ↑ production (e.g., hemolysis) or ↓ excretion. Subtypes are as follows:

- **Conjugated (direct) hyperbilirubinemia:** Always pathologic.
- **Unconjugated (indirect) hyperbilirubinemia:** May be physiologic or pathologic. See Table 2.13-9 for differentiating characteristics.
- **Kernicterus:** A complication of unconjugated hyperbilirubinemia that results from irreversible bilirubin deposition in the basal ganglia, pons, and cerebellum. It typically occurs at levels of > 20 mg/dL and can be fatal. Risk factors include prematurity, asphyxia, and sepsis.

TABLE 2.13-7. Viral Exanthems

DISEASE	CAUSE	CHARACTERISTICS	COMPLICATIONS
Erythema infectiosum (fifth disease)	Parvovirus B19	**Prodrome:** None; fever is often absent or low grade. **Rash:** "**Slapped-cheek**" erythematous rash; erythematous, pruritic, maculopapular rash starts on the arms and spreads to the trunk and legs; **worse with fever and sun exposure.**	Arthritis, hemolytic anemia, encephalopathy. Congenital infection associated with fetal hydrops and death. Aplastic crisis may be precipitated in children with ↑ RBC turnover (e.g., sickle cell anemia, hereditary spherocytosis) or in those with ↓ RBC production (e.g., severe iron deficiency anemia).
Measles	Paramyxovirus	**Prodrome:** Low-grade fever with cough, coryza, and conjunctivitis (the "**three C's**"); Koplik's spots (small irregular red spots with central gray specks) appear on the buccal mucosa after 1–2 days. **Rash:** Erythematous, maculopapular rash spreads from the head toward the feet.	**Common:** Otitis media, pneumonia, laryngotracheitis. **Rare:** Subacute sclerosing panencephalitis.
Rubella	Rubella virus	**Prodrome:** Asymptomatic or tender, generalized lymphadenopathy. **Rash:** Erythematous, tender maculopapular rash and slight fever. Polyarthritis may be seen in adolescents.	Encephalitis, thrombocytopenia (rare complication of postnatal infection). Congenital infection is associated with congenital anomalies.
Roseola infantum	HHV-6	**Prodrome:** Acute onset of high fever (> 40°C); no other symptoms for 3–4 days. **Rash: Maculopapular rash appears as fever breaks** (begins on the trunk and quickly spreads to the face and extremities) and often lasts < 24 hours.	**Febrile seizures** may occur as a result of rapid fever onset.
Varicella	Varicella-zoster virus (VZV)	**Prodrome:** Mild fever, anorexia, and malaise precede rash by 24 hours. **Rash:** Generalized, pruritic, "**teardrop**" vesicular rash begins on the trunk and spreads to the periphery; **lesions are often at different stages of healing.** Infectious from 24 hours before eruption until lesions crust over.	Progressive varicella with meningoencephalitis and hepatitis occurs in immune-compromised children. Congenital infection associated with congenital anomalies.
Varicella zoster	VZV	**Prodrome:** Reactivation of varicella infection; starts as pain along an affected sensory nerve. **Rash:** Pruritic "teardrop" vesicular rash in a **dermatomal distribution.** Uncommon unless immunocompromised.	Encephalopathy, aseptic meningitis, pneumonitis, thrombotic thrombocytopenic purpura, Guillain-Barré syndrome, cellulitis, arthritis.
Hand-foot-and-mouth disease	Coxsackie A	**Prodrome:** Fever, anorexia, oral pain. **Rash: Oral ulcers;** maculopapular **vesicular rash** on hands, feet, and sometimes buttocks.	None (self-limited).

HIGH-YIELD FACTS

PEDIATRICS

TABLE 2.13-8.   Selected Congenital Malformations

MALFORMATION	PRESENTATION/DIAGNOSIS/TREATMENT
Tracheoesophageal fistula	Tract between the trachea and esophagus. Associated with defects such as esophageal atresia and **VACTERL** anomalies (**V**ertebral, **A**nal, **C**ardiac, **T**racheal, **E**sophageal, **R**enal, **L**imb). **Presentation:** Polyhydramnios in utero, ↑ oral secretions, inability to feed, gagging, respiratory distress. **Diagnosis:** CXR after NG tube placement identifies esophageal atresia. The presence of air in the GI tract is suggestive; confirm with bronchoscopy. **Treatment:** Surgical repair.
Congenital diaphragmatic hernia	GI tract segments protrude through the diaphragm into the thorax; 90% are posterior left (Bochdalek). **Presentation:** Respiratory distress (from **pulmonary hypoplasia and pulmonary hypertension), sunken abdomen, bowel sounds over left hemithorax.** **Diagnosis:** Ultrasound in utero; confirmed by postnatal CXR. **Treatment:** High-frequency ventilation or extracorporeal membrane oxygenation to manage pulmonary hypertension; surgical repair.
Gastroschisis	Herniation of the intestine through the abdominal wall next to the umbilicus (usually on the right) with no sac. **Presentation:** Polyhydramnios in utero; often premature; associated with GI stenoses or atresia. **Treatment: A surgical emergency!** Single-stage closure is possible in only 10% of cases.
Omphalocele	Herniation of abdominal viscera through the abdominal wall at umbilicus **into a sac covered by peritoneum and amniotic membrane.** **Presentation:** Polyhydramnios in utero; often premature; associated with other GI and cardiac defects. **Treatment:** C-section can prevent sac rupture; **if sac is intact, postpone surgical correction** until the patient is fully resuscitated. Keep the sac covered/stable with petroleum and gauze. Intermittent NG suction to prevent abdominal distention.
Duodenal atresia	Complete or partial failure of the duodenal lumen to recanalize during gestational weeks 8–10. **Presentation:** Polyhydramnios in utero; **bilious emesis** within hours **after first feeding; associated with Down syndrome** and other cardiac/GI anomalies (e.g., annular pancreas, malrotation, imperforate anus). **Diagnosis:** Abdominal radiographs show **"double-bubble" sign** (air bubbles in the stomach and duodenum) proximal to the site of atresia. **Treatment:** Surgical repair.
Meckel's diverticulum	Vestigial remnant of the omphalomesenteric duct **(the most common congenital GI tract anomaly).** **Rule of 2's: 2** times as many males affected; **2** feet from the ileocecal valve (most common); **2** types of mucosa (gastric, pancreatic); **2**% of people affected. **Presentation:** Painless rectal bleeding (most common), intestinal obstruction from intussusception or volvulus, painful diverticulitis (often mistaken for appendicitis). **Diagnosis:** Meckel's scan (for ectopic gastric mucosa; uses IV **technetium pertechnetate,** which is preferentially taken up by gastric mucosa).
Hirschsprung's disease (congenital aganglionic megacolon)	Absence of autonomic innervation of bowel wall; inadequate relaxation and peristalsis → intestinal obstruction. **Presentation:** Abdominal distention, bilious vomiting, **failure to pass meconium** in the first 24 hours of life. **Diagnosis: Barium enema** reveals dilated proximal segment and narrowed distal segment. **Rectal biopsy** with lack of ganglion cells is confirmatory. **Treatment:** Colostomy prior to corrective surgery allows for pelvic growth and normalization of dilated bowel.

TABLE 2.13-9. Differentiating Physiologic and Pathologic Jaundice

PHYSIOLOGIC JAUNDICE	PATHOLOGIC JAUNDICE
Not present until 72 hours after birth.	Present in the first 24 hours of life.
Bilirubin ↑ < 5 mg/dL/day.	Bilirubin ↑ > 0.5 mg/dL/hour.
Bilirubin peaks at < 14–15 mg/dL.	Bilirubin ↑ to >15 mg/dL.
Direct bilirubin is < 10% of total.	Direct bilirubin is >10% of total.
Resolves by one week in term infants and two weeks in preterm infants.	Persists beyond one week in term infants and two weeks in preterm infants.

HISTORY/PE

- Ask if the child is **breast or formula fed.**
- Look for intrauterine drug exposure and a family history of hemoglobinopathies, enzyme deficiencies, or RBC defects.
- Note abdominal distention, delayed passage of meconium, **light-colored stools, dark urine,** low Apgar scores, weight loss, and vomiting.
- Kernicterus presents with lethargy, poor feeding, a high-pitched cry, hypertonicity, and seizures.
- Jaundice may follow a **cephalopedal progression** as bilirubin concentration ↑.
- Look for infection, congenital malformations, cephalohematomas, bruising, pallor, petechiae, and hepatomegaly.
- The differential includes the following:
  - **Conjugated:** Extrahepatic cholestasis (biliary atresia, choledochal cysts), intrahepatic cholestasis (neonatal hepatitis, inborn errors of metabolism, TPN cholestasis), ToRCHeS infections.
  - **Unconjugated:** Physiologic jaundice, hemolysis, breast milk jaundice, ↑ enterohepatic circulation (e.g., GI obstruction), disorders of bilirubin metabolism, sepsis.

DIAGNOSIS

- Obtain a CBC with peripheral blood smear, blood typing of mother and infant (for **ABO or Rh incompatibility**), Coombs' test, and bilirubin levels.
- For direct hyperbilirubinemia, check LFTs, bile acids, blood cultures, sweat test, and tests for aminoacidopathies and α_1-antitrypsin deficiency.
- A jaundiced neonate who is febrile, hypotensive, and/or tachypneic needs a full sepsis workup and ICU monitoring.

TREATMENT

- Treat underlying causes (e.g., infection).
- Treat unconjugated hyperbilirubinemia with **phototherapy** (mild elevations) or **exchange transfusion** (severe elevations). Start phototherapy earlier (10–15 mg/dL) for preterm infants. Phototherapy with conjugated hyperbilirubinemia can → skin bronzing.

A jaundiced neonate with abnormal vital signs requires a full workup for sepsis.

Respiratory Distress Syndrome (RDS)

The most common cause of respiratory failure in **preterm infants** (affects > 70% of infants born at 28–30 weeks' gestation). **Surfactant deficiency** → poor lung compliance and atelectasis. Risk factors include maternal DM, male sex, and the second born of twins.

HISTORY/PE

Presents in the **first 48–72 hours of life** with **a respiratory rate > 60/min**, progressive **hypoxemia**, cyanosis, **nasal flaring, intercostal retractions,** and **expiratory grunting.**

DIAGNOSIS

- Check ABGs, CBC, and blood cultures to rule out infection.
- Diagnosis is based mainly on characteristic CXR findings:
  - **RDS:** Bilateral diffuse atelectasis → a **"ground-glass"** appearance and air bronchograms.
  - **Transient tachypnea of the newborn:** Retained amniotic fluid → prominent perihilar streaking in interlobular fissures.
  - **Meconium aspiration:** Coarse, irregular infiltrates; hyperexpansion and pneumothoraces.
- **Congenital pneumonia:** Nonspecific patchy infiltrates; neutropenia, tracheal aspirate, and Gram stain suggest the diagnosis.

TREATMENT

- **Continuous positive airway pressure (CPAP)** or intubation and mechanical **ventilation.**
- **Artificial surfactant** administration ↓ mortality.
- Pretreat mothers at risk for preterm delivery with **corticosteroids;** monitor fetal lung maturity via **lecithin-sphingomyelin ratio** and phosphatidylglycerol.

COMPLICATIONS

Persistent PDA and bronchopulmonary dysplasia. Retinopathy of prematurity, intraventricular hemorrhage, and necrotizing enterocolitis are complications of treatment.

NEUROLOGY

Cerebral Palsy

A range of **nonprogressive**, nonhereditary disorders of movement and posture; the most common movement disorder in children. In most cases the cause is unknown, but it often results from perinatal neurologic insult. Risk factors include prematurity, perinatal asphyxia, intrauterine growth retardation, early infection or trauma, brain malformation, and neonatal cerebral hemorrhage. Categories include the following:

- **Pyramidal (spastic):** Spastic paresis of any or all limbs. Accounts for 75% of cases. Mental retardation is present in up to 90%.
- **Extrapyramidal (nonspastic):** A result of damage to extrapyramidal tracts. Subtypes are **ataxic** (difficulty coordinating purposeful movements), **choreoathetoid,** and **dystonic** (uncontrollable jerking, writhing, or posturing). Abnormal movements worsen with stress and disappear during sleep.

HISTORY/PE

- May be associated with **seizure** disorder, behavioral disorder, hearing or vision impairment, **learning disabilities,** and **speech deficits.**
- Affected limbs may show **hyperreflexia,** pathologic reflexes (e.g., Babinski), ↑ **tone/contractures,** weakness, and/or underdevelopment.
- Toe walking and scissor gait are common. Hip dislocations and scoliosis may occur.

DIAGNOSIS

Clinical impression. EEG may be useful in patients with seizures.

TREATMENT

- Special education, physical therapy, braces, and surgical release of contractures may help.
- Treat spasticity with **diazepam, dantrolene, or baclofen.** Baclofen pumps and posterior rhizotomy may alleviate severe contractures.

Febrile Seizures

Usually occur in children between **six months and six years** of age who have **no evidence of intracranial infection or other cause.** Risk factors include a **rapid ↑ in temperature** and a history of febrile seizures in a close relative.

HISTORY/PE

- Seizures usually **occur during onset of fever** and may be the first sign of an underlying illness (e.g., otitis media, **roseola**).
- Classified as simple or complex:
    - **Simple:** A short-duration (< 15 minutes), **generalized seizure** with one seizure in a 24-hour period. High fever (> 39°C) and fever onset within hours of the seizure are typical.
    - **Complex:** A long-duration (> 15 minutes), **focal seizure** with > 1 seizure in a 24-hour period. Low-grade fever for several days before seizure onset may be present.

DIAGNOSIS

- Focus on finding a source of infection. **LP is indicated if there are clinical signs of CNS infection** (e.g., altered consciousness, meningismus, tense/bulging anterior fontanelle) after ruling out ↑ ICP.
- No lab studies are needed if presentation is consistent with febrile seizures in children > 18 months of age.
- For atypical presentations, obtain electrolytes, serum glucose, blood cultures, UA, and CBC with differential.
- The utility of **EEG and MRI** in evaluating **complex febrile seizures** is controversial.

Perform LP if CNS infection is suspected in a patient with a febrile seizure.

TREATMENT

- Use **antipyretic therapy** (avoid aspirin owing to the risk of Reye's syndrome) and treat any underlying illness. Note that antipyretic therapy does not ↓ the occurrence of febrile seizures.
- For complex seizures, perform a thorough neurologic evaluation. Chronic anticonvulsant therapy (e.g., diazepam or phenobarbital) may be necessary.

Patients with complex febrile seizures may require chronic anticonvulsant therapy.

COMPLICATIONS

Febrile seizures will recur in 30% of children. For simple seizures, there is **no** ↑ **risk of epilepsy** or developmental, intellectual, or growth abnormalities. Patients with **complex** seizures have a 10% risk of developing epilepsy.

Neuroblastoma

An **embryonal tumor of neural crest cell origin.** More than half of patients are < 2 years of age. Associations include neurofibromatosis and Hirschsprung's disease, as well as the N-myc oncogene.

HISTORY/PE

- Lesions may occur anywhere in the body (e.g., abdomen, mediastinum).
- Symptoms vary with location and may include a **nontender abdominal mass** (may cross the midline), **Horner's syndrome, hypertension,** or cord compression (from a paraspinal tumor).
- Patients may have anemia, FTT, and fever.
- Site-specific metastases may → **proptosis** and **periorbital bruising** ("raccoon eyes"), **subcutaneous tumor nodules,** bone pain with pancytopenia (from bone marrow infiltration), and **opsoclonus/myoclonus** ("dancing eyes, dancing feet").

DIAGNOSIS

Check abdominal CT and 24-hour urinary catecholamines for ↑ **VMA** and **HVA.** Assess disease extent with CXR, bone scan, CBC, LFTs, BUN/creatinine, and coagulation panel.

> **Top childhood cancers:**
>
> 1. Leukemia (ALL)
> 2. CNS tumors
> 3. Lymphoma
> 4. Neuroblastoma

TREATMENT

- Localized tumors are usually cured with **excision.**
- Chemotherapy and adjunctive radiation may be used for tumor spread beyond the organ of origin.

Wilms' Tumor

A **renal tumor of embryonal origin** that is the most common renal tumor in children. Usually seen in children 2–4 years of age. Associated with a family history, Beckwith-Wiedemann syndrome (hemihypertrophy, macroglossia, visceromegaly), neurofibromatosis, and **WAGR** syndrome (**W**ilms', **A**niridia, **G**enitourinary abnormalities, mental **R**etardation).

HISTORY/PE

- Patients may have nausea, emesis, bone pain, dysuria, polyuria, weight loss, **hematuria** (usually microscopic), **fever,** and **hypertension.**
- The most common finding is a **painless abdominal/flank mass** (does not cross the midline).

Wilms' tumor is associated with aniridia and hemihypertrophy.

DIAGNOSIS

- **Abdominal CT or ultrasound** shows a solid **intrarenal mass.**
- Assess for metastases with CXR, chest CT, CBC, LFTs, and BUN/creatinine.

TREATMENT

- **Transabdominal nephrectomy** and **postsurgical chemotherapy.**
- Flank irradiation is used in some cases.
- Prognosis is generally good but depends on staging and histology.

HIGH-YIELD FACTS IN

Psychiatry

Generalized Anxiety Disorder

- **Chronic, excessive anxiety or worry** about **activities or life** → significant impairment or distress.
- The male-to-female ratio is 1:2; clinical onset is usually in the early 20s.
- **Hx/PE:** Anxiety on most days (≥ 6 months) and ≥ 3 somatic symptoms (restlessness, fatigue, difficulty concentrating, irritability, muscle tension, disturbed sleep).
- **Rx:** Lifestyle changes, psychotherapy, medication. SSRIs, venlafaxine, and buspirone are most often used (see Table 2.14-1). Benzodiazepines may be used for immediate symptom relief. Patient education is essential.

Obsessive-Compulsive Disorder (OCD)

- Characterized by obsessions and/or compulsions that → significant distress and dysfunction in social or personal areas. Typically presents in late adolescence or early adulthood.
- Often a chronic condition that is difficult to treat.
- **Hx/PE:**
  - **Obsessions:** Persistent, unwanted, and **intrusive ideas, thoughts, impulses, or images** that → marked anxiety or distress (e.g., contamination, fear of harm to oneself or loved ones) and occur despite the patient's attempts to prevent them.
  - **Compulsions: Repeated mental acts or behaviors** that neutralize anxiety from obsessions (e.g., hand washing, elaborate rituals for ordinary tasks, counting, excessive checking).
  - Patients **recognize these as excessive and irrational products of their own minds.**
- **Rx:** Pharmacotherapy (clomipramine or SSRIs; see Table 2.14-1) and cognitive-behavioral therapy (CBT) using exposure and response prevention/desensitization. Patient education is imperative.

TABLE 2.14-1. Anxiolytic Medications

NAME	INDICATIONS	SIDE EFFECTS
SSRIs (fluoxetine, sertraline, paroxetine, citalopram, escitalopram)	Generalized anxiety disorder, OCD, PTSD.	Nausea, GI upset, somnolence.
Buspirone	Generalized anxiety disorder, OCD, PTSD.	Seizures with chronic use. No tolerance, dependence, or withdrawal.
β-blockers	Performance anxiety, PTSD.	Bradycardia, hypotension.
Benzodiazepines	Anxiety, insomnia, alcohol withdrawal, muscle spasm.	↓ sleep duration. Risk of abuse, tolerance, and dependence.
Flumazenil	Antidote to benzodiazepine intoxication.	Resedation. Nausea, dizziness, vomiting, pain at injection site.

Panic Disorder

- Characterized by recurrent, unexpected panic attacks.
- Common among females in their 20s. **Agoraphobia** is present in 30–50% of cases.
- Hx/PE:
  - **Panic attacks:** Discrete periods of intense fear or discomfort in which at least four of the following symptoms develop abruptly and peak within 10 minutes: chest pain, **palpitations, diaphoresis,** nausea, tachypnea, trembling, dizziness, **fear of dying** or "going crazy," and depersonalization.
  - **One or more months** of concern about having additional attacks or significant behavior change as a result of the attacks.
- **Rx:** CBT, respiratory training, antidepressants (e.g., SSRIs, TCAs). Benzodiazepines (e.g., clonazepam) may be used for immediate relief, but avoid long-term use in light of their potential for addiction and for the development of tolerance (see Table 2.14-1).

Phobias (Social and Specific)

- Defined as follows:
  - **Social phobia:** Characterized by marked anxiety provoked by **social or performance situations** in which embarrassment may occur. It may be specific (e.g., public speaking) or general (e.g., social interaction) and often begins in adolescence.
  - **Specific phobia:** Anxiety is provoked by exposure to a **feared object or situation** (e.g., animals, heights, airplanes). Most cases begin in childhood.
- **Hx/PE:** Excessive or unreasonable fear and/or avoidance of an object or situation that is persistent and → significant distress or impairment. A related history of traumatic events or panic attacks may be present.
- **Rx:**
  - Desensitization through incremental exposure to the feared object or situation.
  - Other options include relaxation and breathing techniques; hypnosis; and supportive, family, and insight-oriented psychotherapy.
  - SSRIs, low-dose benzodiazepines, or β-blockers (for performance anxiety) may be used for social phobia (see Table 2.14-1).

Post-traumatic Stress Disorder (PTSD)

- Follows exposure to an extreme traumatic stressor (e.g., assault, combat, witnessing a violent crime) that evoked intense fear, helplessness, or horror.
- Hx/PE:
  - **Reexperiencing of the event** (e.g., nightmares), **avoidance** of stimuli associated with the trauma, **numbed responsiveness** (e.g., detachment, anhedonia), and ↑ **arousal** (e.g., hypervigilance, exaggerated startle) are characteristic.
  - Symptoms must persist for > **1 month.**
  - Survivor guilt, irritability, poor concentration, amnesia, personality change, sleep disturbance, substance abuse, depression, and suicidality may be present.
- **Rx:** SSRIs are first line; buspirone is occasionally helpful (see Table 2.14-1). Short-term agents **targeting anxiety** include β-blockers, benzodiazepines, and α₂-agonists (e.g., clonidine). **CBT** and **support groups** are also effective.

DEMENTIAS:

Degenerative diseases (Parkinson's, Huntington's)

Endocrine (thyroid, parathyroid, pituitary, adrenal)

Metabolic (alcohol, electrolytes, vitamin B_{12} deficiency, glucose, hepatic, renal, Wilson's disease)

Exogenous (heavy metals, carbon monoxide, drugs)

Neoplasia

Trauma (subdural hematoma)

Infection (meningitis, encephalitis, endocarditis, syphilis, HIV, prion diseases, Lyme disease)

Affective disorders (pseudodementia)

Stroke/**S**tructure (vascular dementia, ischemia, vasculitis, normal pressure hydrocephalus)

Dementia

An acquired impairment in **cognitive** functioning with **global deficits, especially memory loss**. Prevalence is highest in people > 85 years of age. The course is typically chronic and progressive. The most common causes are **Alzheimer's disease** (50%) and **multi-infarct dementia** (25%). Other causes are outlined in the mnemonic **DEMENTIAS**.

HISTORY/PE

Diagnostic criteria include **memory impairment and ≥ 1** of the following:

- Aphasia.
- Apraxia.
- Agnosia.
- **Impaired executive function** in the presence of a **clear sensorium.**
- Symptoms may worsen at night (**"sundowning"**).
- Personality, mood, and behavior changes are common.
- Insomnia and aggression are common caregiver complaints about the patient.

DIAGNOSIS

- A careful history and physical is critical. Serial mini-mental status exams should be performed.
- Rule out treatable causes of dementia; obtain CBC, RPR, CMP, TFTs, HIV, B_{12}/folate, ESR, and UA.
- Table 2.14-2 outlines key characteristics distinguishing dementia from delirium.

TREATMENT

- Insomnia and aggression often necessitate nursing home placement. Provide **environmental cues** and a rigid structure to the patient's daily life.
- Low-dose **antipsychotics** may be used for agitation. **Avoid benzodiazepines,** which may worsen disinhibition and confusion.
- Adequate support for the caregiver is imperative.

TABLE 2.14-2. Delirium vs. Dementia

	DELIRIUM	DEMENTIA
Level of attention	Impaired (fluctuating).	Usually alert.
Onset	Acute.	Gradual.
Course	Fluctuating from hour to hour.	Progressive deterioration.
Consciousness	Clouded.	Intact.
Hallucinations	Present (often visual or tactile).	Usually absent unless disease is very advanced.
Prognosis	Reversible.	Irreversible.

Delirium

A **transient disturbance of consciousness** with **altered cognition** that is not attributable to dementia and develops over a short period of time (usually hours to days). Children, the elderly, and hospitalized patients (**e.g., ICU psychosis**) are particularly susceptible. Major causes are outlined in the mnemonic **I WATCH DEATH**.

HISTORY/PE

- Presents with acute onset of **waxing and waning consciousness** and **perceptual disturbances** (hallucinations, illusions, delusions).
- Anxiety, paranoia, or combativeness may be present.
- Also characterized by ↓ attention span and short-term memory; reversed sleep-wake cycle; and ↑ symptoms at night.

DIAGNOSIS

- Check vitals, pulse oximetry, and glucose; perform physical and neurologic exams.
- Note recent medications (narcotics or benzodiazepines), substance use, prior episodes, medical problems, signs of organ failure, and infection (**occult UTI is common in the elderly;** check UA).
- Laboratory and radiologic studies to identify a possible underlying cause.

TREATMENT

- Treat underlying causes (delirium is often reversible).
- Normalize fluids and electrolytes.
- **Optimize the sensory environment.**
- Use low-dose **antipsychotics** (e.g., haloperidol) for agitation and psychotic symptoms.
- Use **physical restraints** if necessary to prevent harm to the patient or others.

MOOD DISORDERS

Major Depressive Disorder

A unipolar mood disorder characterized by ≥ 1 major depressive episodes (MDEs). The **male-to-female ratio is 1:2.** Onset may be at any age but usually occurs in the mid-20s; in the elderly, prevalence ↑ with age. **Chronic illness and stress** ↑ risk. **Untreated MDEs typically last ≥ 4 months,** and the risk of recurrence is 60% after one MDE. Up to 15% of patients die by suicide.

HISTORY/PE

Diagnosis requires **depressed mood or loss of interest/pleasure AND ≥ 5 signs/symptoms** from the **SIG E CAPS** mnemonic nearly every day **for a two-week period.** Table 2.14-3 outlines disorders that may be mistaken for depression. Selected depression subtypes include the following:

- **Psychotic features:** Typically **mood-congruent** delusions/hallucinations.
- **Postpartum:** Occurs within one month postpartum; has a 10% incidence and a high risk of recurrence.
- **Atypical:** Weight gain, hypersomnia, rejection sensitivity.

TABLE 2.14-3. **Differential of Major Depression**

DISEASE	DISTINGUISHING FEATURES
Mood disorder due to a medical condition	Hypothyroidism, Parkinson's disease, stroke, CNS neoplasm.
Substance-induced mood disorder	Illicit drugs, alcohol. Symptoms usually resolve after detoxification.
Adjustment disorder with depressed mood	A constellation of symptoms resembling an MDE, but in the context of a recent life stressor.
Normal bereavement	Occurs after loss of a loved one. No severe impairment/suicidality; usually resolves in one year, but varies with cultural norms.
Dysthymia	Milder, chronic depression for < 2 years; often resistant to treatment.

Cheese and red wine can precipitate a hypertensive crisis when consumed while a patient is on an MAOI.

Psychotherapy and antidepressant treatment are more effective together than either treatment alone.

Symptoms of mania—

DIG FAST

Distractibility
Insomnia (↓ need for sleep)
Grandiosity (↑ self-esteem)/more **G**oal directed
Flight of ideas (or racing thoughts)
Activities/psychomotor Agitation
Sexual indiscretions
Talkativeness

■ **Seasonal:** Recurrent fall and winter depression; treat with bright-light therapy +/− antidepressants.
■ **Double depression:** MDE in a dysthymic patient.

TREATMENT

■ **Pharmacotherapy:** Effective in 50–70% of patients. Allow 2–4 weeks for effect; treat for ≥ 6 months (see Table 2.14-4).
■ **Electroconvulsive therapy (ECT):**
  ■ Safe, highly effective, often lifesaving therapy that is reserved for refractory or psychotic depression.
  ■ May also be used for acute mania and acute psychosis; usually requires 6–12 treatments.
  ■ Adverse effects include postictal confusion, arrhythmias, headache, and **retrograde amnesia.**
■ Contraindications include recent MI/stroke, intracranial mass, seizure disorder, and high anesthetic risk (a relative contraindication).
■ **Psychotherapy:** Psychotherapy combined with antidepressants is more **effective than either treatment alone.** Cognitive, behavioral, and interpersonal therapies are among the techniques with proven efficacy.

Bipolar Disorders

Prevalence is approximately 1%, and the male-to-female ratio is 1:1. A family history of bipolar illness significantly ↑ risk. Average age of onset is 20, and the frequency of mood episodes tends to ↑ with age. Up to 10–15% of those affected die by suicide. Subtypes are as follows:

■ **Bipolar I: At least one manic or mixed episode** (usually requiring hospitalization) that may alternate with MDEs or hypomanic episodes.
■ **Bipolar II: At least one MDE and one hypomanic episode** (less intense than mania). Patients do not meet the criteria for full manic or mixed episodes.
■ **Rapid cycling:** Four or more episodes (MDE, manic, mixed, or hypomanic) in one year.
■ **Cyclothymic:** Chronic and less severe, with alternating periods of hypomania and moderate depression.

TABLE 2.14-4. Indications and Side Effects of Common Antidepressants

NAME	INDICATIONS	SIDE EFFECTS
SSRIs Fluoxetine Sertraline Paroxetine Citalopram Escitalopram	First-line therapy for depression. Anxiety disorders.	Sexual side effects. ↓ appetite, insomnia, headache, tremor. **Serotonin syndrome** (fever, myoclonus, mental status changes, cardiovascular collapse) can occur if used with MAOIs.
Atypicals Bupropion Venlafaxine Mirtazapine Nefazodone Trazodone	First-line therapy for depression owing to **lack of sexual side effects.** Other indications include OCD, chronic pain, and migraine. Trazodone is also used as a sleep aid as well as for erectile dysfunction.	**Bupropion:** ↓ seizure threshold; no sexual side effects. **Venlafaxine:** Diastolic hypertension. **Mirtazapine:** Weight gain, sedation. **Nefazodone:** Sedation, headache, dry mouth. **Trazodone:** Highly sedating; priapism.
TCAs Nortriptyline Desipramine Amitriptyline Imipramine	Depression.	**Lethal** with overdose owing to cardiac conduction arrhythmias. **Anticholinergic** effects (dry mouth, constipation, urinary retention).
MAOIs Tranylcypromine Phenelzine	Depression.	Hypertensive crisis if taken with high-**tyramine** foods (cheese, red wine). Sexual side effects.

HISTORY/PE

- The mnemonic **DIG FAST** outlines the clinical presentation of mania.
- Patients may report excessive spending or sexual activity, reckless behaviors, and/or psychotic features.
- Antidepressant use may trigger manic episodes.

DIAGNOSIS

- A manic episode is ≥ 1 week (or less if the patient is hospitalized) of **persistently elevated, expansive, or irritable mood** plus **three DIG FAST symptoms.**
- Symptoms are not due to a substance or medical condition and → significant functional impairment.
- Hypomania is similar but does not → marked functional impairment and is of shorter duration.

TREATMENT

- **Acute mania:** Antipsychotics (see Table 2.14-5) and mood stabilizers (see Table 2.14-6). Benzodiazepines may be useful in refractory agitation.
- **Bipolar depression:** Mood stabilizers +/– antidepressants. **Start mood stabilizers first** to avoid inducing mania. ECT may be used to treat refractory cases.

> TCA toxicity–
>
> **Tri-C's:**
>
> **C**onvulsions
> **C**oma
> **C**ardiac arrhythmias

Chronic lithium use can → hypothyroidism and nephrotoxicity. Lamotrigine can → a life-threatening skin rash.

TABLE 2.14-5. **Antipsychotic Medications**

NAME	INDICATIONS	SIDE EFFECTS
Typical antipsychotics Haloperidol Droperidol Fluphenazine Thioridazine Chlorpromazine	Psychotic disorders and acute agitation.	**Extrapyramidal symptoms** (EPS). **Hyperprolactinemia.** **Anticholinergic effects:** Dry mouth, urinary retention, constipation. Seizures. **Neuroleptic malignant syndrome:** Fever, muscle rigidity, autonomic instability, clouded consciousness.
Atypical antipsychotics Clozapine Risperidone Quetiapine Olanzapine Ziprasidone Aripiprazole	Currently first-line treatment for schizophrenia. Clozapine is reserved for treatment resistance and severe tardive dyskinesia. Benefits are fewer EPS and anticholinergic effects.	Weight gain, type 2 diabetes mellitus, somnolence, QTc prolongation. **Clozapine: Agranulocytosis** requiring weekly CBC monitoring.

TABLE 2.14-6. **Mood Stabilizers**

NAME	INDICATIONS	SIDE EFFECTS
Lithium	1° mood stabilizer. Used for acute mania (in combination with antipsychotics); prophylaxis of mania and depression in bipolar disorders; and augmentation of depression treatment.	Thirst, polyuria, tremor, weight gain, hypothyroidism. Nephrotoxicity, ataxia, dysarthria, delirium, nausea, diarrhea, seizures. Narrow therapeutic window.
Carbamazepine	Second-line mood stabilizer, anticonvulsant.	Nausea, skin rash, leukopenia, AV block, respiratory depression, coma. Rarely, aplastic anemia (monitor CBC biweekly). Stevens-Johnson syndrome.
Valproic acid	Most widely used drug for bipolar disorder; also used for acute mania. No proven effect for prophylaxis, but still used for this purpose.	GI, tremor, sedation, ataxia, alopecia, weight gain. Rarely, pancreatitis, thrombocytopenia, fatal hepatotoxicity, and agranulocytosis.
Lamotrigine	Mood stabilizer in treatment-refractory patients.	Ataxia, blurred vision, GI distress. Stevens-Johnson syndrome.

HIGH-YIELD FACTS

PSYCHIATRY

Characterized by chronically inadequate maladaptive traits that affect most aspects of one's life (see the mnemonic **MEDIC**). Onset is in early adulthood. Impairment in baseline functioning encompasses a broad range of situations throughout the patient's life; these are defined under Axis II (Axis I disorders are considered a clinical syndrome that is a distinct departure from premorbid functioning). Specific disorders are outlined in Table 2.14-7.

DIAGNOSIS

- Rule out Axis I disorders.
- Ask about attitudes, mood variability, activities, and reaction to stress. Patients have chronic problems dealing with responsibilities, roles, and stressors. They also have difficulty understanding the cause of their problems as well as difficulty changing their behavior patterns.

TREATMENT

- **Psychotherapy** is the mainstay of therapy.
- **Pharmacotherapy** is reserved for cases of comorbid mood, anxiety, or psychotic disorders.

> **Characteristics of personality disorders—**
>
> **MEDIC**
>
> **M**aladaptive
> **E**nduring
> **D**eviates from cultural norms
> **I**nflexible
> **C**auses impairment in social functioning

TABLE 2.14-7. Signs and Symptoms of Personality Disorders

CLUSTER	DISORDERS	CHARACTERISTICS	CLINICAL DILEMMA/STRATEGY
Cluster A: **"weird"**	Paranoid	Distrustful, suspicious; interpret others' motives as malevolent.	Patients are suspicious and distrustful of doctors and rarely seek medical attention.
	Schizoid	Isolated, detached "loners." Restricted emotional expression.	Be clear, honest, noncontrolling, and nondefensive. Avoid humor. Maintain emotional distance.
	Schizotypal	Odd behavior, perceptions, appearance. Magical thinking, ideas of reference.	
Cluster B: **"wild"**	Borderline	Unstable mood/relationships, feelings of emptiness. Impulsive.	Patients change the rules, demand attention, and feel they are special.
	Histrionic	Excessively emotional and attention seeking. Sexually provocative.	Will manipulate staff and doctor ("splitting").
	Narcissistic	Grandiose, need admiration, sense of entitlement. Lack empathy.	Be firm: Stick to treatment plan. Be fair: Do not be punitive or derogatory.
	Antisocial	Violate rights of others, social norms, laws. Impulsive. Lack remorse.	Be consistent: Do not change rules.
Cluster C: **"worried and wimpy"**	Obsessive-compulsive	Preoccupied with perfectionism, order, control. Inflexible morals, values.	Patients are controlling and may sabotage their treatment. Words may be inconsistent with actions.
	Avoidant	Socially inhibited, rejection sensitive. Fear being disliked or ridiculed.	Avoid power struggles. Give clear recommendations, but do not push
	Dependent	Submissive, clingy, need to be taken care of. Difficulty making decisions.	patients into decisions.

HIGH-YIELD FACTS

PSYCHIATRY

Schizophrenia

Characterized by hallucinations, delusions, disordered thoughts, behavioral disturbances, and disrupted social functioning in a clear sensorium. Prevalence is approximately 1%; the male-to-female ratio is 1:1. **Peak onset is earlier in males (ages 18–25)** than in **females (ages 25–35).** Schizophrenia in first-degree relatives ↑ risk. Etiologic theories focus on neurotransmitter abnormalities such as dopamine dysregulation (frontal hypoactivity, limbic hyperactivity) and brain abnormalities on CT and MRI. **Ten percent of those affected commit suicide.** Subtypes are as follows:

- **Paranoid:** Delusions (often persecuting the patient) and/or hallucinations are present. Cognitive function is usually preserved. Associated with the best overall prognosis.
- **Disorganized:** Speech and behavior patterns are highly disordered with flat affect. Carries the worst prognosis.
- **Catatonic:** Psychomotor disturbance with ≥ 2 of the following: excessive motor activity, immobility, extreme negativism, mutism, waxy flexibility, echolalia, or echopraxia.

HISTORY/PE

- Two or more of the following are present continuously for **≥ 6 months** with **social or occupational dysfunction:**
  - ⊕ **symptoms:** Hallucinations (most often auditory), delusions, disorganized speech and behavior.
  - ⊖ **symptoms:** Flat affect, ↓ emotional reactivity, poverty of speech, lack of purposeful actions.
- The differential includes the following:
  - **Schizophreniform disorder:** Symptoms of schizophrenia with a duration of < 6 months.
  - **Schizoaffective disorder:** Combines the symptoms of schizophrenia with a major affective disorder (major depressive disorder or bipolar disorder).

TREATMENT

- **Antipsychotics** (see Table 2.14-5) and hospitalization during psychotic episodes.
- Supportive psychotherapy and training in social skills may help.
- ⊖ symptoms may be more difficult to treat. Treatment has the disadvantage of extrapyramidal side effects (see Table 2.14-8).

Attention-Deficit Hyperactivity Disorder (ADHD)

A persistent pattern of excessive inattention and/or hyperactivity/impulsivity. More common in males; typically presents between ages 3 and 13. Often shows a familial pattern.

HISTORY/PE

Diagnosis requires **≥ 6 symptoms** from each category for **≥ 6 months** in **at least two settings** → significant social and academic impairment. Some symptoms must be present in patients **before age seven.**

The 4 A's of schizophrenia:

Associations (loose)
Affect (flat)
Autism (self-preoccupation, noncommunication)
Ambivalence

Evolution of EPS:

4 hours: Acute dystonia
4 days: Akinesia
4 weeks: Akathisia
4 months: Tardive dyskinesia

TABLE 2.14-8. Extrapyramidal Symptoms and Treatment

EPS	Description	Treatment
Acute dystonia	Involuntary muscle contraction or spasm (e.g., torticollis, oculogyric crisis).	Give an anticholinergic (benztropine) or diphenhydramine. To prevent, give prophylactic benztropine and antipsychotic.
Akathisia	Subjective/objective restlessness.	↓ neuroleptic and try β-blockers (propranolol). Benzodiazepines or anticholinergics may help.
Dyskinesia	Pseudoparkinsonism (e.g., shuffling gait, cogwheel rigidity).	Give an anticholinergic (benztropine) or dopamine agonist (amantadine). Decrease dose of neuroleptic or discontinue (if tolerated).
Tardive dyskinesia	Stereotypic oral-facial movements. Likely from dopamine receptor sensitization. Often irreversible (50%).	Discontinue or ↓ dose of neuroleptic, attempt treatment with more appropriate drugs, and consider changing neuroleptic (e.g., to clozapine or risperidone). **Giving anticholinergics or decreasing neuroleptic may initially worsen tardive dyskinesia.**

- **Inattention: Poor attention span** for schoolwork/play; poor attention to detail or careless mistakes; does not listen when spoken to; has **difficulty following instructions or finishing tasks;** loses items needed to complete tasks; forgetful and **easily distracted.**
- **Hyperactivity/impulsivity:** Fidgets; leaves seat in classroom; runs around inappropriately; cannot play quietly; talks excessively, **does not wait turn; interrupts others.**

Children must exhibit ADHD symptoms in two or more settings (e.g., home and school).

TREATMENT

- Initial treatment may be nonpharmacologic (e.g., behavior modification). Sugar and food additives are **not** considered etiologic factors.
- Pharmacologic treatment includes the following:
  - **Psychostimulants: Methylphenidate** (beware of abuse potential), dextroamphetamine. Adverse effects include insomnia, irritability, ↓ appetite, tic exacerbation, and ↓ growth velocity (normalizes when medication is stopped).
  - **Antidepressants** (e.g., SSRIs, nortriptyline, bupropion) and α_2-agonists (e.g., **clonidine**).

Autism Spectrum Disorders

More common in males. May be associated with **tuberous sclerosis and fragile X syndrome.** Symptom severity and IQ vary widely.

HISTORY/PE

- Characterized by abnormal or **impaired social interaction and communication** together with **restricted activities and interests,** evident **before age three.**

- Patients fail to develop normal social behaviors (e.g., social smile, eye contact) and lack interest in relationships.
- Language development is delayed or absent.
- Children show **stereotyped speech and behavior** (e.g., hand flapping) and restricted interests.
- Other pervasive developmental disorders include the following:
    - **Asperger's syndrome:** An autism-like disorder **without marked language or cognitive delays.**
    - **Rett's disorder:** A genetic neurodegenerative disorder of females with progressive impairment (e.g., language, coordination) **after five months of normal development.**
    - **Childhood disintegrative disorder:** Severe developmental **regression** after < 2 years of normal development.

TREATMENT

- Intensive special education, **behavioral management,** and symptom-targeted medications.
- Family support and counseling are crucial.

Conduct disorder is seen in
Children.

Conduct Disorders

- More common in males and in patients with a history of abuse.
- Hx/PE:
    - Repetitive, persistent pattern of **violating the basic rights of others** or age-appropriate **societal norms or rules** for ≥ 1 year. Behaviors may be **aggressive** (e.g., rape, robbery) or **nonaggressive** (e.g., stealing, lying).
    - **Oppositional defiant disorder** is a pattern of **negativistic, defiant, disobedient, and hostile behavior** toward authority figures (e.g., losing temper, arguing) for ≥ 6 months.
    - May progress to antisocial personality disorder.
- **Rx:** Individual and family therapy.

Antisocial personality disorder
is seen in Adults.

Learning Disabilities

- Occurs more frequently in males and in those of low SES; often has a familial pattern.
- Hx/PE:
    - **Academic functioning is substantially below that expected for age, intelligence, and education** as measured by standardized test achievement in reading, mathematics, or written expression.
    - Learning problems significantly interfere with schooling and daily activities.
    - Always rule out physical disorders (e.g., deafness) and social factors (e.g., non–English speakers).
- **Rx:** Interventions include **remedial classes** or **individualized learning strategies.**

Mental Retardation

- Associated with male gender, chromosomal abnormalities, congenital infections, teratogens, and inborn errors of metabolism.
- Hx/PE:
    - Significantly subaverage intellectual functioning (**an IQ of < 70**) with **deficits in adaptive functioning** (e.g., hygiene, social skills) and onset before the age of 18.

- Levels of severity are **mild** (IQ 50–70; **85% of cases**), moderate (IQ 35–49), severe (IQ 20–34), and profound (IQ < 20).
- **Rx:** Family counseling and support; speech and language therapy; occupational/physical therapy; behavioral intervention; educational assistance.

Tourette's Syndrome

- More common in males; shows a genetic predisposition. **Associated with ADHD, learning disorders, and OCD.**
- **Hx/PE:** Begins prior to age 18. Characterized by **multiple motor** (e.g., blinking, grimacing) and **vocal** (e.g., grunting, coprolalia) **tics** occurring many times per day, recurrently, for > 1 year.
- **Rx:** Treatments include haloperidol, pimozide, or clonidine. Counseling can aid in social adjustment and coping. Stimulants can worsen or precipitate tics.

MISCELLANEOUS DISORDERS

Substance Abuse/Dependence

Distinguish substance abuse from dependence as follows:

- **Substance abuse** requires ≥ 1 of the following in one year:
    - **Failure to fulfill responsibilities.**
    - Use in **physically hazardous** situations.
    - **Legal problems** during the time of substance use.
- **Substance dependence** requires ≥ 1 of the following in one year:
    - **Tolerance** and using progressively larger amounts to obtain the same desired effect.
    - **Withdrawal** symptoms when not taking the substance.
    - Failed **attempts to abstain** from the substance.
    - Significant time spent obtaining the substance.
    - Isolation from life activities.

DIAGNOSIS/TREATMENT

- Substance use is often denied or underreported, so seek out collateral information from family and friends.
- Check urine and blood toxicology screens, LFTs, and serum EtOH level.
- Management of intoxication for selected drugs is described in Table 2.14-9.

Alcoholism

- Occurs more often in **males** (4:1) and in those 21–34 years of age, although the incidence in women is rising. Also associated with a ⊕ family history.
- **Hx/PE:** See Table 2.14-9 for the symptoms of intoxication and withdrawal. Look for palmar erythema or telangiectasias as well as other signs and symptoms of end-organ complications.
- **Dx:** Screen with the **CAGE** questionnaire. Monitor vital signs for evidence of withdrawal. Lab tests may reveal ↑ LFTs, LDH, HDL, and MCV.
- **Rx:**
    - Rule out medical complications; correct electrolyte abnormalities.
    - Start **benzodiazepine taper** for withdrawal symptoms.

More than 15% of the U.S. adult population has a serious substance use problem.

Features of substance dependence—

WITHDraw IT

≥ 3 of 7 within a 12-month period:
Withdrawal
Interest or Important activities given up or reduced
Tolerance
Harm (physical and psychosocial) with continued use
Desire to cut down/control
Intended time/amount exceeded
Time spent obtaining/using the substance is ↑

TABLE 2.14-9. **Signs and Symptoms of Substance Abuse**

DRUG	INTOXICATION	WITHDRAWAL
Alcohol	Disinhibition, emotional lability, slurred speech, ataxia, aggression, hypoglycemia, blackouts (retrograde amnesia), coma.	Tremor, tachycardia, hypertension, malaise, nausea, seizures, DTs, agitation, hallucinations.
Opioids	CNS depression, nausea, vomiting, constipation, **pupillary constriction,** seizures, respiratory depression (life threatening in overdose). Naloxone/naltrexone will block opioid receptors and reverse effects (beware of antagonist clearing before opioid, particularly with long-acting opioids such as methadone).	Anxiety, insomnia, anorexia, diaphoresis, dilated pupils, fever, rhinorrhea, piloerection, nausea, stomach cramps, diarrhea, yawning.
Amphetamines	Psychomotor agitation, impaired judgment, hypertension, **pupillary dilation,** tachycardia, fever, euphoria, prolonged wakefulness/attention, arrhythmias, delusions, hallucinations. Can give haloperidol for severe agitation and symptom-targeted medications (e.g., antiemetics, NSAIDs).	Post-use "crash" with anxiety, lethargy, headache, stomach cramps, hunger, fatigue, depression/dysphoria, sleep disturbance.
Cocaine	Psychomotor agitation, euphoria, impaired judgment, tachycardia, **pupillary dilation,** hypertension, paranoia, angina, hallucinations, sudden death. Treat with haloperidol for severe agitation and symptom-targeted medications.	Post-use "crash" with hypersomnolence, depression, malaise, severe craving, suicidality.
Phencyclidine hydrochloride (PCP)	Belligerence, psychosis, violence, impulsiveness, psychomotor agitation, fever, tachycardia, **vertical/horizontal nystagmus,** ataxia, delirium. Give benzodiazepines for severe symptoms; otherwise reassure.	Recurrence of intoxication symptoms due to reabsorption in the GI tract; sudden onset of severe, random violence.
LSD	Marked anxiety or depression, delusions, visual hallucinations, flashbacks, pupillary dilation. Give benzodiazepines or traditional antipsychotics for severe symptoms.	
Marijuana	Euphoria, slowed sense of time, impaired judgment, social withdrawal, increased appetite, dry mouth, conjunctival injection, hallucinations, anxiety, paranoia, amotivational syndrome.	
Barbiturates	Low safety margin, respiratory depression.	Anxiety, seizures, delirium, life-threatening cardiovascular collapse.
Benzodiazepines	Interactions with alcohol, amnesia, ataxia, somnolence, mild respiratory depression.	Rebound anxiety, seizures, tremor, insomnia, hypertension, tachycardia.
Caffeine	Restlessness, insomnia, diuresis, muscle twitching, arrhythmias.	Headache, lethargy, depression, weight gain.
Nicotine	Restlessness, insomnia, anxiety, arrhythmias.	Irritability, headache, anxiety, weight gain, craving, tachycardia.

- Give **multivitamins and folic acid; administer thiamine** before glucose (which depletes thiamine) to prevent Wernicke's encephalopathy.
- Give anticonvulsants to patients with a seizure history.
- Group therapy, disulfiram, or naltrexone can aid patients with dependence.
- **Complications: GI bleeding, pancreatitis, liver disease,** DTs, alcoholic hallucinosis, peripheral neuropathy, Wernicke's encephalopathy, Korsakoff's psychosis.

Anorexia Nervosa

- Risk factors include female gender, low self-esteem, and high SES. Also associated with OCD, major depressive disorder, and careers such as modeling, gymnastics, ballet, and running.
- Hx/PE:
  - **Refusal to maintain normal body weight;** intense **fear of weight gain;** distorted body image **(patients perceive themselves as fat); amenorrhea.**
  - Patients **restrict** (e.g., fasting, excessive exercise) or **binge and purge** (through vomiting, laxatives, and diuretics).
  - Signs and symptoms include **lanugo,** dry skin, bradycardia, lethargy, hypotension, and cold intolerance.
- **Dx:** Measure height and weight; check CBC, electrolytes, endocrine tests, and ECG. Perform a **psychiatric evaluation** to screen for comorbid conditions.
- **Rx:**
  - Initially, monitor caloric intake to stabilize weight; then focus on **weight gain.**
  - Hospitalize if necessary to restore nutritional status and correct electrolyte imbalances.
  - Once the patient is medically stable, initiate individual, family, and group **psychotherapy.** Treat comorbid depression and anxiety.
- **Complications:** Mitral valve prolapse, arrhythmias, hypotension, bradycardia, amenorrhea (missing three consecutive cycles), nephrolithiasis, osteoporosis, multiple stress fractures, pancytopenia, thyroid abnormalities. Mortality from **suicide** or medical complications is > **10%.**

Bulimia Nervosa

- More common among women; associated with low self-esteem and OCD.
- Hx/PE: Diagnostic criteria are as follows:
  - At least two times a week for ≥ 3 months, patients have episodes of **binge eating** and **compensatory behaviors** that include **purging** or **fasting.**
  - Patients are usually **ashamed** and conceal their behaviors.
  - **Signs** include **dental enamel erosion, enlarged parotid glands,** and **scars on the dorsal hand surfaces** (from inducing vomiting). Patients usually have normal body weight.
- **Rx:** Psychotherapy focuses on behavior modification and body image. **Antidepressants** are effective for both depressed and nondepressed patients.

Sexual Disorders

Sexual disorders fall into three categories:

- **Paraphilias:** Abnormal expressions of one's sexuality ranging from nearly normal practices to harmful or destructive behaviors to oneself or others.

Bulimic patients tend to be more disturbed by their behavior than anorexics and are more easily engaged in therapy. Anorexic patients deny health risks associated with their behavior, making them resistant to treatment.

Sexual excitement is derived from unique exposures to certain situations, individuals, or objects. Found almost exclusively in men. See Table 2.14-10 for specific examples.

- **Gender identity disorders: Strong, persistent cross-gender identification** and **discomfort with one's assigned sex** in the absence of intersexual disorders. Associated with depression, substance abuse, and personality disorders.
- **Sexual dysfunction:** Problems in sexual **arousal, desire, orgasm, or pain** with sexual intercourse. Prevalence is 30%. One-third of cases are attributable to biological factors and another third to psychological factors.

Somatoform and Factitious Disorders

Patients often present with **medically unexplained symptoms,** generally with varying etiologies.

- **Somatoform disorders:** Patients have **no conscious control over symptoms.** The five main categories are outlined in Table 2.14-11.
- **Factitious disorders:** Symptom production allows patients to receive 2° **gain from assuming the sick role. Patients fabricate symptoms or cause self-injury to assume the sick role (1° gain).** More common in men; Munchausen syndrome is an example in **health care workers.**
- **Malingering:** Patients **intentionally cause** or feign symptoms for 2° **gain** of **financial benefit** or housing.

Sexual and Physical Abuse

- Most frequently affects women < 35 years of age who fill the following criteria:
  - Are experiencing marital discord and are substance abusers or have a partner who is a substance abuser; or
  - Are pregnant or of low SES or have obtained a restraining order.
- Victims of childhood abuse are more like to become adult victims of abuse.

Sexual abusers are usually male and are often known to the victim (often family members).

TABLE 2.14-10. **Features of Common Paraphilias**

Disorder	Clinical Manifestations
Exhibitionism	Sexual arousal from exposing one's genitals to a stranger.
Pedophilia	Urges or behaviors involving sexual activities with children.
Voyeurism	Observing unsuspecting persons unclothed or involved in sex.
Fetishism	Use of nonliving objects (often clothing) for sexual arousal.
Transvestic fetishism	Cross-dressing for sexual arousal.
Frotteurism	Touching or rubbing against a nonconsenting person.
Sexual sadism	Sexual arousal from inflicting suffering.
Sexual masochism	Sexual arousal from being hurt, humiliated, or threatened.

TABLE 2.14-11. Somatoform Disorders

Somatization disorder	Multiple, chronic symptoms from different organ systems. Frequent clinical contacts and/or surgeries. Significant functional impairment. Male-to-female ratio is 1:20. Manage with regular appointments.
Conversion disorder	Symptoms or deficits of voluntary motor or sensory function (e.g., blindness, seizure) suggest a condition incompatible with medical processes. Close temporal relationship to stress or intense emotion. More common in young females and in lower socioeconomic and less educated groups.
Hypochondriasis	Preoccupation with or fear of having a serious disease despite medical reassurance. Causes significant distress/impairment. Often history of prior physical disease. Men and women are equally affected. Onset in adulthood.
Body dysmorphic disorder	Preoccupation with imagined physical defect or abnormality causes significant distress/impairment. Often presents to dermatologists or plastic surgeons. Slight female predominance. May be associated with depression, and SSRIs may help.
Pain disorder	Intensity or profile of pain symptoms is inconsistent with physiologic processes. More common in females. May be associated with depression.

- Hx/PE:
  - Patients typically have **multiple somatic complaints, frequent ER visits, and unexplained injuries** with **delayed medical treatment**. They may also **avoid eye contact** or act afraid or hostile.
  - Children may exhibit precocious sexual behavior, **genital or anal trauma, STDs,** UTIs, and psychiatric problems.
  - Other clues include a partner who answers questions for the patient or refuses to leave the exam room.
- Rx: Provide **medical care,** emotional **support, and counseling;** educate the patient about **support services** and refer appropriately. **Documentation** is crucial.

Suicide is the third leading cause of death (after homicide and accidents) among 15- to 24-year-olds in the United States.

Suicidality

- Risk factors include psychiatric disorders (major depression, presence of psychotic symptoms), recent severe stressors, and a family suicide history (see the mnemonic **SAD PERSONS**). Women are more likely to attempt suicide, whereas men are more likely to succeed by virtue of their ↑ use of more lethal methods.
- Dx:
  - Perform a comprehensive psychiatric evaluation.
  - Ask about family history, previous attempts, ambivalence toward death, and hopelessness.
  - Ask directly about suicidal ideation, intent, and plan, and look for available means.
- Rx: A patient who endorses suicidality requires emergent inpatient hospitalization even against his will. Suicide risk ↑ after antidepressant therapy is initiated because a patient's energy to act on suicidal thoughts may return before depressed mood lifts.

> **Risk factors for suicide—**
>
> **SAD PERSONS**
>
> **S**ex (male)
> **A**ge (older)
> **D**epression
> **P**revious attempt
> **E**thanol/substance abuse
> **R**ational thought
> **S**ickness (chronic illness)
> **O**rganized plan
> **N**o spouse
> **S**ocial support lacking

Pulmonary

Causes of restrictive lung disease—

PAINT

Pleural (fibrosis, effusions, empyema, pneumothorax)

Alveolar (edema, hemorrhage, pus)

Interstitial lung disease (idiopathic pulmonary fibrosis), **I**nflammatory (sarcoid, bronchiolitis obliterans with organizing pneumonia), **I**diopathic

Neuromuscular (myasthenia, phrenic nerve palsy, myopathy)

Thoracic wall (kyphoscoliosis, obesity, ascites, pregnancy, ankylosing spondylitis)

Figure 2.15-1 contrasts obstructive with restrictive lung disease. The etiologies of restrictive lung disease are shown in the mnemonic **PAINT**.

Interstitial Lung Disease

The classic type of restrictive lung disease; characterized by interstitial thickening of the alveolar walls → dilated terminal/respiratory bronchioles (cystic spaces). Causes include idiopathic pulmonary fibrosis, collagen vascular disease, granulomatous disorders, and pneumoconiosis.

HISTORY/PE

Presents with **shallow, rapid breathing;** dyspnea with exercise; and nonproductive **cough.** Patients may have cyanosis, inspiratory squeaks, fine or "Velcro" crackles, finger clubbing, or right heart failure.

DIAGNOSIS

- **CXR:** Reticular pattern that is more pronounced at the bases; honeycomb pattern (severe disease).
- ↓ TLC, ↓ FVC, ↓ DL_{CO}, normal FEV_1/FVC. Serum markers of connective tissue diseases should be obtained if clinically indicated.

TREATMENT

Supportive. Avoid exposure to the causative agent. Some inflammatory diseases respond to **steroids.**

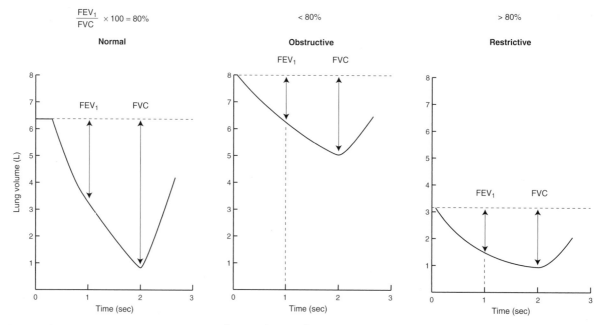

Note: Obstructive lung volumes > normal (↑ TLC, ↑ FRC, ↑ RV); restrictive lung volumes < normal. In both obstructive and restrictive, FEV_1 and FVC are reduced, but in obstructive, FEV_1 is more dramatically reduced, resulting in a ↓ FEV_1/FVC ratio.

FIGURE 2.15-1.   Obstructive vs. restrictive lung disease.

Systemic Sarcoidosis

A systemic rheumatologic disease of unknown etiology characterized by **noncaseating granulomas**. Most commonly found in **black females** and Norwegians; most often arises in the third or fourth decade of life.

HISTORY/PE

A multisystem disorder that commonly presents with **fever, cough, malaise,** weight loss, dyspnea, and **arthritis.** The lungs, liver, eyes, skin (erythema nodosum), nervous system, heart, and kidney may be affected. Symptoms may be GRUELING (see mnemonic).

DIAGNOSIS

- **CXR**: Bilateral hilar lymphadenopathy, usually with interstitial infiltrate.
- **Biopsy**: Transbronchial or video-assisted thoracoscopic biopsy reveals **noncaseating granulomas.**
- **PFTs**: ↓ volumes and diffusion capacity.
- **Other findings**: ↑ **serum ACE levels** (neither sensitive nor specific), **hypercalcemia,** hypercalciuria, ↑ alkaline phosphatase (with liver involvement), lymphopenia, cranial nerve defects, arrhythmias.

TREATMENT

Systemic **corticosteroids.**

Hypersensitivity Pneumonitis

- Risk factors include environmental exposure to antigens → alveolar thickening and granulomas. Types and etiologies are listed in Table 2.15-1.
- Hx/PE:
    - **Acute**: Dyspnea, fever, shivering, cough starting 4–6 hours after exposure.
    - **Chronic**: Progressive dyspnea; exam reveals fine bilateral rales.
- **Dx**: CXR is normal or shows miliary nodular infiltrate (acute); fibrosis is seen in the upper lobes (chronic).
- **Rx**: Avoid ongoing exposure; give steroids to ↓ inflammation.

Drugs associated with interstitial lung disease include busulfan, nitrofurantoin, amiodarone, bleomycin, radiation, and long-term high O_2 concentration (e.g., ventilators).

Features of sarcoid—

GRUELING

Granulomas
Rheumatoid arthritis (it is not really rheumatoid)
Uveitis
Erythema nodosum
Lymphadenopathy
Interstitial fibrosis
Negative TB test
Gammaglobulinemia

TABLE 2.15-1. Antigens of Hypersensitivity Pneumonitis

DISORDER	ANTIGEN
Farmer's lung	Spores of actinomycetes from moldy hay
Bird fancier's lung	Antigens from feathers, excreta, serum
Mushroom worker's lung	Spores of actinomycetes from compost
Malt worker's lung	Spores of *Aspergillus clavatus*
Grain handler's lung	Grain weevil dust
Bagassosis	Spores of actinomycetes from sugarcane
Air conditioner lung	Spores of actinomycetes from air conditioners

Pneumoconiosis

- Risk factors include prolonged occupational exposure and inhalation of small dust particles.
- Hx/PE/Dx: Table 2.15-2 outlines the findings and diagnostic criteria associated with common pneumoconioses.
- Rx: Supportive therapy and supplemental O_2.

The causes of obstructive lung disease are described in the mnemonic **ABCT**.

Asthma

Reversible airway obstruction 2° to bronchial **hyperreactivity**, airway **inflammation, mucous plugging,** and **smooth muscle hypertrophy.**

TABLE 2.15-2. **Pneumoconioses**

	HISTORY	DIAGNOSIS	COMPLICATIONS
Asbestosis	Work involving manufacture of tile or brake linings, insulation, construction, demolition, or building maintenance. Presents 15–20 years after initial exposure.	**CXR:** Linear opacities at lung bases and pleural plaques. **Biopsy:** Asbestos bodies.	↑ risk of mesothelioma and lung cancer; worse in smokers.
Coal mine disease	Work in underground coal mines.	**CXR:** Small nodular opacities (< 1 cm) in upper lung zones. **Spirometry:** Consistent with restrictive disease.	Progressive massive fibrosis.
Silicosis	Work in mines or quarries or with glass, pottery, silica.	**CXR:** Small (< 1 cm) nodular opacities in upper lung zones. **Eggshell calcifications. Spirometry:** Consistent with restrictive disease.	↑ risk of TB; need annual TB skin test. Progressive massive fibrosis.
Berylliosis	Work in high-technology fields such as aerospace, nuclear, and electronics plants; ceramics industries; foundries; plating facilities; dental material sites; and dye manufacturing.	**CXR:** Diffuse infiltrates; hilar adenopathy.	Requires chronic steroid treatments.

HISTORY/PE

Presents with **cough**, dyspnea, **episodic wheezing**, and/or chest tightness. Symptoms often worsen at night or early in the morning. Male gender and older age are additional historical risk factors. Exam reveals tachypnea, tachycardia, ↓ breath sounds, **wheezing, prolonged expiratory duration** (↓ I/E ratio), ↓ O_2 saturation (late sign), hyperresonance, **accessory muscle use**, and possible pulsus paradoxus.

DIAGNOSIS

- **ABG: Mild hypoxia** and **respiratory alkalosis.** Normalizing PCO_2 in an acute exacerbation warrants close observation (may indicate fatigue and impending respiratory failure).
- **Spirometry/PFTs:** Peak flow is **diminished** acutely; ↓ FEV_1, ↑ residual volume.
- **CBC:** Eosinophilia.
- **CXR:** Hyperinflation.
- **Methacholine challenge:** Tests for bronchial hyperresponsiveness; allows definitive diagnosis. Should be performed ≥ 3 months following an acute episode.

TREATMENT

In general, avoid allergens or any potential exacerbating factor. Management is as follows (see also Tables 2.15-3 and 2.15-4):

- **Acute:** O_2, bronchodilating agents (β-agonists are first-line therapy), ipratropium (never use alone), inhaled **steroids.** Intubation for severe cases.

Asthma triggers include allergens, URIs, cold air, exercise, and stress. Beware— all that wheezes is not asthma. Asthma should be suspected in children with multiple episodes of croup and URIs associated with dyspnea.

Medications for treating asthma exacerbations—

ASTHMA

Albuterol
Steroids
Theophylline
Humidified O_2
Magnesium
Antileukotrienes

TABLE 2.15-3. Common Asthma Medications and Their Mechanisms

Nonspecific β-agonists	**Isoproterenol:** Relaxes bronchial smooth muscle ($β_2$). Adverse effect is tachycardia ($β_1$).
$β_2$-agonists	**Albuterol:** Relaxes bronchial smooth muscle ($β_2$). Use during acute exacerbation. **Salmeterol:** Long-acting agent for prophylaxis.
Methylxanthines	**Theophylline:** Likely causes bronchodilation by inhibiting phosphodiesterase, thereby ↓ cAMP hydrolysis. The usage is limited because of narrow therapeutic index (cardiotoxicity, neurotoxicity).
Muscarinic antagonists	**Ipratropium:** Competitive block of muscarinic receptors, preventing bronchoconstriction.
Cromolyn	Prevents release of mediators from mast cells. Effective only for the prophylaxis of asthma. Not effective during an acute asthmatic attack. Toxicity is rare.
Corticosteroids	**Beclomethasone, prednisone:** Inhibit the synthesis of virtually all cytokines. Inactivate NF-κB, the transcription factor that induces the production of TNFα, among other inflammatory agents. First-line therapy for chronic asthma.
Antileukotrienes	**Zileuton:** A 5-lipoxygenase pathway inhibitor. Blocks conversion of arachidonic acid to leukotrienes. **Zafirlukast:** Blocks leukotriene receptors.

TABLE 2.15-4. Medications for Chronic Treatment of Asthma

TYPE	SYMPTOMS (DAY/NIGHT)	FEV₁	MEDICATIONS
Severe persistent	Continual Frequent	60%	High-dose inhaled corticosteroids + long-acting inhaled β_2-agonists. Possible PO steroids. PRN short-acting bronchodilator.
Moderate persistent	Daily 1 night/week	60–80%	Low- to medium-dose inhaled corticosteroids + long-acting inhaled β_2-agonists. PRN short-acting bronchodilator.
Mild persistent	2/week but < 1/day > 2 nights/month	≥ 80%	Low-dose inhaled corticosteroids. PRN short-acting bronchodilator.
Mild intermittent	≤ 2 days/week ≤ 2 nights/month	80%	No daily medications. PRN short-acting bronchodilator.

- **Chronic:** Measure lung function (FEV_1, peak flow, ABG) to guide management. Administer regularly inhaled **bronchodilators** and/or steroids, systemic **steroids**, cromolyn, or **theophylline. Montelukast** and other leukotriene antagonists are oral adjuncts to inhalant therapy.

Bronchiectasis

A disease caused by cycles of infection and inflammation in the bronchi/bronchioles that → permanent fibrosis, remodeling, and **dilatation of bronchi.**

HISTORY/PE

- Presents with frequent bouts of yellow or green **sputum** accompanied by **cough,** dyspnea, and possible hemoptysis and halitosis.
- Associated with a history of pulmonary infections (e.g., *Pseudomonas, Haemophilus,* TB), hypersensitivity (allergic bronchopulmonary aspergillosis), CF, immunodeficiency, aspiration, autoimmune disease (e.g., rheumatoid arthritis, SLE), or IBD.
- Exam reveals rales, wheezes, rhonchi, purulent mucus, and occasional hemoptysis.

DIAGNOSIS

- **CXR:** ↑ bronchovascular markings; **tram lines** (parallel lines outlining dilated bronchi as a result of peribronchial inflammation and fibrosis); areas of **honeycombing.**
- **High-resolution CT: Dilated airways** and ballooned cysts at the end of the bronchus (mostly lower lobes). Spirometry shows a ↓ FEV_1/FVC ratio.

TREATMENT

- Antibiotics for bacterial infections; consider inhaled corticosteroids.
- Maintain bronchopulmonary hygiene (cough control, postural drainage, chest physiotherapy).
- Consider lobectomy or lung transplantation for severe disease.

> **Differential diagnosis—**
>
> **BRONCHIECTASIS**
>
> **B**ronchial cyst
> **R**epeated gastric acid aspiration
> **O**r due to foreign bodies
> **N**ecrotizing pneumonia
> **C**hemical corrosive substances
> **H**ypogamma-globulinemia
> **I**mmotile cilia syndrome
> **E**osinophilia (pulmonary)
> **C**ystic fibrosis
> **T**uberculosis (1°) or *Mycobacterium avium-intracellulare*
> **A**topic bronchial asthma
> **S**treptococcal pneumonia
> **I**n Young's syndrome
> **S**taphylococcal pneumonia

Chronic Obstructive Pulmonary Disease (COPD)

Characterized by ↓ lung function with airflow obstruction. Generally due to chronic bronchitis or emphysema, which are distinguished as follows:

- **Chronic bronchitis:** Productive cough ≤ 3 months per year for two consecutive years.
- **Emphysema:** Terminal airway destruction that may be due to **smoking** (centrilobular) or to α_1-**antitrypsin deficiency** (panlobular).

HISTORY/PE

- Symptoms are minimal or nonspecific until the disease is advanced (> 50% of lung function is lost).
- Presents as follows:
  - **Emphysema ("pink puffer"): Dyspnea, pursed lips,** minimal cough, ↓ breath sounds, late hypercarbia/hypoxia. Pure emphysematous patients tend to have less reactive airways between exacerbations.
  - **Chronic bronchitis ("blue bloater"): Productive cough;** cyanosis with mild dyspnea; patients are often overweight with peripheral edema, rhonchi, and early hypercarbia/hypoxia. Look for barrel chest, use of accessory chest muscles, JVD, end-expiratory **wheezing,** or muffled breath sounds.

DIAGNOSIS

- **CXR:** ↓ lung markings with flat diaphragms, **hyperinflated lungs,** and a thin-appearing heart and mediastinum. Parenchymal **bullae** or subpleural **blebs** (pathognomonic of emphysema) are also seen (see Figure 2.15-2).

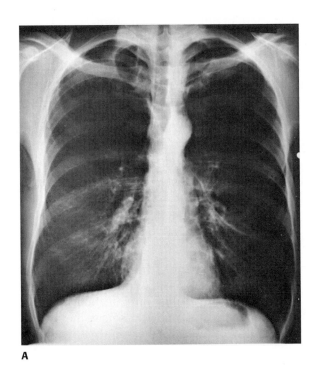
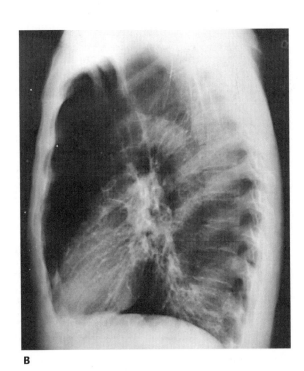

A   B

FIGURE 2.15-2. **Chronic obstructive pulmonary disease.**

Note the hyperinflated and hyperlucent lungs, flat diaphragms, increased AP diameter, narrow mediastinum, and large upper bullae on (A) AP and (B) lateral CXRs. (Reproduced, with permission, from Stobo JD et al. *The Principles and Practice of Medicine,* 23rd ed. Stamford, CT: Appleton & Lange, 1997:135.)

347

- **PFTs:** $\downarrow$ FEV_1/FVC, normal or $\downarrow$ FVC, normal or $\uparrow$ TLC (emphysema, asthma).
- **ABG:** Hypoxemia with **acute respiratory acidosis** ($\uparrow$ P_{CO_2}).
- **Blood cultures:** Obtain if the patient is febrile.
- **Gram stain and sputum culture:** Obtain if fever or productive cough is present.

TREATMENT

- **Acute exacerbations:** O_2, inhaled β-agonists (albuterol) and **anticholinergics** (ipratropium), IV steroids, **antibiotics.** Severe cases may benefit from noninvasive ventilation.
- **Chronic:** **Smoking cessation**, supplemental O_2, inhaled β-agonists, anticholinergics, steroids. Give pneumococcal and **flu vaccines.**

ACUTE RESPIRATORY FAILURE

Hypoxemia

- Causes include right-to-left shunt, hypoventilation, low inspired O_2 content (important only at altitudes), **ventilation-perfusion (V/Q) mismatch,** and **diffusion impairment.**
- **Hx/PE:** Findings depend on etiology. $\downarrow$ HbO_2 saturation, cyanosis, tachypnea, shortness of breath, pleuritic chest pain, and altered mental status are possible.
- **Dx:**
  - **Pulse oximetry:** Demonstrates $\downarrow$ HbO_2 saturation.
  - **CXR:** To rule out ARDS, atelectasis, or an infiltrative process (e.g., pneumonia) and to look for signs of pulmonary embolism.
  - **ABGs:** To evaluate PaO_2 and to calculate the **alveolar-arterial (A-a) gradient** ($[(P_{atm} - 47) \times F_{IO_2}] - [(PaCO_2/0.8) - PaO_2]$). An $\uparrow$ A-a gradient suggests a V/Q mismatch or a diffusion impairment. Figure 2.15-3 summarizes the approach toward hypoxemic patients.
- **Rx:**
  - Based on the underlying etiology.
  - O_2 (before initiating evaluation).
  - **If the patient is on a ventilator:** $\uparrow$ O_2 saturation by $\uparrow$ F_{IO_2}, $\uparrow$ **positive end-expiratory pressure (PEEP),** or $\uparrow$ I/E ratio.
  - **Hypercapnic patients:** $\uparrow$ minute ventilation ($\uparrow$ tidal volume or $\uparrow$ respiratory rate).

Acute Respiratory Distress Syndrome (ARDS)

Acute respiratory failure with refractory **hypoxemia,** $\downarrow$ **lung compliance,** and **noncardiogenic pulmonary edema.** The pathogenesis is thought to be endothelial injury. Commonly occurs with sepsis, aspiration, infection, multiple blood transfusions, inhaled/ingested toxins, trauma, multiorgan failure, or shock. Overall mortality is > 50%.

HISTORY/PE

Presents with acute-onset (12–48 hours) tachypnea, dyspnea, tachycardia, fever, cyanosis, labored breathing, diffuse high-pitched rales, and hypoxemia

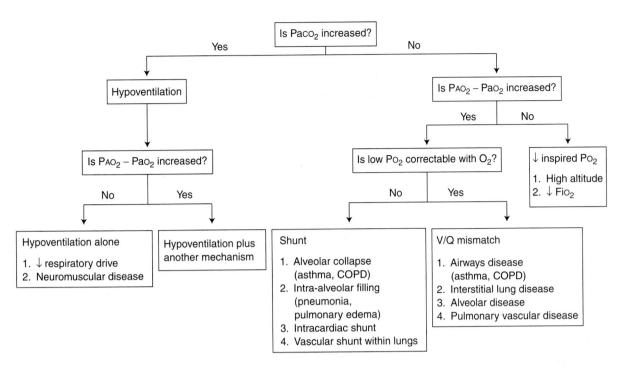

FIGURE 2.15-3. Determination of the mechanism of hypoxia.

(Reproduced, with permission, from Kasper DL et al (eds). *Harrison's Principles of Internal Medicine*, 16th ed. New York: McGraw-Hill, 2005.)

in the setting of one of the systemic inflammatory causes or exposure. Additional findings are as follows:

- **Phase 1 (acute injury):** Normal physical exam; respiratory alkalosis.
- **Phase 2 (6–48 hours):** Hyperventilation, hypocapnia, widening A-a oxygen gradient.
- **Phase 3:** Acute respiratory failure, tachypnea, dyspnea, ↓ lung compliance, scattered rales, diffuse chest infiltrates on CXR (see Figure 2.15-4).
- **Phase 4:** Severe hypoxemia unresponsive to therapy; ↑ intrapulmonary shunting; metabolic and respiratory acidosis.

> **ARDS diagnosis:**
>
> **A**cute onset
> **R**atio (Pao_2/Fio_2) ≤ 200
> **D**iffuse infiltration
> **S**wan-Ganz wedge
>   pressure < 18 mmHg

DIAGNOSIS

The criteria for ARDS diagnosis (according to the American-European Consensus Conference definition) are as follows:

- Acute onset of respiratory distress.
- **Pao_2/Fio_2 ratio ≤ 200 mmHg.**
- Bilateral pulmonary infiltrates on CXR.
- **No evidence of cardiac origin** (normal capillary wedge pressure = 18 mmHg).

TREATMENT

There is no standard successful treatment. **Treat the underlying disease and maintain adequate perfusion and O_2 delivery to the organs.** Use mechanical ventilation with low tidal volumes and PEEP (because of ↓ lung compliance). Goal oxygenation is Fio_2 < 0.6, Pao_2 < 60 mmHg, and Sao_2 > 90%; the objective is to minimize further airway trauma from high pressure.

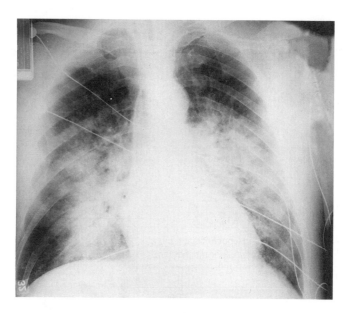

FIGURE 2.15-4. **AP chest radiograph demonstrating a diffuse alveolar filling pattern due to ARDS.**

(Reproduced, with permission, from Kasper DL et al (eds). *Harrison's Principles of Internal Medicine*, 16th ed. New York: McGraw-Hill, 2005:1497.)

The main disorder of the pulmonary vasculature is pulmonary hypertension, which is defined as a mean $P_{PA} > 25$ mmHg (normal = 15 mmHg). Causes include left heart failure, mitral valve disease, and ↑ resistance in the pulmonary veins, including hypoxic vasoconstriction.

PULMONARY VASCULAR DISEASE

Pulmonary Hypertension/Cor Pulmonale

- Causes include diseases of the heart (left heart failure → right heart failure, mitral disease); problems with the pulmonary vessels (1° pulmonary hypertension, thromboembolic disease); or problems with the lung parenchyma → hypoxic vasoconstriction → right heart failure (COPD).
- **Hx/PE:**
  - Dyspnea on exertion, fatigue, lethargy, chest pain, edema, abdominal distention, syncope with exertion.
  - Associated with a history of COPD, sickle cell anemia, emphysema, and pulmonary emboli.
  - Presents with a loud, palpable S2 (often split), systolic ejection murmur, S4, or parasternal heave.
- **Dx:** CXR shows enlargement of central pulmonary arteries; ECG shows RVH.
- **Rx:** Supplemental O_2, diuretics, vasodilators, or digoxin. Treatment is dependent on etiology.

Pulmonary Thromboembolism

Occlusion of the pulmonary vasculature by a blood clot. Ninety-five percent of emboli originate from DVTs in the deep leg veins. Often → pulmonary infarction, right heart failure, and hypoxemia. **Virchow's triad** consists of the following:

- **Stasis:** Immobility, CHF, obesity, surgery, ↑ central venous pressure.
- **Endothelial injury:** Trauma, surgery, recent fracture, previous DVT.
- **Hypercoagulable states:** Pregnancy/postpartum, OCP use, coagulation disorders (e.g., protein C/protein S deficiency, factor V Leiden), malignancy, severe burns.

HISTORY/PE

- Presents with sudden-onset dyspnea, **pleuritic chest pain, low-grade fever,** cough, and hemoptysis (rarely).
- **Pulmonary embolism:**
    - Hypoxia and hypocarbia with resulting respiratory alkalosis.
    - Tachypnea, tachycardia, fever.
    - Loud P2; prominent jugular a waves with right heart failure.
- **Venous thrombosis:** Unilateral swelling; Homans' sign (calf pain on forced dorsiflexion); cords on the calf.

DIAGNOSIS

- **ABG:** Respiratory alkalosis (due to hyperventilation) with $Po_2 < 80$ mmHg.
- **CXR:** Usually normal, but may show atelectasis, pleural effusion, **Hampton's hump** (a wedge-shaped infarct), or **Westermark's sign** (oligemia in the embolized lung zone).
- **ECG:** Not diagnostic; most commonly reveals **sinus tachycardia.** The classic triad of **S1Q3T3**—acute right heart strain with an S wave in lead I, a Q wave in lead III, and an inverted T wave in lead III—is uncommon.
- **V/Q scan:** May reveal segmental areas of mismatch. Results are reported with a designated probability of pulmonary embolism (low, indeterminate, high) and are interpreted on the basis of clinical suspicion.
- **Helical (spiral) CT with IV contrast:** Sensitive for pulmonary embolism in the proximal pulmonary arteries, but less so in the distal segmental arteries.
- **Angiogram:** Gold standard, but more invasive and rarely done (see Figure 2.15-5).

Dyspnea, tachycardia, and a normal CXR in a hospitalized and/or bedridden patient should raise suspicion of pulmonary embolism.

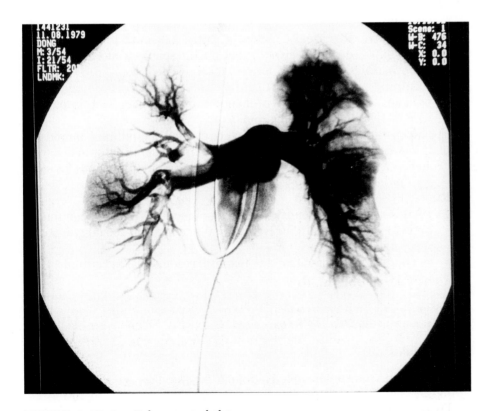

FIGURE 2.15-5. Pulmonary embolus.

A large filling defect in the pulmonary artery is evident on pulmonary angiogram.

- **D-dimer:** Sensitive but not specific in patients at risk for DVT or pulmonary embolism.
- **Venous ultrasound of the lower extremity:** Can detect a clot that may have given off the pulmonary embolism.

TREATMENT

- **Heparin:** Bolus and then weight-based continuous infusion (or low-molecular-weight heparin [LMWH]).
- **Warfarin:** For long-term anticoagulation, usually given for 3–6 months unless the underlying predisposing factor persists (then given indefinitely). Follow INR (goal = 2–3).
- **IVC filter:** Indicated if anticoagulation is contraindicated or if the patient has recurrent emboli while anticoagulated.
- **Thrombolysis:** Indicated only in severe cases with right heart failure.
- **DVT prophylaxis:** Treat bedridden medical patients and surgical patients; use **low-dose SQ heparin**, LMWH, intermittent pneumatic compression of the lower extremities (less effective), and **early ambulation (most effective)**.

SLEEP-DISORDERED BREATHING

Obstructive Sleep Apnea

- Risk factors include **male** gender, **obesity, sedative use for sleep,** nasal obstruction, hypothyroidism, macroglossia, micrognathia, and acromegaly.
- **Hx/PE:** Snoring, gasping for air while sleeping, insomnia, **daytime hypersomnolence,** hypertension (systemic and pulmonary), cor pulmonale. Normal PFTs. Obstructive sleep apnea is distinguished from central sleep apnea as follows:
  - **Obstructive:** Recurrent episodes of partial or complete closure of the upper airway during sleep with continued respiratory efforts. **Anatomic abnormalities** of the upper airway are a possible cause.
  - **Central:** Episodic cessation of airflow and respiratory efforts due to loss of central drive. The cause is unknown, but it is often seen in patients with CHF or CNS disease.
- **Dx:** Sleep studies (polysomnography) document the number of arousals, obstructions, and episodes of ↓ O_2 saturation; distinguish obstructive from central apnea; and identify possible movement disorders, seizures, or other sleep disorders.
- **Rx:**
  - Early treatment is essential. Options include weight loss or continuous positive airway pressure (CPAP). Avoid alcohol and sedating/hypnotic medications.
  - In children, most cases are due to tonsillar/adenoidal hypertrophy (corrected surgically).

NEOPLASMS OF THE LUNGS

Lung Nodules

- **Hx/PE:** Often asymptomatic. There may be chronic cough, dyspnea, and shortness of breath. Always inquire about smoking and exposure history.
- **Dx:**
  - **Serial CXRs:** Determine the location, progression, and extent of the nodule.

- **Chest CT:** Determine the nature, extent, and infiltrating nature of the nodule.
- **Characteristics favoring carcinoma:** Age > 45–50; new or larger lesions; absence of calcification or irregular calcification; size > 2 cm; irregular margins.
- **Characteristics favoring a benign lesion:** Age < 35; no change from old films; central/uniform/laminated calcification; smooth margins; size < 2 cm.
- **Rx:** Surgical resection if the lesion is a possible carcinoma; the patient is < 35 years of age; or there is a change in the size or character of the lesion. If not, **repeat study in 3–6 months.**

Lung Cancer

The leading cause of cancer death. Risk factors include tobacco smoke (except for bronchoalveolar carcinoma) and radon or asbestos exposure. Types are as follows:

- **Small cell lung cancer (SCLC):**
    - Highly correlated with **cigarette exposure.**
    - **Central location.**
    - **Neuroendocrine origin;** associated with paraneoplastic syndromes (see Table 2.15-5).
    - Commonly presents with metastases (brain, liver, bone).

TABLE 2.15-5. Paraneoplastic Syndromes of Lung Cancer

CLASSIFICATION	SYNDROME	HISTOLOGIC TYPE
Endocrine/metabolic	Cushing's syndrome	Small cell
	SIADH	Small cell
	Hypercalcemia	Squamous cell
	Gynecomastia	Large cell
Connective tissue	Hypertrophic pulmonary osteoarthropathy	Non–small cell
Neuromuscular	Peripheral neuropathy	Small cell
	Subacute cerebellar degeneration	Small cell
	Myasthenia (Eaton-Lambert syndrome)	Small cell
	Dermatomyositis	All
Cardiovascular	Thrombophlebitis	Adenocarcinoma
	Nonbacterial verrucous endocarditis	Adenocarcinoma
Hematologic	Anemia	All
	DIC	All
	Eosinophilia	All
	Thrombocytosis	All
Cutaneous	Acanthosis nigricans	All
	Erythema gyratum repens	All

- **Non–small cell lung cancer (NSCLC): Less propensity to metastasize.**
    - **Adenocarcinoma:** The most common lung cancer; **peripheral** location.
    - **Bronchoalveolar carcinoma:** Associated with multiple nodules, interstitial infiltration, and prolific sputum production.
- **Squamous cell carcinoma:** Central location; 98% are seen in smokers.
- **Large cell/neuroendocrine carcinomas:** Least common; associated with a poor prognosis.

HISTORY/PE

- Presents with cough, hemoptysis, chest pain, weight loss, and possible abnormalities on respiratory exam (crackles, atelectasis).
- Other findings include **Horner's syndrome** (miosis, ptosis, anhidrosis) in patients with Pancoast's tumor at the apex of the lung, as well as many **paraneoplastic syndromes** (see Table 2.15-5).

DIAGNOSIS

- **CXR** or **lung CT.**
- Fine-needle aspiration (CT guided) or bronchoscopy (biopsy or brushing).
- Thoracoscopic biopsy may be performed, with conversion to open thoracotomy if the lesion is found to be malignant.

TREATMENT

- **SCLC: Not resectable.** Often responds to radiation and chemotherapy initially but always recurs; lower median survival rate than NSCLC. Usually metastasized at the time of diagnosis.
- **NSCLC: Surgical resection** in early stages (IA, IB, IIA, IIB, and possibly IIIA). The extent of resection is based on lesion size; the presence of metastases; and the patient's age, general health, and lung function. Supplement surgery with radiation or chemotherapy (depending on stage). Palliation (radiation and/or chemotherapy) for symptomatic but unresectable disease.

TRAUMA

Pneumothorax

A collection of air in the pleural space that can → pulmonary collapse.

- **1° spontaneous pneumothorax:** Due to rupture of subpleural apical blebs (usually in **tall, thin young males**).
- **2° pneumothorax:** Due to COPD, TB, trauma, *Pneumocystis carinii* pneumonia (PCP), and iatrogenic factors (thoracocentesis, subclavian line placement, positive-pressure mechanical ventilation, bronchoscopy).
- **Tension pneumothorax:** A pulmonary or chest wall defect acts as a **one-way valve,** drawing air into the pleural space during inspiration but trapping air during expiration. Etiologies include penetrating trauma, infection, and positive-pressure mechanical ventilation. Shock and death result unless it is immediately recognized and treated.

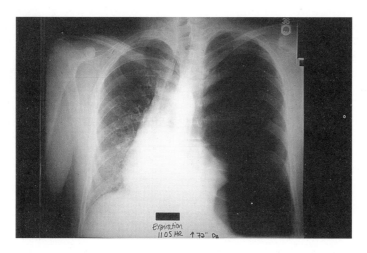

FIGURE 2.15-6. **Tension pneumothorax.**

Note the hyperlucent lung field (1), hyperexpanded lower diaphragm (2), collapsed lung (3), tracheal deviation (4), mediastinal shift (5), and compression of the opposite lung (6) on AP CXR.

HISTORY/PE

- Unilateral pleuritic chest pain and dyspnea.
- Physical exam reveals tachypnea, **diminished or absent breath sounds, hyperresonance,** and ↓ **tactile fremitus.**
- Suspect tension pneumothorax in the presence of respiratory distress, falling O_2 saturation, hypotension, distended neck veins, and **tracheal deviation.**

DIAGNOSIS

CXR shows presence of a visceral pleural line and/or **lung retraction** from the chest wall (best seen in end-expiratory films; see Figure 2.15-6).

TREATMENT

- Small pneumothoraces may reabsorb spontaneously. Supplemental O_2 therapy is helpful.
- Large, symptomatic pneumothoraces require chest tube placement.
- Tension pneumothorax requires immediate needle decompression (second intercostal space at the midclavicular line) followed by a chest tube.

Renal/Genitourinary

In hypernatremia, patients may not drink enough free water to replace insensible losses.

Hypernatremia causes—

the 6 D's:

Diuretics
Dehydration
Diabetes insipidus
Docs (iatrogenic)
Diarrhea
Disease (e.g., kidney, sickle cell)

Hypernatremia

Serum sodium > 145 mEq/L. Usually due to water loss rather than sodium gain.

HISTORY/PE

- Presents with **thirst** (due to hypertonicity) as well as oliguria or polyuria (depending on the etiology).
- **Neurologic symptoms** include mental status changes, weakness, focal neurologic deficits, and seizures.
- Examination reveals **"doughy" skin** and signs of volume depletion.

DIAGNOSIS

- Assess volume status by conducting a clinical exam and measuring urine volume and osmolality.
  - **Hypertonic Na^+ gain:** Due to hypertonic saline/tube feeds or ↑ **aldosterone.**
  - **Pure water loss:** Due to central or nephrogenic **diabetes insipidus (DI)**; characterized by large volumes of dilute urine. Dermal or respiratory-insensible losses.
  - **Hypotonic fluid loss:** Due to ↓ intake, diuretics, intrinsic renal disease, GI losses (**diarrhea**), burns, and osmotic diuresis (mannitol).
- A minimal volume (approximately 500 mL/day) of maximally concentrated urine (> 800 mOsm/kg) suggests adequate renal response without adequate free-water replacement.

TREATMENT

- Treat the underlying causes and replace free-water deficit with hypotonic saline, D5W, or oral water, depending on volume status.
- Correction of chronic hypernatremia (> 36–48 hours) should occur **gradually over 48–72 hours** to prevent neurologic damage 2° to cerebral swelling.

Hyponatremia

Serum sodium < 136 mEq/L.

HISTORY/PE

- May be asymptomatic or may present with **confusion, lethargy,** muscle cramps, hyporeflexia, and nausea.
- Can progress to seizures, coma, or brain stem herniation.

DIAGNOSIS

Hyponatremia can be classified by serum and urine osmolality and by volume status (by clinical exam). Osmolality is classified as follows:

- **High (> 295 mEq/L):** Hyperglycemia, hypertonic infusion (e.g., mannitol).
- **Normal (280–295 mEq/L):** Hypertriglyceridemia, paraproteinemia (pseudohyponatremia).
- **Low (< 280 mEq/L):** Applies to the majority of cases. Hypotonic etiologies are listed in Table 2.16-1.

358

TABLE 2.16-1. **Evaluation and Treatment of Hypotonic Hyponatremia**

VOLUME STATUS	ETIOLOGIES	TREATMENT
Hypervolemic	Renal failure, nephrotic syndrome, cirrhosis, CHF.	Water restriction.
Euvolemic	SIADH, hypothyroidism, renal failure, drugs, psychogenic polydipsia, adrenal insufficiency.	Water restriction.
Hypovolemic	Diuretics, vomiting, diarrhea, third spacing, dehydration.	Replete volume with normal saline.

TREATMENT

- Specific treatments are outlined in Table 2.16-1.
- Chronic hyponatremia (> 72 hours' duration) should be corrected slowly (no more than 0.5–1.0 mEq/L/hr) in order to prevent central pontine myelinolysis (quadriplegia and pseudobulbar palsy).

Hypervolemic hyponatremia is caused by "nephrOSIS, cirrhOSIS, and cardiOSIS."

Hyperkalemia

Serum potassium > 5 mEq/L. Etiologies are as follows:

- **Spurious:** Hemolysis of blood samples, fist clenching during blood draw, extreme leukocytosis or thrombocytosis, rhabdomyolysis.
- **↓ excretion:** Renal insufficiency, drugs (e.g., spironolactone, triamterene, ACEIs, trimethoprim, NSAIDs), mineralocorticoid deficiency/type 4 renal tubular acidosis (RTA).
- **Cellular shifts:** Tissue injury, insulin deficiency, acidosis, drugs (e.g., succinylcholine, digitalis, arginine, β-blockers).
- **Iatrogenic.**

HISTORY/PE

May be asymptomatic or present with nausea, vomiting, **intestinal colic, areflexia, weakness,** flaccid paralysis, and paresthesias.

DIAGNOSIS

- Verify hyperkalemia with a **repeat blood draw.** In the setting of extreme leukocytosis or thrombocytosis, check plasma potassium.
- ECG findings include **tall, peaked T waves;** PR prolongation; wide QRS; and loss of P waves (see Figure 2.16-1). Can progress to **sine waves,** ventricular fibrillation, and cardiac arrest.

Treatment of hyperkalemia—

C BIG K

Calcium
Bicarbonate
Insulin
Glucose
Kayexalate

TREATMENT

- Values of > 6.5 mEq/L or ECG changes (especially PR prolongation or wide QRS) require emergent treatment.
- The mnemonic **C BIG K** summarizes the treatment of hyperkalemia.
  - First give **calcium gluconate** for cardiac cell membrane stabilization.
  - Give **bicarbonate and/or insulin and glucose** to temporarily shift potassium into cells.
  - β-agonists promote cellular reuptake of potassium.
  - **Kayexalate** and loop diuretics (e.g., furosemide) to remove potassium from the body.
  - Dialysis for patients with renal failure or for severe, refractory cases.

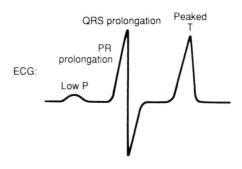

FIGURE 2.16-1. **Hyperkalemia.**

Electrocardiographic manifestations include peaked T waves, PR prolongation, and a widened QRS complex. (Reproduced, with permission, from Cogan MG. *Fluid and Electrolytes*, 1st ed. Stamford, CT: Appleton & Lange, 1991:170.

Hypokalemia

Serum potassium < 3.6 mEq/L. Etiologies are as follows:

Hypokalemia is usually due to renal or GI losses.

- **Transcellular shifts:** Insulin, β_2-agonists, alkalosis, familial hypokalemic periodic paralysis.
- **GI losses:** Diarrhea, chronic laxative abuse, vomiting, NG suction.
- **Renal losses:** Diuretics (e.g., loop or thiazide), 1° mineralocorticoid excess or 2° hyperaldosteronism, ↓ circulating volume, Bartter's syndrome, drugs (e.g., gentamicin, amphotericin), DKA, hypomagnesemia, type 1 RTA (defective distal H^+ secretion).

HISTORY/PE

Fatigue, **muscle weakness or cramps, ileus,** hyporeflexia, paresthesias, rhabdomyolysis, ascending paralysis.

DIAGNOSIS

- Twenty-four-hour or spot urine potassium may distinguish renal from GI losses.
- ECG may show **T-wave flattening, U waves** (an additional wave after the T wave), and ST-segment depression → AV block and subsequent cardiac arrest.
- Consider RTA in the setting of metabolic acidosis.

TREATMENT

- Treat the underlying disorder.
- Oral and/or IV **potassium repletion.**
- Replace magnesium, as this deficiency makes potassium repletion difficult.
- Monitor ECG and plasma potassium levels frequently during replacement.

Hypercalcemia

Serum calcium > 10.2 mg/dL. The most common causes are **hyperparathyroidism and malignancy** (e.g., breast cancer, squamous cell cancers, multiple myeloma). Other causes are summarized in the mnemonic **CHIMPANZEES.**

> *Causes of hypercalcemia—*
>
> **CHIMPANZEES**
>
> **C**alcium
>   supplementation
> **H**yperparathyroidism
> **I**atrogenic (e.g.,
>   thiazides)/**I**mmobility
> **M**ilk-alkali syndrome
> **P**aget's disease
> **A**ddison's
>   disease/**A**cromegaly
> **N**eoplasm
> **Z**ollinger-Ellison
>   syndrome (e.g.,
>   MEN I)
> **E**xcess vitamin A
> **E**xcess vitamin D
> **S**arcoidosis and other
>   granulomatous
>   disease

May present with **bones** (fractures), **stones** (kidney stones), abdominal **groans** (anorexia, constipation), and **psychiatric overtones** (weakness, fatigue, altered mental status).

DIAGNOSIS

Order an ECG (may show a **short QT interval**), total/ionized calcium, albumin, phosphate, PTH, PTHrP (parathyroid hormone–related peptide), and vitamin D.

TREATMENT

- **IV hydration** followed by **furosemide** to ↑ calcium excretion.
- Calcitonin, bisphosphonates (e.g., pamidronate), glucocorticoids, and dialysis are used for severe or refractory cases. **Avoid thiazide diuretics,** which ↑ tubular reabsorption of calcium.

Loops (furosemide) Lose calcium.

Hypocalcemia

Serum calcium < 8.5 mg/dL. Etiologies include hypoparathyroidism (postsurgery, idiopathic), malnutrition, hypomagnesemia, acute pancreatitis, vitamin D deficiency, and pseudohypoparathyroidism.

HISTORY/PE

- Presents with **abdominal muscle cramps,** dyspnea, **tetany, perioral and acral paresthesias,** and convulsions.
- Facial spasm elicited from tapping of the facial nerve (**Chvostek's sign**) and carpal spasm after arterial occlusion by a BP cuff (**Trousseau's sign**) are classic findings.

DIAGNOSIS

- Order an ionized Ca^{2+}, Mg^+, PTH, albumin, and possibly calcitonin. If the patient is post-thyroidectomy, review the operative note to determine the number of parathyroid glands removed.
- ECG may show a **prolonged QT interval.**

TREATMENT

- Treat the underlying disorder.
- Magnesium repletion.
- Administer oral **calcium supplements;** IV calcium for severe symptoms.

Serum calcium may be falsely low in hypoalbuminemia.

The classic case of hypocalcemia is a patient who develops cramps and tetany following thyroidectomy.

Hypomagnesemia

Serum magnesium < 1.5 mEq/L. Etiologies are as follows:

- ↓ **intake:** Malnutrition, malabsorption, short bowel syndrome, total parenteral nutrition (TPN).
- ↑ **loss:** Diuretics, diarrhea, vomiting, hypercalcemia, drugs (amphotericin), alcoholism.
- **Miscellaneous: DKA,** pancreatitis.

HIGH-YIELD FACTS

RENAL/GENITOURINARY

HISTORY/PE

- Symptoms are generally related to concurrent hypocalcemia and hypokalemia; they include anorexia, nausea, vomiting, muscle cramps, and weakness.
- At very low levels, symptoms include hyperactive reflexes, paresthesias, irritability, confusion, lethargy, seizures, and arrhythmias.

DIAGNOSIS

- Labs may show concurrent hypocalcemia and hypokalemia.
- ECG may show prolonged PR and QT intervals.

TREATMENT

- IV and oral supplements.
- Hypokalemia and hypocalcemia will not correct without magnesium correction.

↑ *anion gap—*

caused by **MUDPILES**

Methanol
Uremia
DKA
Paraldehyde
Intoxication
Lactic acidosis
Ethylene glycol
Salicylates

ACID-BASE DISORDERS

See Figure 2.16-2 for a diagnostic algorithm for acid-base disorders.

ACUTE RENAL FAILURE (ARF)

An abrupt ↓ in renal function → the retention of creatinine and BUN. ↓ urine output (i.e., oliguria, defined as < 500 cc/day) is not required for ARF. ARF is categorized as follows (see also Table 2.16-2):

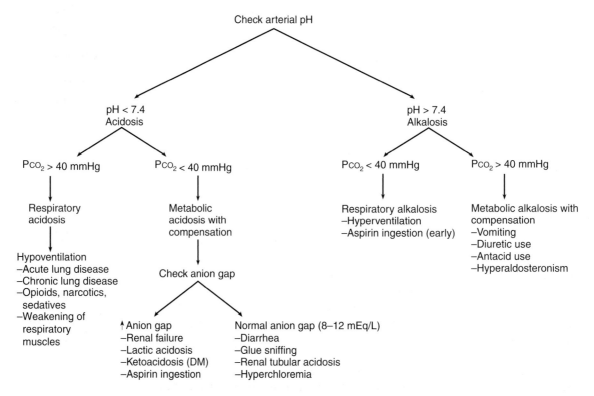

FIGURE 2.16-2. **Diagnostic algorithm for acid-base disorders.**

TABLE 2.16-2. Causes of Acute Renal Failure

PRERENAL	RENAL (INTRINSIC)	POSTRENAL
Hypovolemia (hemorrhage, dehydration, burns)	Acute tubular necrosis (ATN)	Prostate disease
Cardiogenic shock	Acute/allergic interstitial nephritis	Nephrolithiasis
Sepsis	Glomerulonephritis	Pelvic tumors
Anaphylaxis	Thromboembolism	Recent pelvic surgery
Drugs		Retroperitoneal fibrosis
Renal artery stenosis		
Cirrhosis with ascites (hepatorenal syndrome)		

- **Prerenal:** ↓ renal perfusion.
- **Intrinsic:** Injury within the nephron unit.
- **Postrenal:** Urinary outflow obstruction. Generally, both kidneys must be obstructed in order to → a significant ↑ in BUN and creatinine.

HISTORY/PE

- Symptoms of **uremia** include malaise, fatigue, confusion, oliguria, anorexia, and nausea.
- Examination may show **pericardial rub, asterixis, hypertension,** ↓ urine output, and ↑ respiratory rate (compensation of metabolic acidosis or from pulmonary edema 2° to volume overload).
- Category-specific symptoms are as follows:
  - **Prerenal:** Thirst, orthostatic hypotension, tachycardia, ↓ skin turgor, dry mucous membranes, reduced axillary sweating, stigmata of comorbid conditions.
  - **Intrinsic:** Drug exposure history (aminoglycosides, NSAIDs); contrast or toxin (e.g., myoglobin, myeloma protein).
  - **Acute interstitial nephritis:** Fever, arthralgias, and a pruritic, erythematous rash. Methicillin is the classic association.
    - **Atheroemboli:** Subcutaneous nodules, livedo reticularis, digital ischemia.
    - **Glomerulonephritis:** Oliguria, edema, hypertension.
  - **Postrenal:** Prostatic disease, suprapubic pain, distended bladder and flank pain.

DIAGNOSIS

- Check serum electrolytes. Examine the urine for RBCs, WBCs, casts (see Table 2.16-3), and **urine eosinophils.**
- An $Fe_{Na} < 1\%$, a $U_{Na} < 20$, a specific gravity > 1.020, or a BUN/creatinine ratio > 20 suggests a prerenal etiology.
- A urinary catheter and renal ultrasound can help rule out obstruction. Ultrasound can also identify kidneys that are ↓ in size, as occurs with chronic renal failure.
- In patients with oliguria, the Fe_{Na} can help identify prerenal failure and distinguish it from intrinsic renal disease.
- Obtain a renal biopsy only when the cause of intrinsic renal disease is unclear.

Patients with ARF may have a normal urine volume.

Renal ischemia, toxins, hemoglobinuria, or myoglobinuria may → ATN.

$Fe_{Na} < 1\%$ indicates the kidneys are trying to conserve sodium, suggesting a prerenal etiology.

URINE SEDIMENT	ETIOLOGY	CLASSIFICATION
Hyaline casts	Normal finding, but ↑ amount suggests volume depletion	Prerenal
Red cell casts, dysmorphic red cells	Glomerulonephritis	Intrinsic
White cells, eosinophils	Allergic interstitial nephritis, atheroembolic disease	Intrinsic
Granular casts, renal tubular cells, "muddy-brown cast"	ATN	Intrinsic
White cells, white cell casts	Pyelonephritis	Postrenal

Indications for urgent dialysis—

AEIOU

Acidosis
Electrolyte abnormalities (hyperkalemia)
Ingestions (salicylates, theophylline, methanol, barbiturates, lithium, ethylene glycol)
Overload (fluid)
Uremic symptoms (pericarditis, encephalopathy, bleeding, nausea, pruritus, myoclonus)

Think nephritic syndrome if the patient has hematuria, hypertension, and oliguria.

TREATMENT

- Balance fluids and electrolytes.
- In acute or allergic interstitial nephritis, adjust or discontinue offending medications.
- Dialyze if indicated (see the mnemonic **AEIOU**).

COMPLICATIONS

- Chronic renal failure may result, requiring dialysis to prevent the buildup of K^+, H^+, **and toxic metabolites.**
- Patients who are dialysis dependent are at ↑ risk for a number of diseases, including CAD.

DIURETICS

Table 2.16-4 summarizes the actions and side effects of commonly used diuretics.

GLOMERULAR DISEASE

Nephritic Syndrome

A disorder of glomerular inflammation, also called glomerulonephritis. Proteinuria may be present but is usually < 1.5 g/day. Causes are summarized in Table 2.16-5.

HISTORY/PE

The classic findings are oliguria, macroscopic/microscopic hematuria (smoky-brown urine), hypertension, and **edema.**

DIAGNOSIS

- UA shows hematuria and possibly mild proteinuria.
- Patients have a ↓ GFR with elevated BUN and creatinine. Complement, ANA, ANCA, and anti-GBM antibody levels should be measured to determine the underlying etiology.
- Renal biopsy may be useful for histologic evaluation.

TABLE 2.16-4. Mechanism of Action and Side Effects of Diuretics

TYPE	DRUGS	SITE OF ACTION	MECHANISM OF ACTION	SIDE EFFECTS
Carbonic anhydrase inhibitors	Acetazolamide	Proximal convoluted tubule.	Inhibits carbonic anhydrase, ↑ H^+ reabsorption, blocks Na^+/H^+ exchange.	Hyperchloremic metabolic acidosis, sulfa allergy.
Osmotic agents	Mannitol, urea	Entire tubule.	↑ tubular fluid osmolarity.	Pulmonary edema, due to CHF and anuria.
Loop agents	Furosemide, ethacrynic acid, bumetanide, torsemide	Ascending loop of Henle.	Inhibits $Na^+/K^+/2\ Cl^-$ transporter.	Water loss, metabolic alkalosis, ↓ K^+, ↓ **Ca^{2+}**, **ototoxicity**, sulfa allergy (e.g., except ethacrynic acid, hyperuricemia).
Thiazide agents	Hydrochlorothiazide, chlorothiazide	Distal convoluted tubule.	Inhibits Na^+/Cl^- transporter.	Water loss, metabolic alkalosis, ↓ **Na^+**, ↓ K^+, ↑ glucose, ↑ **Ca^{2+}**, ↑ uric acid, sulfa allergy, pancreatitis.
K^+-sparing agents	Spironolactone, triamterene, amiloride	Cortical collecting tubule.	Aldosterone receptor antagonist (spironolactone), block sodium channel (triamterene, amiloride).	Metabolic acidosis, ↑ K^+, antiandrogenic effects, including gynecomastia (spironolactone).

TREATMENT

- Treat hypertension, fluid overload, and uremia with salt and water restriction, diuretics, and, if necessary, dialysis.
- **Corticosteroids** are useful in reducing glomerular inflammation in some cases.

Nephrotic Syndrome

Defined as **proteinuria (≥ 3.5 g/day), generalized edema, hypoalbuminemia,** and **hyperlipidemia.** Approximately one-third of all cases are the result of systemic diseases such as DM, SLE, or amyloidosis. Causes are summarized in Table 2.16-6.

HISTORY/PE

- Presents with **generalized edema** and **foamy urine.** In severe cases, dyspnea and ascites may develop.
- Patients have ↑ susceptibility to infection as well as a predisposition to hypercoagulable states with an ↑ risk for venous thrombosis and pulmonary embolism.

Proteinuria, hypoalbuminemia, edema, hyperlipidemia, and hyperlipiduria are due to the initial ↑ permeability of the glomerulus to protein.

TABLE 2.16-5. Causes of Nephritic Syndrome

	DESCRIPTION	HISTORY/PE	LABS/HISTOLOGY	TREATMENT/PROGNOSIS
Immune complex				
Postinfectious glomerulo-nephritis	Often associated with a recent group A β-hemolytic **streptococcal infection** (within two weeks).	Oliguria, edema, hypertension, smoky-brown urine.	Low serum C3, ↑ **ASO titer, lumpy-bumpy immuno-fluorescence.**	Supportive. Almost all children and most adults have a complete recovery.
IgA nephropathy (Berger's disease)	**Most common type;** associated with upper respiratory or GI infections. Commonly seen in young men; may be seen in Henoch-Schönlein purpura.	Episodic gross hematuria or persistent microscopic hematuria.	Normal C3.	Glucocorticoids for select patients; ACEIs in patients with proteinuria. Some 20% of cases progress to end-stage renal disease.
Pauci-immune				
Wegener's granulomatosis	Granulomatous inflammation of the respiratory tract and kidney with necrotizing vasculitis.	Fever, weight loss, hematuria, hearing disturbances, respiratory and sinus symptoms. Cavitary pulmonary lesions bleed and → **hemoptysis.**	Presence of **c-ANCA** (cell-medicated immune response). Renal biopsy shows segmental necrotizing glomerulonephritis with few immunoglobulin deposits on immuno-fluorescence.	High-dose corticosteroids and cytotoxic agents. Patients tend to have frequent relapses.
Anti-GBM disease				
Goodpasture's syndrome	Glomerulonephritis with pulmonary hemorrhage; peak incidence in men in their mid-20s.	**Hemoptysis,** dyspnea, possible respiratory failure.	**Linear anti-GBM deposits** on immuno-fluorescence; iron deficiency anemia; hemosiderin-filled macrophages in sputum; pulmonary infiltrates on CXR.	Plasma exchange therapy, pulsed steroids. May progress to end-stage renal disease.
Alport's syndrome	Hereditary glomerulonephritis; presents in boys 5–20 years of age.	Asymptomatic hematuria associated with **nerve deafness** and eye disorders.	GBM splitting on electron microscopy.	Progresses to renal failure. Anti-GBM nephritis may recur after transplant.

HIGH-YIELD FACTS

RENAL/GENITOURINARY

TABLE 2.16-6.   Causes of Nephrotic Syndrome

	DESCRIPTION	HISTORY/PE	LABS/HISTOLOGY	TREATMENT/PROGNOSIS
Minimal change disease	The most common cause of nephritic syndrome in children. Idiopathic etiology; 2° causes include NSAIDs and hematologic malignancies.	Tendency toward infections and thrombotic events.	Light microscopy appears **normal;** electron microscopy shows **fusion of epithelial foot processes** with lipid-laden renal cortices.	Steroids; excellent prognosis.
Focal segmental glomerular sclerosis	Idiopathic, IV drug use, HIV infection, obesity.	The typical patient is a young black male with uncontrolled hypertension.	Microscopic hematuria; biopsy shows sclerosis in capillary tufts.	Prednisone, cytotoxic therapy.
Membranous nephropathy	**The most common nephropathy in Caucasian adults.** 2° causes includes solid tumor malignancy (especially in patients > 60 years of age) and immune complex disease.	Associated with HBV, syphilis, **malaria,** and gold.	**"Spike-and-dome"** appearance due to granular deposits of IgG and C3 at the basement membrane.	Prednisone and cytotoxic therapy for severe disease.
Diabetic nephropathy	Two characteristic forms: diffuse hyalinization and nodular glomerulosclerosis **(Kimmelstiel-Wilson lesions).**	Generally have long-standing, poorly controlled DM with evidence of retinopathy or neuropathy.	Thickened GBM; ↑ **mesangial matrix.**	Tight control of blood sugar; ACEIs for type 1 DM and ARBs for type 2 DM.
Lupus nephritis	Classified as WHO types I–VI. Both nephrotic and nephritic. The severity of renal disease often determines overall prognosis.	Proteinuria or RBCs on UA may be found during evaluation of SLE patients.	Mesangial proliferation; subendothelial immune complex deposition.	Prednisone and cytotoxic therapy may ↓ disease progression.
Renal amyloidosis	1° (plasma cell dyscrasia) and 2° (infectious or inflammatory) are the most common.	Patients may have multiple myeloma or a chronic inflammatory disease (e.g., rheumatoid arthritis, TB).	Fat pad biopsy; seen with **Congo red stain; apple-green** birefringence under polarized light.	Prednisone and melphalan. Bone marrow transplant may be used for multiple myeloma.

HIGH-YIELD FACTS

RENAL/GENITOURINARY

TABLE 2.16-6. Causes of Nephrotic Syndrome (continued)

	DESCRIPTION	HISTORY/PE	LABS/HISTOLOGY	TREATMENT/PROGNOSIS
Membranoproliferative nephropathy	Can also be nephritic syndrome. Type I is associated with HCV, cryoglobulinemia, lupus, and subacute bacterial endocarditis.	Slow progression to renal failure.	"Tram-track," double-layered basement membrane. Type I has subendothelial deposits and mesangial deposits; all three types have low serum C3; type II by way of C3 nephritic factor.	Corticosteroids and cytotoxic agents may help.

DIAGNOSIS

- UA shows **proteinuria** ($\geq$ 3.5 g/day) and lipiduria.
- Blood chemistry shows $\downarrow$ **albumin** (< 3 g/dL) and hyperlipidemia.
- Evaluation should include workup for 2° causes.
- Renal biopsy is used to definitively diagnose the underlying etiology.

TREATMENT

- **Protein and salt restriction,** diuretic therapy, antihyperlipidemics.
- **ACEIs** $\downarrow$ proteinuria and diminish the progression of renal disease in patients with diabetic nephropathy.
- Vaccinate with 23-polyvalent pneumococcus vaccine (PPV23), as patients are at $\uparrow$ risk of *Streptococcus pneumoniae* infection.

NEPHROLITHIASIS

Renal calculi. Stones are most commonly calcium oxalate but may also be calcium phosphate, struvite, uric acid, or cystine (see Table 2.16-7). Risk factors include a $\oplus$ family history, **low fluid intake,** gout, post-colectomy/ileostomy, specific enzyme disorders, RTA (due to alkaline urinary pH), and hyperparathyroidism. Most common in older males.

HISTORY/PE

- **Acute onset of severe, colicky flank pain** that may **radiate to the testes or vulva** and is associated with nausea and vomiting.
- Patients are unable to get comfortable and shift position frequently (as opposed to those with peritonitis, who lie still).

DIAGNOSIS

- UA may show gross or **microscopic hematuria** (15% do not have hematuria) and an **altered urine pH.**
- Obtain an AXR in patients with known radiopaque stones and possibly a **renal ultrasound** to look for obstruction as well as for pregnant patients, in whom radiation should be avoided.

TABLE 2.16-7. Types of Nephrolithiasis

TYPE	FREQUENCY	ETIOLOGY AND CHARACTERISTICS	TREATMENT
Calcium oxalate/ calcium phosphate	83%	Most common causes are **idiopathic hypercalciuria,** elevated urine uric acid 2° to diet, and 1° hyperparathyroidism. Alkaline urine. Radiopaque.	Hydration, thiazide diuretic.
Struvite (Mg-NH$_4$-PO$_4$)	9%	"Triple phosphate stones." Associated with urease-producing organisms (e.g., *Proteus*). Form staghorn calculi. Alkalne urine. Radiopaque.	Hydration; treat UTI if present.
Uric acid	7%	Associated with gout and high purine turnover states. Acidic urine (pH < 5.5). **Radiolucent.**	Hydration; alkalinize urine with citrate, which is converted to HCO$_3^-$ in the liver; dietary purine restriction and allopurinol.
Cystine	1%	Due to a defect in renal transport of certain amino acids (COLA—cystine, ornithine, lysine, and arginine). **Hexagonal crystals.** Radiopaque.	Hydration, alkalinize urine, penicillamine.

- Noncontrast abdominal CT scans may diagnose stones and other causes of flank pain.
- An **IVP** can be used to confirm the diagnosis if there is a lack of contrast filling below the stone.

TREATMENT

- **Hydration and analgesia** are the initial treatment.
- Kidney stones < 5 mm in diameter can pass through the urethra; stones < 3 cm in diameter can be treated with **extracorporeal shock-wave lithotripsy (ESWL)** or percutaneous nephrolithotomy.
- Preventive measures include hydration; additional prophylaxis is dependent on stone composition.

POLYCYSTIC KIDNEY DISEASE (PCKD)

Characterized by the presence of renal cysts as well as by cysts in the spleen, liver, and pancreas. The two major forms are as follows:

- **Autosomal dominant:**
  - Most common.
  - Usually asymptomatic until patients are > 30 years of age.
  - One-half of autosomal-dominant PCKD patients will have end-stage renal disease requiring dialysis by age 60.
  - Associated with an ↑ risk of cerebral aneurysm, especially in patients with a ⊕ family history.
- **Autosomal recessive:** Less common but more severe. Presents in infants and young children with renal failure, liver fibrosis, and portal hypertension; may → death in the first few years of life.

HISTORY/PE

- **Pain and hematuria** are the most common presenting symptoms. Sharp, localized pain may result from cyst rupture, infection, or passage of renal calculi.
- Additional findings include **hypertension, hepatic cysts, cerebral berry aneurysms,** diverticulosis, and mitral valve prolapse.
- Patients may have large, palpable kidneys on abdominal exam.

DIAGNOSIS

Based on ultrasound or CT scan. Multiple bilateral cysts will be present throughout the renal parenchyma, and renal enlargement will be visualized.

TREATMENT

- **Prevent complications and ↓ the rate of progression to end-stage renal disease.** Early management of UTIs is critical to prevent renal cyst infection. BP control is necessary to reduce hypotension-induced renal damage.
- Dialysis and renal transplantation are used to manage patients with end-stage renal disease.

RENAL TUBULAR ACIDOSIS (RTA)

A net ↓ in either tubular H^+ secretion or HCO_3^- reabsorption that → a **non–anion gap metabolic acidosis.** There are three main types of RTA; **type IV (distal) is the most common form** (see Table 2.16-8).

TABLE 2.16-8. Types of RTA

	TYPE I (DISTAL)	TYPE II (PROXIMAL)	TYPE IV (DISTAL)
Defect	H^+ secretion.	HCO_3^- reabsorption.	Aldosterone deficiency or resistance → defects in Na^+ reabsorption, H^+ and K^+ excretion.
Serum K^+	High or low.	Low.	High.
Urinary pH	> 5.3.	5.3 initially; < 5.3 once serum is acidic.	< 5.3.
Etiologies (most common)	Hereditary, amphotericin, cirrhosis, autoimmune disorders, sickle cell disease, lithium.	Hereditary, carbonic anhydrase inhibitors, Fanconi's syndrome, multiple myeloma.	Hyporeninemic hypoaldosteronism; chronic kidney disease from DM, hypertension, and HIV.
Treatment	Potassium citrate.	Potassium citrate.	Furosemide, fludrocortisone, and low-potassium diet in patients with aldosterone deficiency.
Complications	Nephrolithiasis.	Rickets, osteomalacia.	Hyperkalemia.

- Retrograde projection of urine from the bladder to the ureters and kidneys. Often caused by insufficient tunneling of ureters into submucosal bladder tissue → ineffective restriction of retrograde urine flow during bladder contraction. Classified as follows:
  - **Mild reflux (grades I–II):** No ureteral or renal pelvic dilatation. Often resolves spontaneously.
  - **Moderate to severe reflux (grade III–V):** Ureteral dilatation with associated calyceal blunting in severe cases
- Hx/PE: Patients present with **recurrent UTIs.**
- Dx: Perform a **voiding cystourethrogram** to detect abnormalities at ureteral insertion sites and to classify the grade of reflux. All children < 7 years of age presenting with their first UTI should undergo a voiding cystourethrogram to screen for reflux.
- Rx: Treat infections aggressively. Treat mild reflux with daily prophylactic antibiotics until reflux resolves at puberty. Ureteral implantation may be considered in severe reflux. Inadequate treatment can → progressive renal scarring and end-stage renal disease.

Failure to concentrate urine through central or nephrogenic dysfunction of ADH. Subtypes are as follows:

- **Central DI:** The posterior pituitary fails to secrete ADH. Causes include **tumor,** ischemia (Sheehan's syndrome), traumatic cerebral injury, infection, and autoimmune disorders.
- **Nephrogenic DI:** The kidneys fail to respond to circulating ADH. Causes include renal diseases and drugs (e.g., **lithium,** demeclocycline).

HISTORY/PE

- Presents with **polydipsia, polyuria,** and **persistent thirst** with dilute urine.
- Patients may present with hypernatremia and dehydration, but if given unlimited access to water, they are typically normonatremic.

DIAGNOSIS

- During a **water deprivation test,** patients excrete a high volume of dilute urine.
- Desmopressin acetate (DDAVP) challenge:
  - **Central DI:** DDAVP (a synthetic analog of ADH) challenge will ↓ **urine output and ↑ urine osmolarity.**
  - **Nephrogenic DI:** DDAVP challenge will not significantly ↓ urine output.
- MRI may show a pituitary or hypothalamic mass in central DI.

TREATMENT

- Treat the underlying cause.
- **Central DI:** Administer DDAVP intranasally.
- **Nephrogenic DI:** Salt restriction and ↑ water intake are the 1° treatment. Thiazide diuretics are used to promote mild volume depletion and to stimulate proximal reabsorption of salt and water.

For unknown reasons, patients with DI prefer ice-cold beverages.

A common cause of euvolemic hyponatremia that results from **nonosmotically stimulated ADH release.**

HISTORY/PE

Associated with **CNS disease** (e.g., head injury, tumor), **pulmonary disease** (e.g., sarcoid, pneumonia), ectopic tumor production/paraneoplastic syndrome (e.g., small cell carcinoma), drugs (e.g., antipsychotics, antidepressants), or surgery.

Fluid restriction is the cornerstone of SIADH treatment.

DIAGNOSIS

- Diagnose on the basis of a urine osmolality > 50–100 mOsm/kg with concurrent serum hyposmolarity in the absence of a physiologic reason for ↑ ADH (e.g., CHF, cirrhosis, hypovolemia).
- **Urinary sodium ≥ 20 mEq/L** demonstrates that the patient is not hypovolemic.

TREATMENT

- **Restrict fluid** and address the underlying cause.
- If hyponatremia is severe (< 110 mEq/L) or the patient is significantly symptomatic (e.g., comatose, seizing), cautiously give hypertonic saline.
- **Demeclocycline** can help normalize serum sodium by antagonizing the action of ADH in the collecting duct.
- Chronic correction depends on treatment of the underlying disorder.

Enlargement of the prostate that is a normal part of the aging process and is seen in **> 80% of men by age 80.** Most commonly presents in men **> 50 years of age.**

BPH most commonly occurs in the central zone of the prostate and may not be detected on exam.

HISTORY/PE

- In BPH, the enlarged prostate may → obstructive and irritative symptoms.
  - **Obstructive:** Hesitancy, weak stream, intermittent stream, incomplete emptying, urinary retention, bladder fullness.
  - **Irritative:** Nocturia, daytime frequency, urge incontinence, opening hematuria.
- On DRE, the prostate is uniformly enlarged with a rubbery texture. If the prostate is hard or has irregular lesions, suspect cancer.

DIAGNOSIS

- Potentially dangerous causes of urinary symptoms must be ruled out before BPH is diagnosed.
- **DRE** to screen for masses; if findings are suspicious, evaluate for prostate cancer.
- **UA and urine culture** to rule out infection and hematuria.
- **Creatinine levels** to rule out obstructive uropathy and renal insufficiency.
- PSA testing and cystoscopy are not recommended for longitudinal BPH monitoring.

TREATMENT

- **Reassurance** for mild symptoms.
- **Medical therapy** with α-blockers (terazosin) and 5α-reductase inhibitors (finasteride) to reduce mild to moderate symptoms.
- Transurethral resection of the prostate (TURP) or open prostatectomy for patients with moderate to severe symptoms.

The major side effect of α-blockers is orthostatic hypotension.

PROSTATE CANCER

The **most common cancer in men** and the **second leading cause of cancer death** in men (after lung cancer). Risk factors include advanced age and a ⊕ family history.

HISTORY/PE

- Usually **asymptomatic,** but may present with obstructive urinary symptoms (e.g., **urinary retention,** a ↓ in the force of the urine stream) as well as with lymphedema due to obstructing metastases, constitutional symptoms, and **back pain due to bone metastases.**
- DRE may reveal a **palpable nodule** or an area of induration. Early carcinoma is usually not detectable on exam.
- A tender prostate suggests prostatitis.

DIAGNOSIS

- Suggested by clinical findings and/or a markedly ↑ **PSA** (> 4 ng/mL)
- Definitive diagnosis is made with **ultrasound-guided transrectal biopsy.**
- Tumors are graded by the **Gleason histologic system,** which sums the scores (from 1 to 5) of the two most dysplastic samples (10 is the highest grade).
- Look for metastases with CXR and **bone scan.**

Elevated PSA may be due to BPH, prostatitis, UTI, prostatic trauma, or carcinoma.

TREATMENT

- Treatment is controversial, as many cases of prostate cancer are slow to progress. Treatment choice is based on the aggressiveness of the tumor and the patient's mortality risk.
- **Watchful waiting** may be the best approach for elderly patients with low-grade tumors.
- **Radical prostatectomy** and **radiation therapy** (e.g., brachytherapy or external beam) are associated with an ↑ risk of incontinence and/or impotence.
- **PSA,** while controversial as a screening test, is used to follow patients post-treatment to evaluate for disease recurrence.
- Treat metastatic disease with **androgen ablation** (e.g., GnRH agonists, orchiectomy, flutamide) and chemotherapy.

An annual DRE after the age of 50 is the recommended screening method for prostate cancer.

PREVENTION

- All males > 50 years of age should have an **annual DRE.** Screening should begin earlier in African-American males and in those with a first-degree relative with prostate cancer.
- Screening with PSA is common, but its utility is controversial.

Differential for hematuria—

S2I3T3

Strictures
Stones
Infection
Inflammation
Infarction
Tumor
Trauma
TB

BLADDER CANCER

The second most common urologic cancer and **the most frequent malignant tumor of the urinary tract**; usually a **transitional cell carcinoma.** Most prevalent in men during the sixth and seventh decades. Risk factors include smoking, diets rich in meat and fat, schistosomiasis, chronic treatment with cyclophosphamide, and exposure to aniline dye (a benzene derivative).

HISTORY/PE

- **Gross hematuria** is the most common presenting symptom.
- Other urinary symptoms, such as frequency, urgency, and dysuria, can also occur, but most patients are asymptomatic in the early stages of disease.

DIAGNOSIS

- **Cystoscopy with biopsy is diagnostic.**
- **UA** often shows hematuria (macro- or microscopic); cytology may show dysplastic cells.
- **IVP** can examine the upper urinary tract as well as defects in bladder filling.
- MRI, CT, and bone scan are important tools with which to define invasion and metastases.

TREATMENT

Treatment depends on the extent of spread beyond the bladder mucosa.

- **Carcinoma in situ:** Intravesicular chemotherapy.
- **Superficial cancers:** Complete transurethral resection or intravesicular chemotherapy with mitomycin-C or BCG (the vaccine for TB).
- **Large, high-grade recurrent lesions:** Intravesicular chemotherapy.
- **Invasive cancers without metastases:** Radical cystectomy or radiotherapy for patients who are deemed poor candidates for radical cystectomy or with unresectable local disease.
- **Patients with distant metastases:** Chemotherapy alone.

RENAL CELL CARCINOMA

An adenocarcinoma from tubular epithelial cells that → 80–90% of all malignant tumors of the kidney. Can spread along the renal vein to the IVC and metastasize to lung and bone. Risk factors include male **gender, smoking, obesity, acquired cystic kidney disease in end-stage renal disease,** and von Hippel–Lindau disease.

The classic triad of renal cell carcinoma is hematuria, flank pain, and a palpable flank mass.

HISTORY/PE

- Presents with the triad of **hematuria, flank pain,** and a **palpable flank mass.**
- Many patients have **fever** or other constitutional symptoms. Varicocele is seen in men.
- **Anemia is common at presentation, but polycythemia** due to ↑ erythropoietin production may be seen in 5–10% of patients.

DIAGNOSIS

Ultrasound and/or CT to characterize the renal mass (usually complex cysts or solid tumor).

TREATMENT

- **Surgical resection** may be curative in localized disease.
- Response rates from chemotherapy are only 15–30%.

TESTICULAR CANCER

A heterogeneous group of neoplasms. Some 95% of testicular tumors derive from **germ cells,** and **virtually all are malignant. Cryptorchidism** is associated with an ↑ risk of neoplasia in both testes. **Klinefelter's syndrome** is also a risk factor. Testicular cancer is the most common malignancy in men 25–34 years of age.

History/PE

- Patients most often present with **painless enlargement of the testes.**
- Most testicular cancers occur between the ages of 15 and 30, but seminomas have a peak incidence between 40 and 50 years of age.

Diagnosis

- **Testicular** ultrasound.
- CXR and abdominal/pelvic CT to evaluate for metastasis.
- **Tumor markers** are useful in diagnosis and in monitoring treatment response.
    - β-hCG is always elevated in choriocarcinoma and is elevated in 10% of seminomas.
    - α-fetoprotein (AFP) is often elevated in nonseminomatous germ cell tumors, particularly endodermal sinus (yolk sac) tumors.

Treatment

- Radical orchiectomy.
- Seminomas are **exquisitely radiosensitive** and also respond to chemotherapy.
- Platinum-based chemotherapy is used for nonseminomatous germ cell tumors.

CRYPTORCHIDISM

- Failure of the testes to fully descend into the scrotum.
- Prematurity is a risk factor.
- **Hx:** Bilateral cryptorchidism is associated with oligospermia and infertility.
- **PE:** Testes **cannot be manipulated into the scrotal sac** with gentle pressure (vs. retracted testes) and may be palpated anywhere along the inguinal canal or in the abdomen.
- **Rx:** **Orchiopexy** after age one (in all but 1% of males, the testes will descend by that age) but before age five (to preserve fertility). If it is discovered later in life, treat with orchiectomy to avoid the risk of testicular cancer.

ERECTILE DYSFUNCTION (ED)

Found in 10–25% of middle-aged and elderly men; has a significant impact on the well-being of affected individuals. Pathophysiologically classified as failure to initiate (e.g., psychological, endocrinologic, neurologic), failure to

β-*hCG = choriocarcinoma.*

AFP = endodermal sinus
tumor.

fill (e.g., arteriogenic), or failure to store (e.g., veno-occlusive dysfunction). Risk factors include **DM, atherosclerosis, medications** (e.g., β-blockers, SSRIs), hypertension, heart disease, surgery or radiation for prostate cancer, and spinal cord injury.

HISTORY/PE

- Because patients rarely volunteer this complaint, physicians should make a specific inquiry.
- Ask about risk factors, **medication use,** recent life changes, and psychological stressors.
- The distinction between psychological and organic ED is based on the presence of **nocturnal or early-morning erections** (if present, it is nonorganic) and on **situation dependence** (i.e., occurring with only one partner).
- Evaluate for **neurologic dysfunction** (e.g., anal tone, lower extremity sensation) and for **hypogonadism** (e.g., small testes, loss of 2° sexual characteristics).

DIAGNOSIS

- **Testosterone and gonadotropin levels** may be abnormal.
- Check prolactin, as elevated **prolactin** can → ↓ androgen activity.

TREATMENT

- Patients with psychological ED may benefit from psychotherapy or sex therapy involving discussion and exercises with the appropriate partner.
- Oral **sildenafil (Viagra) and vardenafil (Levitra)** are phosphodiesterase-5 (PDE5) inhibitors that → prolonged action of cGMP-mediated smooth muscle relaxation and ↑ blood flow in the corpora cavernosa. PDE5 inhibitors are effective for a broad range of etiologies.
- **Testosterone** is a useful therapy for patients with hypogonadism of testicular or pituitary origin; it is discouraged for patients with normal testosterone levels.
- Vacuum pumps, intracavernosal injections, and surgical implantation of semirigid or inflatable penile prostheses are alternatives for patients who fail PDE5 therapy.

Selected Topics in Emergency Medicine

Aspects of a pain history—

OPQRST

Onset
Precipitating factors
Quality
Radiation
Symptoms
Temporal
   course/**T**reatment
   modalities

If the patient remembers the exact moment of pain onset, think perforation.

ACUTE ABDOMEN

Acute-onset abdominal pain has many potential etiologies and may require immediate medical or surgical intervention. Sharp, focal pain generally implies a parietal (peritoneal) etiology; dull, diffuse pain is commonly of visceral (organ) origin. Figure 2.17-1 identifies the common causes of acute abdomen.

HISTORY/PE

- Obtain a complete history, including the elements indicated in the mnemonic **OPQRST.**
- Obtain a full gynecologic history for females (including last menstrual period, pregnancy, and any STD symptoms).
- **Perforation** → sudden onset of diffuse, severe pain.
- **Obstruction** → acute onset of severe, radiating, colicky pain.
- **Inflammation** → gradual onset (over 10–12 hours) of constant, ill-defined pain.
- **Associated symptoms:**
  - Anorexia, nausea, vomiting, changes in bowel habits, hematochezia, and melena suggest GI etiologies.
  - Hematuria and costovertebral angle tenderness suggest a GU etiology.
  - If associated with meals, consider mesenteric ischemia, PUD, biliary disease, pancreatitis, or bowel pathology.
  - A family history of abdominal pain may indicate familial Mediterranean fever or acute intermittent porphyria.

DIAGNOSIS

- If peritoneal signs, shock, or impending shock is present, emergent exploratory laparotomy is necessary.

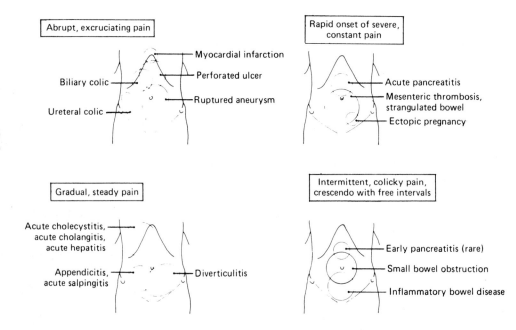

FIGURE 2.17-1.   Acute abdomen.

The location and character of pain are helpful in the differential diagnosis of the acute abdomen. (Reproduced, with permission, from Way LW [ed]. *Current Surgical Diagnosis & Treatment,* 10th ed. Stamford, CT: Appleton & Lange, 1994:444.)

- If the patient is stable, a complete physical exam—including a **rectal exam** and, in women, a **pelvic exam**—is mandatory.
- Obtain electrolytes, LFTs, amylase, lipase, **urine or serum β-hCG**, UA, and a CBC with differential.
- **Radiologic studies:** Consider a KUB, CT, and/or rectal contrast studies. **Avoid PO contrast studies if a complete bowel obstruction is suspected.** In women, ultrasound can be used to evaluate for ectopic pregnancy and ovarian torsion.

TREATMENT

- Hemodynamically unstable patients must have an **emergent exploratory laparotomy.**
- In stable patients, expectant management may include NPO status, NG tube placement, IV fluids, placement of a Foley catheter (to monitor urine output and fluid status), and vital sign monitoring with serial abdominal exams and serial labs.
- Type and cross all unstable patients.

APPENDICITIS

The inciting event is obstruction of the appendiceal lumen with subsequent inflammation and infection. Rising intraluminal pressure → vascular compromise of the appendix, ischemia, necrosis, and possible perforation. Etiologies include hypertrophied lymphoid tissue (55–65%), fecalith (35%), foreign body, tumor (e.g., carcinoid tumor), and parasites.

HISTORY/PE

- Dull periumbilical pain lasting 1–12 hours → sharp RLQ pain at McBurney's point.
- Nausea, vomiting, anorexia ("hamburger sign"), and low-grade fever.
- Psoas, obturator, and Rovsing's signs are insensitive tests that may be ⊕.
- **Perforated appendix:** Partial pain relief is possible, but peritoneal signs (e.g., rebound, guarding, hypotension, ↑ WBC count, fever) will ultimately develop.
- Children, the elderly, pregnant women, and those with retrocecal appendices may have atypical presentations.

DIAGNOSIS

- Clinical impression.
- Look for fever, mild leukocytosis (11,000–15,000 cells/μL) with left shift, and UA with a few RBCs and/or WBCs.
- If the clinical diagnosis is unequivocal, no imaging studies are necessary. Otherwise, studies include the following:
  - **KUB:** Fecalith or loss of psoas shadow.
  - **Ultrasound:** Enlarged, noncompressible appendix.
  - **CT scan with contrast (95–98% sensitive):** Periappendiceal streaking.

TREATMENT

- The patient should be NPO and should receive IV hydration and antibiotics with anaerobic and gram-⊖ coverage.
- Immediate open or laparoscopic appendectomy is the definitive treatment. If appendicitis is not found, complete exploration of the abdomen is performed.

All female patients with an acute abdomen require a pelvic exam and a pregnancy test to rule out PID, ectopic pregnancy, and ovarian torsion.

McBurney's point is located two-thirds of the distance from the anterior superior iliac spine to the umbilicus.

"Hamburger sign": If a patient wants to eat, consider a diagnosis other than appendicitis.

Psoas sign: Passive extension of the hip → RLQ pain.

Obturator sign: Passive internal rotation of the hip → RLQ pain.

Rovsing's sign: Deep palpation of the LLQ → RLQ pain.

- **Perforation:** Administer antibiotics until the patient is afebrile with a normalized WBC count; the wound should be closed by delayed 1° closure.
- **Abscess:** Treat with broad-spectrum antibiotics and percutaneous drainage; an elective appendectomy should be performed 6–8 weeks later.

AORTIC DISRUPTION

Aortic disruption is often associated with first and second rib and sternal fractures.

A **rapid deceleration injury** that is most commonly seen after high-speed motor vehicle accidents (MVAs), ejection from vehicles, and falls from heights. Since complete aortic rupture is rapidly fatal (85% die at the scene), trauma patients with an aortic disruption injury usually have a contained hematoma within the adventitia. Laceration is most common at the ligamentum arteriosum. **Always suspect aortic disruption if there are sternal or first and second rib fractures.**

DIAGNOSIS

- **Immediate CXR:** Reveals **widened mediastinum (> 8 cm), loss of aortic knob, pleural cap,** deviation of the trachea to the right, and depression of the left main stem bronchus.
- CT evaluation and/or transesophageal echocardiography (TEE) prior to surgery.
- **Aortography is the gold standard for evaluation.**

TREATMENT

Basic trauma management (ABCs); emergent surgery for defect repair.

BURNS

Use the "rule of 9's" to estimate %BSA:

Head and each arm = 9%

Back and chest each = 18%

Each leg = 18%

Perineum = 1%

The **second leading cause of death in children.** Categorized by depth of tissue destruction.

- **First degree:** Only the epidermis is involved. The area is painful and erythematous, but blisters are not present, and capillary refill is intact.
- **Second degree:** The epidermis and partial thickness of the dermis are involved. The area is painful, and blisters are present.
- **Third degree:** The epidermis, full thickness of the dermis, and potentially deeper tissues are involved. The area is painless, white, and charred.

HISTORY/PE

- Patients may present with obvious skin wounds, but significant deep destruction may not be visible, especially with electrical burns.
- Perform a thorough airway and lung exam.

DIAGNOSIS

- Assess the ABCs. If airway compromise is impending, intubate.
- Be vigilant for shock, inhalation injury, and carbon monoxide poisoning.
- Evaluate the percentage of body surface area (%BSA) involved.

Parkland formula: Fluids for the first 24 hours = 4 × patient's weight in kg × %BSA. Give 50% of fluids over the first eight hours and the remaining 50% over the following 16 hours.

TREATMENT

- Supportive measures; tetanus and stress ulcer prophylaxis.
- For second- and third-degree burns, fluid repletion using the **Parkland formula** is critical; adjust repletion on the basis of additional insensible losses to maintain at least 1 cc/kg/hr of urine output.

- Topical silver sulfadiazine and mafenide may be used prophylactically; however, there is no proven benefit associated with the use of PO/IV antibiotics or steroids.

COMPLICATIONS

Shock and superinfection, with the latter most likely due to *Pseudomonas*.

CARDIAC LIFE SUPPORT BASICS

Table 2.17-1 summarizes the basic management of cardiac arrhythmias in an acute setting.

PELVIC FRACTURES

Most commonly occur after traumas such as MVAs. Require immediate attention by the orthopedist owing to their life-threatening potential.

DIAGNOSIS

- Possible unstable pelvis upon compression.
- Pelvic x-rays may confirm the fracture; in a stable patient, a CT scan of the pelvis will better define the extent of injury.
- If hypotension and shock are present, an exsanguinating hemorrhage is likely. In the field, MAST (military antishock trousers; rarely used today) can be used to maintain adequate BP and organ perfusion.

> **Possible causes of PEA—**
>
> **the 5 H's and 5 T's**
>
> **H**ypovolemia
> **H**ypoxia
> **H**ydrogen ion: Acidosis
> **H**yper/**H**ypo: K⁺, other metabolic
> **H**ypothermia
> **T**ablets: Drug OD, ingestion
> **T**amponade: Cardiac
> **T**ension pneumothorax
> **T**hrombosis: Coronary
> **T**hrombosis: Pulmonary embolism

TABLE 2.17-1. **Management of Cardiac Arrhythmias**

ARRHYTHMIA	TREATMENT
Asystole	Epinephrine, atropine.
Ventricular fibrillation	Desynchronized shock with 200, 300, and 360 J → epinephrine **or** Vasopressin → shock → lidocaine **or** Amiodarone → shock → procainamide or magnesium.
Ventricular tachycardia	If unstable and pulseless, desynchronized shock. If stable, give lidocaine or amiodarone.
Pulseless electrical activity (PEA)	Identify and treat the underlying cause. Consider epinephrine and/or atropine.
Atrial fibrillation/flutter	If unstable, shock starting at 100 J. If stable, control rate (using calcium channel blockers, digoxin, or β-blockers), convert rhythm (if < 48 hours, convert electrically or chemically; if > 48 hours, anticoagulate or perform TEE prior to conversion) and anticoagulate.
Supraventricular tachycardia (SVT)	Control rate with maneuvers such as Valsalva, carotid sinus massage, or cold stimulus. If resistant, consider adenosine.
Bradycardia	If symptomatic, give atropine and consider dopamine or dobutamine. If Mobitz II or third-degree heart block is present, place a transvenous pacemaker.

TREATMENT

- Consider embolization of bleeding vessels, emergent external pelvic fixation, or, in a hemodynamically stable patient, internal fixation.
- Pelvic injuries can be associated with urethral injury.
    - Make note of **blood at the urethral meatus; a high-riding, "ballotable" prostate;** or **lack of a prostate.**
    - If present, a **retrograde urethrogram** must be performed to rule out injury before a Foley catheter is placed.
- Never explore a pelvic or retroperitoneal hematoma. Follow with serial hemoglobin and hematocrit.

PENETRATING WOUNDS

Evaluation and treatment depend on the location and extent of the injury.

Neck

- Intubate early.
- Treatment varies according to zone (see Figure 2.17-2).
    - **Zone 1:** Aortography.
    - **Zone 2:** Surgically explore the injury if the platysma is penetrated. In some ERs, angiography and triple endoscopy (tracheobronchoscopy and esophagoscopy) are also being used for injuries to this zone.
    - **Zone 3:** Aortography and triple endoscopy.

Chest

- Unstable patients with penetrating thoracic injuries require immediate **intubation** and bilateral **chest tubes.** Thoracotomy may be necessary if the patient remains unstable despite resuscitative efforts.
- Leave any impaled objects in place until the patient is taken to the OR, as such objects may tamponade further blood loss.

Leave any impaled objects in place until the patient is taken to the OR.

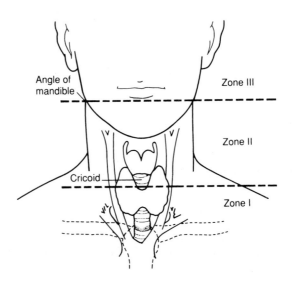

FIGURE 2.17-2.   Zones of the neck.

(Reproduced, with permission, from Way LW [ed]. *Current Surgical Diagnosis & Treatment,* 10th ed. Stamford, CT: Appleton & Lange, 1994:223.)

- Beware of pneumothorax, hemothorax, cardiac tamponade, aortic disruption, diaphragmatic tear, and esophageal injury.
- If a previously stable chest trauma patient suddenly dies, suspect **air embolism.**

Suspect air embolism when a previously stable chest trauma patient suddenly dies.

Abdomen

- The absence of pain does not rule out an abdominal injury.
- Gunshot wounds require immediate exploratory laparotomy.
- Stab wounds or blunt injury in a hemodynamically unstable patient or in a patient with peritoneal signs or evisceration requires immediate exploratory laparotomy.
- Stab wounds or blunt injury in a hemodynamically stable patient warrants a CT scan or focused abdominal sonography for trauma (FAST scan).
- The **spleen** is the **most common abdominal organ injured in blunt trauma.** Suspect splenic injury if there are left lower rib fractures.

Musculoskeletal

- If there is no neurovascular injury on exam, debride and repair. If vascular injury is suspected, do an arteriogram first.
- **Early wound irrigation** and **tissue debridement,** not antibiotic therapy, are the most important steps in the treatment of contaminated wounds. However, do administer antibiotics and tetanus prophylaxis.

POSTOPERATIVE FEVER

- Remember the mnemonic "Wind, Water, Walking, Wounds, and Wonder drugs."
- ↓ the risk of postoperative fever with incentive spirometry, pre- and postoperative antibiotics when indicated, short-term Foley catheter use, early ambulation, and DVT prophylaxis (e.g., anticoagulation, compression stockings).
- Fevers before postoperative day 3 are unlikely to be infectious unless *Clostridium* or β-hemolytic streptococci are involved.

> **The 5 W's of post-operative fever:**
>
> **W**ind: Atelectasis, pneumonia
> **W**ater: UTI
> **W**alking: DVT
> **W**ounds: Wound infection, abscess
> **W**onder drugs: Drug reaction

SHOCK

Defined as **inadequate perfusion to maintain vital organ function.** The multiple etiologies are differentiated by their cardiovascular effects and treatment options (see Table 2.17-2).

TOXICOLOGY

Carbon Monoxide Poisoning

A **hypoxemic poisoning syndrome** seen in patients who have been exposed to automobile exhaust, smoke inhalation, barbecues, or old appliances in poorly ventilated locations.

HISTORY/PE

- Hypoxemia, **cherry-red skin,** confusion, **headaches.** Coma or seizures occur in severe cases.

HIGH-YIELD FACTS

EMERGENCY MEDICINE

383

TABLE 2.17-2. Types of Shock

TYPE OF SHOCK[a]	MAJOR CAUSES	CARDIAC OUTPUT	PCWP[b]	PVR[c]	TREATMENT
Hypovolemic	Trauma, blood loss, inadequate fluid repletion, third spacing, burns.	↓	↓	↑	Replete with isotonic solution (e.g., LR or NS) and blood in a 3:1 (fluid-to-blood) ratio.
Cardiogenic	Tension pneumothorax, CHF, cardiac tamponade, arrhythmia, structural heart disease (severe mitral regurgitation, VSD), MI (> 40% of LV function).	↓	↑	↑	Identify the cause and treat if possible. Give pressors such as **dobutamine** and, if necessary, dopamine or norepinephrine.
Septic	Bacteremia, especially gram-⊖ organisms.	↑	↓	↓	Administer fluid and antibiotics. Consider a Swan-Ganz catheter. Give dopamine or norepinephrine.
Anaphylactic	Bee stings, medication, food allergies.	↑	↓	↓	Give diphenhydramine. If severe, administer 1:1000 epinephrine.

[a] Type of shock = neurogenic shock, which is characterized by hypotension with bradycardia and differs from Cushing's triad (↑ ICP), which involves hypertension with bradycardia.

[b] PCWP = pulmonary capillary wedge pressure.

[c] PVR = peripheral vascular resistance.

- Chronic low-level exposure may cause **flulike symptoms** with generalized myalgias, nausea, and headaches.
- **Suspect smoke inhalation** in the presence of **singed nose hairs, facial burns, hoarseness, wheezing,** or **carbonaceous sputum.**

DIAGNOSIS

- Check an ABG and serum carboxyhemoglobin level (normal is < 5% in nonsmokers and < 10% in smokers).
- Perform laryngoscopy or bronchoscopy if smoke inhalation is suspected.
- Check an ECG in the elderly and in patients with a history of cardiac disease.

TREATMENT

- Treat with 100% O_2.
- Use **hyperbaric O_2** for pregnant patients, those with neurologic symptoms, or those with severely ↑ carboxyhemoglobin to facilitate displacement of carbon monoxide from hemoglobin.
- Patients with **smoke inhalation** may require early intubation, since upper airway edema can rapidly → complete obstruction.

Common Drug Interactions/Reactions

Table 2.17-3 outlines drug interactions and reactions that are commonly encountered in a clinical setting.

TABLE 2.17-3. Drug Interactions and Reactions

INTERACTION/REACTION	DRUGS
Induction of P-450 enzymes	Barbiturates, phenytoin, carbamazepine, rifampin.
Inhibition of P-450 enzymes	Cimetidine, ketoconazole, INH.
Metabolism by P-450 enzymes	Benzodiazepines, amide anesthetics, metoprolol, propranolol, nifedipine, phenytoin, quinidine, theophylline, warfarin, barbiturates.
↑ risk of digoxin toxicity	Quinidine, cimetidine, amiodarone, calcium channel blockers.
Competition for albumin-binding sites	Warfarin, ASA, phenytoin.
Blood dyscrasias	Ibuprofen, quinidine, methyldopa, chemotherapeutic agents.
Hemolysis in G6PD-deficient patients	Sulfonamides, INH, ASA, ibuprofen, nitrofurantoin, primaquine.
Gynecomastia	Cimetidine, ketoconazole, spironolactone.
Stevens-Johnson syndrome	Ethosuximide, sulfonamides.
Photosensitivity	Tetracycline, amiodarone, sulfonamides.
Drug-induced SLE	Procainamide, hydralazine, INH, penicillamine.

Drug Overdose

Table 2.17-4 summarizes antidotes and treatments for substances commonly encountered in overdoses and intoxications.

Major Drug Side Effects

Table 2.17-5 outlines the major side effects of select drugs.

Management of Drug Withdrawal

Table 2.17-6 summarizes common drug withdrawal symptoms and treatment.

HIGH-YIELD FACTS

EMERGENCY MEDICINE

TABLE 2.17-4. Specific Antidotes

TOXIN	ANTIDOTE/TREATMENT
Acetaminophen	*N*-acetylcysteine.
Acid/alkali ingestion	Upper endoscopy to evaluate for stricture.
Anticholinesterases, organophosphates	Atropine, pralidoxime.
Antimuscarinic/anticholinergic agents	Physostigmine.
Arsenic, mercury, gold	Succimer, dimercaprol.
β-blockers	Glucagon.
Barbiturates (phenobarbital)	Urine alkalinization, dialysis, activated charcoal.
Benzodiazepines	Flumazenil.
Black widow bite	Calcium gluconate.
Carbon monoxide	100% O_2, hyperbaric O_2.
Copper, arsenic, lead, gold	Penicillamine.
Cyanide	Nitrite, sodium thiosulfate.
Digitalis	Stop digitalis, normalize K^+, lidocaine (for torsades), anti-digitalis Fab.
Heparin	Protamine sulfate.
Iron salts	Deferoxamine.
Lead	Succimer, CaEDTA, dimercaprol.
Methanol, ethylene glycol (antifreeze)	EtOH, fomepizole, dialysis.
Methemoglobin	Methylene blue.
Opioids	Naloxone.
Phencyclidine hydrochloride (PCP)	NG suction.
Salicylates	Urine alkalinization, dialysis, activated charcoal.
TCAs	Sodium bicarbonate for QRS prolongation; diazepam or lorazepam for seizures; cardiac monitor for arrhythmias.
Theophylline	Activated charcoal.
tPA, streptokinase	Aminocaproic acid.
Warfarin	Vitamin K, FFP.

TABLE 2.17-5.   Drug Side Effects

DRUG	SIDE EFFECTS
ACEIs	**Cough,** rash, proteinuria, angioedema, taste changes, teratogenic effects.
Amantadine	Ataxia, **livedo reticularis.**
Aminoglycosides	Ototoxicity, nephrotoxicity (acute tubular necrosis).
Amiodarone	Pulmonary fibrosis, peripheral deposition → bluish discoloration, arrhythmias, hypo-/hyperthyroidism, corneal deposition.
Amphotericin	Fever/chills, nephrotoxicity, bone marrow suppression, anemia.
Antipsychotics	Sedation, acute dystonic reaction, akathisia, parkinsonism, tardive dyskinesia, **neuroleptic malignant syndrome.**
Azoles (e.g., fluconazole)	Inhibition of P-450 enzymes.
AZT	Thrombocytopenia, megaloblastic anemia.
β-blockers	Asthma exacerbation, masking of hypoglycemia, impotence.
Benzodiazepines	Sedation, dependence, respiratory depression.
Bile acid resins	GI upset, malabsorption of vitamins and medications.
Calcium channel blockers	Peripheral edema, constipation, cardiac depression.
Carbamazepine	Induction of P-450 enzymes, **agranulocytosis,** aplastic anemia.
Chloramphenicol	**Gray baby syndrome,** aplastic anemia.
Cisplatin	Nephrotoxicity, acoustic nerve damage.
Clonidine	Dry mouth; **severe rebound headache and hypertension.**
Clozapine	Agranulocytosis.
Corticosteroids	Mania (acute), immunosuppression, bone mineral loss, thinning of skin, easy bruising, myopathy (chronic), cataracts.
Cyclophosphamide	Myelosuppression, **hemorrhagic cystitis.**
Digoxin	GI disturbance, **yellow visual changes, arrhythmias** (e.g., junctional tachycardia or SVT).
Doxorubicin	**Cardiotoxicity (cardiomyopathy).**
Ethyl alcohol	Renal dysfunction.
Fluoroquinolones	Cartilage damage in children; Achilles tendon rupture in adults.
Furosemide	Ototoxicity, hypokalemia, nephritis.

HIGH-YIELD FACTS

EMERGENCY MEDICINE

TABLE 2.17-5. Drug Side Effects (continued)

DRUG	SIDE EFFECTS
Gemfibrozil	Myositis, reversible ↑ in LFTs.
Halothane	Hepatotoxicity, **malignant hyperthermia.**
HCTZ	Hypokalemia, hyperuricemia, hyperglycemia.
HMG-CoA reductase inhibitors	Myositis, reversible ↑ in LFTs.
Hydralazine	Drug-induced SLE.
Hydroxychloroquine	Retinopathy.
INH	Peripheral neuropathy **(prevent with pyridoxine/vitamin B₆),** hepatotoxicity, inhibition of P-450 enzymes, seizures with overdose.
MAOIs	**Hypertensive tyramine reaction, serotonin syndrome** (with meperidine).
Methanol	Blindness.
Methotrexate	Hepatic fibrosis, pneumonitis, anemia.
Methyldopa	⊕ Coombs' test, drug-induced SLE.
Metronidazole	Disulfiram reaction, vestibular dysfunction, **metallic taste.**
Niacin	**Cutaneous flushing.**
Nitroglycerin	Hypotension, tachycardia, headache, tolerance.
Penicillin/β-lactams	Hypersensitivity reactions.
Penicillamine	Drug-induced SLE.
Phenytoin	Nystagmus, diplopia, ataxia, **gingival hyperplasia,** hirsutism.
Prazosin	First-dose hypotension.
Procainamide	Drug-induced SLE.
Propylthiouracil	Agranulocytosis.
Quinidine	Cinchonism (headache, tinnitus), thrombocytopenia, arrhythmias (e.g., **torsades de pointes**).
Reserpine	Depression.
Rifampin	Induction of P-450 enzymes; **orange-red body secretions.**
Salicylates	Fever; hyperventilation with **respiratory alkalosis and metabolic acidosis;** dehydration, diaphoresis, hemorrhagic gastritis.

TABLE 2.17-5. **Drug Side Effects (continued)**

DRUG	SIDE EFFECTS
SSRIs	Anxiety, **sexual dysfunction.**
Succinylcholine	**Malignant hyperthermia.**
Tetracyclines	Tooth discoloration, photosensitivity, Fanconi's syndrome.
TCAs	Sedation, coma, anticholinergic effects, seizures and arrhythmias.
Valproic acid	Teratogenicity → neural tube defects.
Vancomycin	Nephrotoxicity, ototoxicity, **"red man syndrome"** (histamine release; not an allergy).
Vinblastine	Severe myelosuppression.
Vincristine	Peripheral neuropathy.

TABLE 2.17-6. **Symptoms and Treatment of Drug Withdrawal**

DRUG	WITHDRAWAL SYMPTOMS	TREATMENT
Alcohol	Tremor (6–12 hours). Tachycardia, hypertension, agitation, seizures (within 48 hours). Hallucinations, **DTs**—severe autonomic instability → tachycardia, hypertension, delirium, and possibly death (within 2–7 days). Mortality is 15–20%.	**Benzodiazepines;** haloperidol for hallucinations; **thiamine,** folate, and multivitamin replacement (do not affect withdrawal, but most alcoholics are deficient).
Barbiturates	Anxiety, seizures, delirium, tremor; cardiac and respiratory depression.	**Benzodiazepines.**
Benzodiazepines	Rebound anxiety, seizures, tremor, insomnia.	**Benzodiazepines.** Monitor for DTs.
Cocaine/amphetamines	Depression, hyperphagia, hypersomnolence.	Supportive treatment. Avoid pure β-blockers (may → unopposed α activity, causing hypertension).
Opioids	Anxiety, insomnia, flulike symptoms, piloerection, fever, rhinorrhea, lacrimation, yawning, nausea, stomach cramps, diarrhea, mydriasis.	Clonidine and/or buprenorphine for moderate symptoms; methadone for severe symptoms. Naltrexone for patients who are drug free for 7–10 days.

HIGH-YIELD FACTS

EMERGENCY MEDICINE

1° survey of a trauma patient—

ABCDE

Airway
Breathing
Circulation
Disability
Exposure

Immediately evaluate trauma patients for tension pneumothorax, cardiac tamponade, open pneumothorax, massive hemothorax, and airway obstruction.

Acute management of a trauma patient can be remembered with the mnemonic **ABCDE**. **Airway patency and adequacy of ventilation take precedence over other treatment.**

1° Survey

- Airway:
  - Start with supplemental O_2 by nasal cannula or face mask for conscious patients. Use a chin-lift or jaw-thrust maneuver to reposition the tongue in an unconscious patient. An oropharyngeal or nasopharyngeal airway may facilitate bag-mask ventilation.
  - Perform intubation in patients with apnea, ↓ mental status, impending airway compromise (e.g., significant maxillofacial trauma or inhalation injury in fires), severe closed-head injuries, or failed bag-mask ventilation.
  - Perform a surgical airway (cricothyroidotomy) in patients who cannot be intubated or in whom there is significant maxillofacial trauma.
  - Maintain cervical spine stabilization/immobilization in trauma patients until the spine is appropriately cleared through exam and radiographic studies. However, **never allow this concern to delay airway management.**
- **Breathing:** Thorough cardiac and pulmonary exams will identify the five thoracic causes of immediate death: **tension pneumothorax, cardiac tamponade, open pneumothorax, massive hemothorax,** and **airway obstruction.**
- Circulation:
  - Place a 16-gauge IV in each antecubital fossa.
  - Isotonic fluids (LR or NS) are repleted in a **3:1 ratio (fluid to blood loss).** Start with a fluid bolus of 1–2 L in adults; then recheck vitals and continue repletion as indicated.
  - For severe intravascular depletion, transfuse with packed RBCs.
- **Disability/Exposure:**
  - Disability (CNS dysfunction) is assessed and quantified with the Glasgow Coma Scale.
  - Exposure requires that the patient is completely disrobed and assessed for injury and temperature status.

2° Survey

- Once the patient is stable, perform a full examination.
- Order a trauma radiology series (AP chest, AP pelvis, and AP/lateral/odontoid C-spine views that adequately visualize the T1 vertebra).
- Place a Foley catheter after urethral injury has been ruled out.
- Order pertinent labs based on the mechanism of injury, suspicion of intoxication or OD, and past medical history.

Table 2.17-7 summarizes the signs and symptoms of key vitamin deficiencies.

TABLE 2.17-7. Vitamin Functions and Deficiencies

VITAMIN	SIGNS/SYMPTOMS OF DEFICIENCY
Vitamin A	Night blindness, dry skin.
Vitamin B$_1$ (thiamine)	Beriberi (polyneuritis, dilated cardiomyopathy, high-output CHF, edema), Wernicke-Korsakoff syndrome.
Vitamin B$_2$ (riboflavin)	Angular stomatitis, cheilosis, corneal vascularization.
Vitamin B$_3$ (niacin)	Pellagra (diarrhea, dermatitis, dementia).
Vitamin B$_5$ (pantothenate)	Dermatitis, enteritis, alopecia, adrenal insufficiency.
Vitamin B$_6$ (pyridoxine)	Convulsions, hyperirritability; required during administration of INH.
Vitamin B$_{12}$ (cobalamin)	Macrocytic, megaloblastic anemia; neurologic symptoms (e.g., optic neuropathy, subacute combined degeneration, paresthesias); glossitis.
Vitamin C	Scurvy (e.g., swollen gums, bruising, anemia, poor wound healing).
Vitamin D	Rickets in children (bending bones), osteomalacia in adults (soft bones), hypocalcemic tetany.
Vitamin E	↑ fragility of RBCs.
Vitamin K	Neonatal hemorrhage; ↑ PT and aPTT, normal BT.
Biotin	Dermatitis, enteritis. Can be caused by ingestion of **raw eggs.**
Folic acid	The **most common vitamin deficiency in the United States.** Sprue; macrocytic, megaloblastic anemia without neurologic symptoms.
Magnesium	Weakness, muscle cramps, exacerbation of hypocalcemic tetany, CNS hyperirritability → tremors, choreoathetoid movement,
Selenium	Keshan disease (cardiomyopathy).

HIGH-YIELD FACTS

EMERGENCY MEDICINE

HIGH-YIELD FACTS

RAPID REVIEW

Classic ECG finding in atrial flutter.	"Sawtooth" P waves
Definition of unstable angina.	Angina is new, is worsening, or occurs at rest
Antihypertensive for a diabetic patient with proteinuria.	ACEI
Beck's triad for cardiac tamponade.	Hypotension, distant heart sounds, and JVD
Drugs that slow AV node transmission.	β-blockers, digoxin, calcium channel blockers
Hypercholesterolemia treatment that → flushing and pruritus.	Niacin
Treatment for atrial fibrillation.	Anticoagulation, rate control, cardioversion
Treatment for ventricular fibrillation.	Immediate cardioversion
Autoimmune complication occurring 2–4 weeks post-MI.	Dressler's syndrome: fever, pericarditis, ↑ ESR
IV drug use with JVD and holosystolic murmur at the left sternal border. Treatment?	Treat existing heart failure and replace the tricuspid valve
Diagnostic test for hypertrophic cardiomyopathy.	Echocardiogram (showing thickened left ventricular wall and outflow obstruction)
A fall in systolic BP of > 10 mmHg with inspiration.	Pulsus paradoxus (seen in cardiac tamponade)
Classic ECG findings in pericarditis.	Low-voltage, diffuse ST-segment elevation
Definition of hypertension.	BP > 140/90 on three separate occasions two weeks apart
Eight surgically correctable causes of hypertension.	Renal artery stenosis, coarctation of the aorta, pheochromocytoma, Conn's syndrome, Cushing's syndrome, unilateral renal parenchymal disease, hyperthyroidism, hyperparathyroidism
Evaluation of a pulsatile abdominal mass and bruit.	Abdominal ultrasound and CT
Indications for surgical repair of abdominal aortic aneurysm.	> 5.5 cm, rapidly enlarging, symptomatic, or ruptured
Treatment for acute coronary syndrome.	Morphine, O_2, sublingual nitroglycerin, ASA, IV β-blockers, heparin
What is the metabolic syndrome?	Abdominal obesity, high triglycerides, low HDL, hypertension, insulin resistance, prothrombotic or proinflammatory states

Appropriate diagnostic test? ■ A 50-year-old male with angina can exercise to 85% of maximum predicted heart rate. ■ A 65-year-old woman with left bundle branch block and severe osteoarthritis has unstable angina.	Exercise stress treadmill with ECG Pharmacologic stress test (e.g., dobutamine echo)
Target LDL in a patient with diabetes.	< 70
Signs of active ischemia during stress testing.	Angina, ST-segment changes on ECG, or ↓ BP
ECG findings suggesting MI.	ST-segment elevation (depression means ischemia), flattened T waves, and Q waves
A young patient has angina at rest with ST-segment elevation. Cardiac enzymes are normal.	Prinzmetal's angina
Common symptoms associated with silent MIs.	CHF, shock, and altered mental status
The diagnostic test for pulmonary embolism.	V/Q scan
An agent that reverses the effects of heparin.	Protamine
The coagulation parameter affected by warfarin.	PT
A young patient with a family history of sudden death collapses and dies while exercising.	Hypertrophic cardiomyopathy
Endocarditis prophylaxis regimens.	Oral surgery—amoxicillin; GI or GU procedures—ampicillin and gentamicin before and amoxicillin after
The 6 P's of ischemia due to peripheral vascular disease.	Pain, pallor, pulselessness, paralysis, paresthesia, poikilothermia
Virchow's triad.	Stasis, hypercoagulability, endothelial damage
The most common cause of hypertension in young women.	OCPs
The most common cause of hypertension in young men.	Excessive EtOH

DERMATOLOGY

"Stuck-on" appearance.	Seborrheic keratosis
Red plaques with silvery-white scales and sharp margins.	Psoriasis
The most common type of skin cancer; the lesion is a pearly-colored papule with a translucent surface and telangiectasias.	Basal cell carcinoma
Honey-crusted lesions.	Impetigo

A febrile patient with a history of diabetes presents with a red, swollen, painful lower extremity.	Cellulitis
⊕ Nikolsky's sign.	Pemphigus vulgaris
⊖ Nikolsky's sign.	Bullous pemphigoid
A 55-year-old obese patient presents with dirty, velvety patches on the back of the neck.	Acanthosis nigricans. Check fasting blood sugar to rule out diabetes
Dermatomal distribution.	Varicella zoster
Flat-topped papules.	Lichen planus
Iris-like target lesions.	Erythema multiforme
A lesion characteristically occurring in a linear pattern in areas where skin comes into contact with clothing or jewelry.	Contact dermatitis
Presents with a herald patch, Christmas-tree pattern.	Pityriasis rosea
A 16-year-old presents with an annular patch of alopecia with broken-off, stubby hairs.	Alopecia areata (autoimmune process)
Pinkish, scaling, flat lesions on the chest and back. KOH prep has a "spaghetti-and-meatballs" appearance.	Pityriasis versicolor
Four characteristics of a nevus suggestive of melanoma.	Asymmetry, border irregularity, color variation, large diameter
Premalignant lesion from sun exposure that can → squamous cell carcinoma.	Actinic keratosis
"Dewdrop on a rose petal."	Lesions of 1° varicella
"Cradle cap."	Seborrheic dermatitis. Treat with antifungals
Associated with *Propionibacterium acnes* and changes in androgen levels.	Acne vulgaris
A painful, recurrent vesicular eruption of mucocutaneous surfaces.	Herpes simplex
Inflammation and epithelial thinning of the anogenital area, predominantly in postmenopausal women.	Lichen sclerosus
Exophytic nodules on the skin with varying degrees of scaling or ulceration; the second most common type of skin cancer.	Squamous cell carcinoma

The most common cause of hypothyroidism.	Hashimoto's thyroiditis
Lab findings in Hashimoto's thyroiditis.	High TSH, low T_4, antimicrosomal antibodies
Exophthalmos, pretibial myxedema, and ↓ TSH.	Graves' disease
The most common cause of Cushing's syndrome.	Iatrogenic steroid administration. The second most common cause is Cushing's disease
A patient presents with signs of hypocalcemia, high phosphorus, and low PTH.	Hypoparathyroidism
"Stones, bones, groans, psychiatric overtones."	Signs and symptoms of hypercalcemia
A patient complains of headache, weakness, and polyuria; exam reveals hypertension and tetany. Labs reveals hypernatremia, hypokalemia, and metabolic alkalosis.	1° hyperaldosteronism (due to Conn's syndrome or bilateral adrenal hyperplasia)
A patient presents with tachycardia, wild swings in BP, headache, diaphoresis, altered mental status, and a sense of panic.	Pheochromocytoma
Should α- or β-antagonists be used first in treating pheochromocytoma?	α-antagonists (phentolamine and phenoxybenzamine)
A patient with a history of lithium use presents with copious amounts of dilute urine.	Nephrogenic diabetes insipidus (DI)
Treatment of central DI.	Administration of DDAVP ↓ serum osmolality and free water restriction
A postoperative patient with significant pain presents with hyponatremia and normal volume status.	SIADH due to stress
An antidiabetic agent associated with lactic acidosis.	Metformin
A patient presents with weakness, nausea, vomiting, weight loss, and new skin pigmentation. Labs show hyponatremia and hyperkalemia. Treatment?	1° adrenal insufficiency (Addison's disease). Treat with replacement glucocorticoids, mineralocorticoids, and IV fluids
Goal hemoglobin A_{1c} for a patient with DM.	< 7.0
Treatment of DKA.	Fluids, insulin, and aggressive replacement of electrolytes (e.g., K^+)
Why are β-blockers contraindicated in diabetics?	They can mask symptoms of hypoglycemia

Bias introduced into a study when a clinician is aware of the patient's treatment type.	Observational bias
Bias introduced when screening detects a disease earlier and thus lengthens the time from diagnosis to death.	Lead-time bias
If you want to know if race affects infant mortality rate but most of the variation in infant mortality is predicted by socioeconomic status, then socioeconomic status is a _____.	Confounding variable
The number of true positives divided by the number of patients with the disease is _____.	Sensitivity
Sensitive tests have few false negatives and are used to rule _____ a disease.	Out
PPD reactivity is used as a screening test because most people with TB (except those who are anergic) will have a ⊕ PPD. Highly sensitive or specific?	Highly sensitive for TB
Chronic diseases such as SLE—higher prevalence or incidence?	Higher prevalence
Epidemics such as influenza—higher prevalence or incidence?	Higher incidence
Cross-sectional survey—incidence or prevalence?	Prevalence
Cohort study—incidence or prevalence?	Incidence and prevalence
Case-control study—incidence or prevalence?	Neither
Describe a test that consistently gives identical results, but the results are wrong.	High reliability, low validity
Difference between a cohort and a case-control study.	Cohort studies can be used to calculate relative risk (RR), incidence, and/or odds ratio (OR). Case-control studies can be used to calculate an OR
Attributable risk?	The incidence rate (IR) of a disease in exposed − the IR of a disease in unexposed
Relative risk?	The IR of a disease in a population exposed to a particular factor ÷ the IR of those not exposed
Odds ratio?	The likelihood of a disease among individuals exposed to a risk factor compared to those who have not been exposed

Number needed to treat?	$1 \div$ (rate in untreated group − rate in treated group)
In which patients do you initiate colorectal cancer screening early?	Patients with IBD; those with familial adenomatous polyposis (FAP)/hereditary nonpolyposis colorectal cancer (HNPCC); and those who have first-degree relatives with adenomatous polyps (< 60 years of age) or colorectal cancer
The most common cancer in men and the most common cause of death from cancer in men.	Prostate cancer is the most common cancer in men, but lung cancer causes more deaths
The percentage of cases within one SD of the mean? Two SDs? Three SDs?	68%, 95.5%, 99.7%
Birth rate?	Number of live births per 1000 population
Fertility rate?	Number of live births per 1000 women 15–44 years of age
Mortality rate?	Number of deaths per 1000 population
Neonatal mortality?	Number of deaths from birth to 28 days per 1000 live births
Postnatal mortality?	Number of deaths from 28 days to one year per 1000 live births
Infant mortality?	Number of deaths from birth to one year of age per 1000 live births (neonatal + postnatal mortality)
Fetal mortality?	Number of deaths from 20 weeks' gestation to birth per 1000 total births
Perinatal mortality?	Number of deaths from 20 weeks' gestation to one month of life per 1000 total births
Maternal mortality?	Number of deaths during pregnancy to 90 days postpartum per 100,000 live births

ETHICS

True or false: Once patients sign a statement giving consent, they must continue treatment.	False. Patients may change their minds at any time. Exceptions to the requirement of informed consent include emergency situations and patients without decision-making capacity
A 15-year-old pregnant girl requires hospitalization for preeclampsia. Should her parents be informed?	No. Parental consent is not necessary for the medical treatment of pregnant minors
A doctor refers a patient for an MRI at a facility he/she owns.	Conflict of interest

Involuntary psychiatric hospitalization can be undertaken for which three reasons?	The patient is a danger to self, a danger to others, or gravely disabled (unable to provide for basic needs)
True or false: Withdrawing life-sustaining care is ethically distinct from withholding sustaining care.	False. Withdrawing and withholding life are the same from an ethical standpoint
When can a physician refuse to continue treating a patient on the grounds of futility?	When there is no rationale for treatment, maximal intervention is failing, a given intervention has already failed, and treatment will not achieve the goals of care
An eight-year-old child is in a serious accident. She requires emergent transfusion, but her parents are not present.	Treat immediately. Consent is implied in emergency situations
Conditions in which confidentiality must be overridden.	Real threat of harm to third parties; suicidal intentions; certain contagious diseases; elder and child abuse
Involuntary commitment or isolation for medical treatment may be undertaken for what reason?	When treatment noncompliance represents a serious danger to public health (e.g., active TB)
A 10-year-old child presents in status epilepticus, but her parents refuse treatment on religious grounds.	Treat because the disease represents an immediate threat to the child's life. Then seek a court order
A son asks that his mother not be told about her recently discovered cancer.	A patient's family cannot require that a doctor withhold information from the patient

GASTROINTESTINAL

Patient presents with sudden onset of severe, diffuse abdominal pain. Exam reveals peritoneal signs and AXR reveals free air under the diaphragm. Management?	Emergent laparotomy to repair perforated viscus, likely stomach
The most likely cause of acute lower GI bleed in patients > 40 years old.	Diverticulosis
Diagnostic modality used when ultrasound is equivocal for cholecystitis.	HIDA scan
Sentinel loop on AXR.	Acute pancreatitis
Risk factors for cholelithiasis.	Fat, female, fertile, forty, flatulent
Inspiratory arrest during palpation of the RUQ.	Murphy's sign, seen in acute cholecystitis

Identify key organisms causing diarrhea:	
▪ Most common organism	*Campylobacter*
▪ Recent antibiotic use	*Clostridium difficile*
▪ Camping	*Giardia*
▪ Traveler's diarrhea	ETEC
▪ Church picnics/mayonnaise	*S. aureus*
▪ Uncooked hamburgers	*E. coli* O157:H7
▪ Fried rice	*Bacillus cereus*
▪ Poultry/eggs	*Salmonella*
▪ Raw seafood	*Vibrio*, HAV
▪ AIDS	*Isospora, Cryptosporidium, Mycobacterium avium* complex (MAC)
▪ Pseudoappendicitis	*Yersinia*
A 25-year-old Jewish male presents with pain and watery diarrhea after meals. Exam shows fistulas between the bowel and skin and nodular lesions on his tibias.	Crohn's disease
Inflammatory disease of the colon with ↑ risk of colon cancer.	Ulcerative colitis
Extraintestinal manifestations of IBD.	Uveitis, ankylosing spondylitis, pyoderma gangrenosum, erythema nodosum, 1° sclerosing cholangitis
Medical treatment for IBD.	5-aminosalicylic acid +/– sulfasalazine and steroids during acute exacerbations
Difference between Mallory-Weiss and Boerhaave tears.	Mallory-Weiss—superficial tear in the esophageal mucosa Boerhaave—full-thickness esophageal rupture
Charcot's triad.	RUQ pain, jaundice, and fever/chills in the setting of ascending cholangitis
Reynolds' pentad.	Charcot's triad plus shock and mental status changes, with suppurative ascending cholangitis
Medical treatment for hepatic encephalopathy.	↓ protein intake, lactulose, neomycin
First step in the management of a patient with acute GI bleed.	Establish the ABCs
A four-year-old child presents with oliguria, petechiae, and jaundice following an illness with bloody diarrhea. Most likely diagnosis and cause?	Hemolytic-uremic syndrome (HUS) due to *E. coli* O157:H7
Post-HBV exposure treatment.	HBV immunoglobulin
Classic causes of drug-induced hepatitis.	TB medications (INH, rifampin, pyrazinamide), acetaminophen, and tetracycline

A 40-year-old obese female with elevated alkaline phosphatase, elevated bilirubin, pruritus, dark urine, and clay-colored stools.	Biliary tract obstruction
Hernia with highest risk of incarceration—indirect, direct, or femoral?	Femoral hernia
A 50-year-old man with a history of alcohol abuse presents with boring epigastric pain that radiates to the back and is relieved by sitting forward. Management?	Confirm the diagnosis of acute pancreatitis with elevated amylase and lipase. Make patient NPO and give IV fluids, O_2, analgesia, and "tincture of time"

HEMATOLOGY/ONCOLOGY

Four causes of microcytic anemia.	**TICS**—**T**halassemia, **I**ron deficiency, anemia of **C**hronic disease, and **S**ideroblastic anemia
An elderly male with hypochromic, microcytic anemia is asymptomatic. Diagnostic tests?	Fecal occult blood test and sigmoidoscopy; suspect colorectal cancer
Precipitants of hemolytic crisis in patients with G6PD deficiency.	Sulfonamides, antimalarial drugs, fava beans
The most common inherited cause of hypercoagulability.	Factor V Leiden mutation
The most common inherited hemolytic anemia.	Hereditary spherocytosis
Diagnostic test for hereditary spherocytosis.	Osmotic fragility test
Pure RBC aplasia.	Diamond-Blackfan anemia
Anemia associated with absent radii and thumbs, diffuse hyperpigmentation, café-au-lait spots, microcephaly, and pancytopenia.	Fanconi's anemia
Medications and viruses that → aplastic anemia.	Chloramphenicol, sulfonamides, radiation, HIV, chemotherapeutic agents, hepatitis, parvovirus B19, EBV
How to distinguish polycythemia vera from 2° polycythemia.	Both have ↑ hematocrit and RBC mass, but polycythemia vera should have normal O_2 saturation and low erythropoietin levels
Thrombotic thrombocytopenic purpura (TTP) pentad?	**Pentad of TTP—"FAT RN":** **F**ever, **A**nemia, **T**hrombocytopenia, **R**enal dysfunction, **N**eurologic abnormalities
HUS triad?	Anemia, thrombocytopenia, and acute renal failure
Treatment for TTP.	Emergent large-volume plasmapheresis, corticosteroids, antiplatelet drugs

Treatment for idiopathic thrombocytopenic purpura (ITP) in children.	Usually resolves spontaneously; may require IVIG and/or corticosteroids
Which of the following are ↑ in DIC: fibrin split products, D-dimer, fibrinogen, platelets, and hematocrit.	Fibrin split products and D-dimer are elevated; platelets, fibrinogen, and hematocrit are ↓.
An eight-year-old boy presents with hemarthrosis and ↑ PTT with normal PT and bleeding time. Diagnosis? Treatment?	Hemophilia A or B; consider desmopressin (for hemophilia A) or factor VIII or IX supplements
A 14-year-old girl presents with prolonged bleeding after dental surgery and with menses, normal PT, normal or ↑ PTT, and ↑ bleeding time. Diagnosis? Treatment?	von Willebrand's disease; treat with desmopressin, FFP, or cryoprecipitate
A 60-year-old African-American male presents with bone pain. Workup for multiple myeloma might reveal?	Monoclonal gammopathy, Bence Jones proteinuria, "punched-out" lesions on x-ray of the skull and long bones
Reed-Sternberg cells	Hodgkin's lymphoma
A 10-year-old boy presents with fever, weight loss, and night sweats. Examination shows anterior mediastinal mass. Suspected diagnosis?	Non-Hodgkin's lymphoma
Microcytic anemia with ↓ serum iron, ↓ total iron-binding capacity (TIBC), and normal or ↑ ferritin.	Anemia of chronic disease
Microcytic anemia with ↓ serum iron, ↓ ferritin, and ↑ TIBC.	Iron deficiency anemia
An 80-year-old man presents with fatigue, lymphadenopathy, splenomegaly, and isolated lymphocytosis. Suspected diagnosis?	Chronic lymphocytic leukemia (CLL)
A late, life-threatening complication of chronic myelogenous leukemia (CML).	Blast crisis (fever, bone pain, splenomegaly, pancytopenia)
Auer rods on blood smear.	Acute myelogenous leukemia (AML)
AML subtype associated with DIC.	M3
Electrolyte changes in tumor lysis syndrome.	↓ Ca^{2-}, ↑ K^-, ↑ phosphate, ↑ uric acid
Treatment for AML M3.	Retinoic acid
A 50-year-old male presents with early satiety, splenomegaly, and bleeding. Cytogenetics show t(9,22). Diagnosis?	CML
Heinz bodies?	Intracellular inclusions seen in thalassemia, G6PD deficiency, and postsplenectomy
An autosomal-recessive disorder with a defect in the GPIIbIIIa platelet receptor and ↓ platelet aggregation.	Glanzmann's thrombasthenia

Virus associated with aplastic anemia in patients with sickle cell anemia.	Parvovirus B19
A 25-year-old African-American male with sickle cell anemia has sudden onset of bone pain. Management of pain crisis?	O_2, analgesia, hydration, and, if severe, transfusion
A significant cause of morbidity in thalassemia patients. Treatment?	Iron overload; use deferoxamine

The three most common causes of fever of unknown origin (FUO).	Infection, cancer, and autoimmune disease
Four signs and symptoms of streptococcal pharyngitis.	Fever, pharyngeal erythema, tonsillar exudate, lack of cough
A nonsuppurative complication of streptococcal infection that is not altered by treatment of 1° infection.	Postinfectious glomerulonephritis
Asplenic patients are particularly susceptible to these organisms.	Encapsulated organisms—pneumococcus, meningococcus, *Haemophilus influenzae, Klebsiella*
The number of bacterial culture on a clean-catch specimen to diagnose a UTI.	10^5 bacteria/mL
Which healthy population is susceptible to UTIs?	Pregnant women. Treat this group aggressively because of potential complications
A patient from California or Arizona presents with fever, malaise, cough, and night sweats. Diagnosis? Treatment?	Coccidioidomycosis. Amphotericin B
Nonpainful chancre.	1° syphilis
A "blueberry muffin" rash is characteristic of what congenital infection?	Rubella
Meningitis in neonates. Causes? Treatment?	Group B strep, *E. coli, Listeria.* Treat with gentamicin and ampicillin
Meningitis in infants. Causes? Treatment?	Pneumococcus, meningococcus, *H. influenzae.* Treat with cefotaxime and vancomycin
What should always be done prior to LP?	Check for ↑ ICP; look for papilledema
CSF findings: ■ Low glucose, PMN predominance ■ Normal glucose, lymphocytic predominance ■ Numerous RBCs in serial CSF samples ■ ↑ gamma globulins	 Bacterial meningitis Aseptic (viral) meningitis Subarachnoid hemorrhage (SAH) MS

Initially presents with a pruritic papule with regional lymphadenopathy and evolves into a black eschar after 7–10 days. Treatment?	Cutaneous anthrax. Treat with penicillin G or ciprofloxacin
Findings in 3° syphilis.	Tabes dorsalis, general paresis, gummas, Argyll Robertson pupil, aortitis, aortic root aneurysms
Characteristics of 2° Lyme disease.	Arthralgias, migratory polyarthropathies, Bell's palsy, myocarditis
Cold agglutinins.	*Mycoplasma*
A 24-year-old male presents with soft white plaques on his tongue and the back of his throat. Diagnosis? Workup? Treatment?	Candidal thrush. Workup should include an HIV test. Treat with nystatin oral suspension
Begin *Pneumocystis carinii* pneumonia (PCP) prophylaxis in an HIV-positive patient at what CD4 count? *Mycobacterium avium-intracellulare* (MAI) prophylaxis?	≤ 200 for PCP (with TMP); ≤ 50–100 for MAI (with clarithromycin/azithromycin)
Risk factors for pyelonephritis.	Pregnancy, vesicoureteral reflux, anatomic anomalies, indwelling catheters, kidney stones
Neutropenic nadir postchemotherapy.	7–10 days
Erythema migrans.	Lesion of 1° Lyme disease
Classic physical findings for endocarditis.	Fever, heart murmur, Osler's nodes, splinter hemorrhages, Janeway lesions, Roth's spots
Aplastic crisis in sickle cell disease.	Parvovirus B19
Ring-enhancing brain lesion on CT with seizures	*Taenia solium* (cysticercosis)
Name the organism:	
▪ Branching rods in oral infection.	*Actinomyces israelii*
▪ Painful chancroid.	*Haemophilus ducreyi*
▪ Dog or cat bite.	*Pasteurella multocida*
▪ Gardener.	*Sporothrix schenckii*
▪ Pregnant women with pets.	*Toxoplasma gondii*
▪ Meningitis in adults.	*Neisseria meningitidis*
▪ Meningitis in elderly.	*Streptococcus pneumoniae*
▪ Alcoholic with pneumonia.	*Klebsiella*
▪ "Currant jelly" sputum.	*Klebsiella*
▪ Infection in burn victims.	*Pseudomonas*
▪ Osteomyelitis from foot wound puncture.	*Pseudomonas*
▪ Osteomyelitis in a sickle cell patient.	*Salmonella*

A 55-year-old man who is a smoker and a heavy drinker presents with a new cough and flulike symptoms. Gram stain shows no organisms; silver stain of sputum shows gram-negative rods. What is the diagnosis?	*Legionella* pneumonia
A middle-aged man presents with acute-onset monoarticular joint pain and bilateral Bell's palsy. What is the likely diagnosis, and how did he get it? Treatment?	Lyme disease, *Ixodes* tick, doxycycline
A patient develops endocarditis three weeks after receiving a prosthetic heart valve. What organism is suspected?	*S. aureus* or *S. epidermidis.*

MUSCULOSKELETAL

A patient presents with pain on passive movement, pallor, poikilothermia, paresthesias, paralysis, and pulselessness. Treatment?	All-compartment fasciotomy for suspected compartment syndrome
Back pain that is exacerbated by standing and walking and relieved with sitting and hyperflexion of the hips.	Spinal stenosis
Joints in the hand affected in rheumatoid arthritis.	MCP and PIP joints; DIP joints are spared
Joint pain and stiffness that worsen over the course of the day and are relieved by rest.	Osteoarthritis
Genetic disorder associated with multiple fractures and commonly mistaken for child abuse.	Osteogenesis imperfecta
Hip and back pain along with stiffness that improves with activity over the course of the day and worsens at rest. Diagnostic test?	Suspect ankylosing spondylitis. Check HLA-B27
Arthritis, conjunctivitis, and urethritis in young men. Associated organisms?	Reactive (Reiter's) arthritis. Associated with *Campylobacter, Shigella, Salmonella, Chlamydia,* and *Ureaplasma*
A 55-year-old man has sudden, excruciating first MTP joint pain after a night of drinking red wine. Diagnosis, workup, and chronic treatment?	Gout. Needle-shaped, negatively birefringent crystals are seen on joint fluid aspirate. Chronic treatment with allopurinol or probenecid
Rhomboid-shaped, positively birefringent crystals on joint fluid aspirate.	Pseudogout
An elderly female presents with pain and stiffness of the shoulders and hips; she cannot lift her arms above her head. Labs show anemia and ↑ ESR.	Polymyalgia rheumatica
An active 13-year-old boy has anterior knee pain. Diagnosis?	Osgood-Schlatter disease

Bone is fractured in fall on outstretched hand.	Distal radius (Colles' fracture)
Complication of scaphoid fracture.	Avascular necrosis
Signs suggesting radial nerve damage with humeral fracture.	Wrist drop, loss of thumb abduction
A young child presents with proximal muscle weakness, waddling gait, and pronounced calf muscles.	Duchenne muscular dystrophy
A first-born female who was born in breech position is found to have asymmetric skin folds on her newborn exam. Diagnosis? Treatment?	Developmental dysplasia of the hip. If severe, consider a Pavlik harness to maintain abduction
An 11-year-old obese, African-American boy presents with sudden onset of limp. Diagnosis? Workup?	Slipped capital femoral epiphyses. AP and frog-leg lateral view
The most common 1° malignant tumor of bone.	Multiple myeloma

NEUROLOGY

Unilateral, severe periorbital headache with tearing and conjunctival erythema.	Cluster headache
Prophylactic treatment for migraine.	β-blockers, Ca^{2+} channel blockers, TCAs
The most common pituitary tumor. Treatment?	Prolactinoma. Dopamine agonists (e.g., bromocriptine)
A 55-year-old patient presents with acute "broken speech." What type of aphasia? What lobe and vascular distribution?	Broca's aphasia. Frontal lobe, left MCA distribution
The most common cause of SAH.	Trauma; the second most common is berry aneurysm
A crescent-shaped hyperdensity on CT that does not cross the midline.	Subdural hematoma—bridging veins torn
A history significant for initial altered mental status with an intervening lucid interval. Diagnosis? Most likely etiology? Treatment?	Epidural hematoma. Middle meningeal artery. Neurosurgical evacuation
CSF findings with SAH.	Elevated ICP, RBCs, xanthochromia
Albuminocytologic dissociation.	Guillain-Barré (↑ protein in CSF with only a modest ↑ in cell count)
Cold water is flushed into a patient's ear, and the fast phase of the nystagmus is toward the opposite side. Normal or pathological?	Normal
The most common 1° sources of metastases to the brain.	Lung, breast, skin (melanoma), kidney, GI tract

May be seen in children who are accused of inattention in class and confused with ADHD.	Absence seizures
The most frequent presentation of intracranial neoplasm.	Headache
The most common cause of seizures in children (2–10 years).	Infection, febrile seizures, trauma, idiopathic
The most common cause of seizures in young adults (18–35 years).	Trauma, alcohol withdrawal, brain tumor
First-line medication for status epilepticus.	IV benzodiazepine
Confusion, confabulation, ophthalmoplegia, ataxia.	Wernicke's encephalopathy due to a deficiency of thiamine
What % lesion is an indication for carotid endarterectomy?	Seventy percent if the stenosis is symptomatic
The most common causes of dementia.	Alzheimer's and multi-infarct
Combined UMN and LMN disorder.	ALS
Rigidity and stiffness with resting tremor and masked facies.	Parkinson's disease
The mainstay of Parkinson's therapy.	Levodopa/carbidopa
Treatment for Guillain-Barré syndrome.	IVIG or plasmapheresis
Rigidity and stiffness that progress to choreiform movements, accompanied by moodiness and altered behavior.	Huntington's disease
A six-year-old girl presents with a port-wine stain in the V2 distribution as well as with mental retardation, seizures, and leptomeningeal angioma.	Sturge-Weber syndrome. Treat symptomatically. Possible focal cerebral resection of affected lobe
Café-au-lait spots on skin.	Neurofibromatosis 1
Hyperphagia, hypersexuality, hyperorality, and hyperdocility.	Klüver-Bucy syndrome (amygdala)
Administer to a symptomatic patient to diagnose myasthenia gravis.	Edrophonium

OBSTETRICS

1° causes of third-trimester bleeding.	Placental abruption and placenta previa
Classic ultrasound and gross appearance of complete hydatidiform mole.	Snowstorm on ultrasound. "Cluster-of-grapes" appearance on gross examination
Chromosomal pattern of a complete mole.	46,XX

Molar pregnancy containing fetal tissue.	Partial mole
Symptoms of placental abruption.	Continuous, painful vaginal bleeding
Symptoms of placenta previa.	Self-limited, painless vaginal bleeding
When should a vaginal exam be performed with suspected placenta previa?	Never
Antibiotics with teratogenic effects.	Tetracycline, fluoroquinolones, aminoglycosides, sulfonamides
Shortest AP diameter of the pelvis.	Obstetric conjugate: between the sacral promontory and the midpoint of the symphysis pubis
Medication given to accelerate fetal lung maturity.	Betamethasone or dexamethasone × 48 hours
The most common cause of postpartum hemorrhage.	Uterine atony
Treatment for postpartum hemorrhage.	Uterine massage; if that fails, give oxytocin
Typical antibiotics for group B streptococcus (GBS) prophylaxis.	IV penicillin or ampicillin
A patient fails to lactate after an emergency C-section with marked blood loss.	Sheehan's syndrome (postpartum pituitary necrosis)
Uterine bleeding at 18 weeks' gestation; no products expelled; membranes ruptured; cervical os open.	Inevitable abortion
Uterine bleeding at 18 weeks' gestation; no products expelled; cervical os closed.	Threatened abortion

GYNECOLOGY

The first test to perform when a woman presents with amenorrhea.	β-hCG; the most common cause of amenorrhea is pregnancy
Term for heavy bleeding during and between menstrual periods.	Menometrorrhagia
Cause of amenorrhea with normal prolactin, no response to estrogen-progesterone challenge, and a history of D&C.	Asherman's syndrome
Therapy for polycystic ovarian syndrome.	Weight loss and OCPs
Medication used to induce ovulation.	Clomiphene citrate
Diagnostic step required in a postmenopausal woman who presents with vaginal bleeding.	Endometrial biopsy

Indications for medical treatment of ectopic pregnancy.	Stable, unruptured ectopic pregnancy of < 3.5 cm at < 6 weeks' gestation
Medical options for endometriosis.	OCPs, danazol, GnRH agonists
Laparoscopic findings in endometriosis.	"Chocolate cysts," powder burns
The most common location for an ectopic pregnancy.	Ampulla of the oviduct
How to diagnose and follow a leiomyoma.	Ultrasound
Natural history of a leiomyoma.	Regresses after menopause
A patient has ↑ vaginal discharge and petechial patches in the upper vagina and cervix.	*Trichomonas* vaginitis
Treatment for bacterial vaginosis.	Oral or topical metronidazole
The most common cause of bloody nipple discharge.	Intraductal papilloma
Contraceptive methods that protect against PID.	OCP and barrier contraception
Unopposed estrogen is contraindicated in which cancers?	Endometrial or estrogen receptor–⊕ breast cancer
A patient presents with recent PID with RUQ pain.	Consider Fitz-Hugh–Curtis syndrome
Breast malignancy presenting as itching, burning, and erosion of the nipple.	Paget's disease
Annual screening for women with a strong family history of ovarian cancer.	CA-125 and transvaginal ultrasound
A 50-year-old woman leaks urine when laughing or coughing. Nonsurgical options?	Kegel exercises, estrogen, pessaries for stress incontinence
A 30-year-old woman has unpredictable urine loss. Examination is normal. Medical options?	Anticholinergics (oxybutynin) or β-adrenergics (metaproterenol) for urge incontinence.
Lab values suggestive of menopause.	↑ serum FSH
The most common cause of female infertility.	Endometriosis
Two consecutive findings of atypical squamous cells of undetermined significance (ASCUS) on Pap smear. Follow-up evaluation?	Colposcopy and endocervical curettage
Breast cancer type that ↑ the future risk of invasive carcinoma in both breasts.	Lobular carcinoma in situ

Nontender abdominal mass associated with elevated VMA and HVA.	Neuroblastoma
The most common type of tracheoesophageal fistula (TEF). Diagnosis?	Esophageal atresia with distal TEF (85%). Unable to pass NG tube
Not contraindications to vaccination.	Mild illness and/or low-grade fever, current antibiotic therapy, and prematurity
Tests to rule out shaken baby syndrome.	Ophthalmologic exam, CT, and MRI
A neonate has meconium ileus.	CF or Hirschsprung's disease
Bilious emesis within hours after the first feeding.	Duodenal atresia
A two-month-old presents with nonbilious projectile emesis. What are the appropriate steps in management?	Correct metabolic abnormalities. Then correct pyloric stenosis with pyloromyotomy
The most common 1° immunodeficiency.	Selective IgA deficiency
An infant has a high fever and onset of rash as fever breaks. What is he at risk for?	Febrile seizures (roseola infantum)
What is the immunodeficiency? ■ A boy has chronic respiratory infections. Nitroblue tetrazolium test is ⊕. ■ A child has eczema, thrombocytopenia, and high levels of IgA. ■ A four-month-old boy has life-threatening *Pseudomonas* infection.	Chronic granulomatous disease Wiskott-Aldrich syndrome Bruton's X-linked agammaglobulinemia
Acute-phase treatment for Kawasaki disease.	High-dose aspirin for inflammation and fever; IVIG to prevent coronary artery aneurysms
Treatment for mild and severe unconjugated hyperbilirubinemia.	Phototherapy (mild) or exchange transfusion (severe)
Sudden onset of mental status changes, emesis, and liver dysfunction after taking aspirin.	Reye's syndrome
A child has loss of red light reflex. Diagnosis?	Suspect retinoblastoma
Vaccinations at a six-month well-child visit.	HBV, DTaP, Hib, IPV, PCV
Tanner stage 3 in a six-year-old female.	Precocious puberty
Infection of small airways with epidemics in winter and spring.	RSV bronchiolitis
Cause of neonatal RDS.	Surfactant deficiency

A condition associated with red "currant-jelly" stools.	Intussusception
A congenital heart disease that cause 2° hypertension.	Coarctation of the aorta
First-line treatment for otitis media.	Amoxicillin × 10 days
The most common pathogen causing croup.	Parainfluenza virus type 1
A homeless child is small for his age and has peeling skin and a swollen belly.	Kwashiorkor (protein malnutrition)
Defect in an X-linked syndrome with mental retardation, gout, self-mutilation, and choreoathetosis.	Lesch-Nyhan syndrome (purine salvage problem with HGPRTase deficiency)
A newborn female has continuous "machinery murmur."	Patent ductus arteriosus (PDA)

PSYCHIATRY

First-line pharmacotherapy for depression.	SSRIs
Antidepressants associated with hypertensive crisis.	MAOIs
Galactorrhea, impotence, menstrual dysfunction, and ↓ libido.	Patient on dopamine antagonist
A 17-year-old female has left arm paralysis after her boyfriend dies in a car crash. No medical cause is found.	Conversion disorder
Name the defense mechanism: ▪ A mother who is angry at her husband yells at her child. ▪ A pedophile enters a monastery. ▪ A woman calmly describes a grisly murder. ▪ A hospitalized 10-year-old begins to wet his bed.	Displacement Reaction formation Isolation Regression
Life-threatening muscle rigidity, fever, and rhabdomyolysis.	Neuroleptic malignant syndrome
Amenorrhea, bradycardia, and abnormal body image in a young female.	Anorexia
A 35-year-old male has recurrent episodes of palpitations, diaphoresis, and fear of going crazy.	Panic disorder
The most serious side effect of clozapine.	Agranulocytosis
A 21-year-old male has three months of social withdrawal, worsening grades, flattened affect, and concrete thinking.	Schizophreniform disorder (diagnosis of schizophrenia requires ≥ 6 months of symptoms)
Key side effects of atypical antipsychotics.	Weight gain, type 2 DM, QT prolongation

A young weight lifter receives IV haloperidol and complains that his eyes are deviated sideways. Diagnosis? Treatment?	Acute dystonia (oculogyric crisis). Treat with benztropine or diphenhydramine
Medication to avoid in patients with a history of alcohol withdrawal seizures.	Neuroleptics
A 13-year-old male has a history of theft, vandalism, and violence toward family pets.	Conduct disorder
A five-month-old girl has ↓ head growth, truncal dyscoordination, and ↓ social interaction.	Rett's disorder
A patient hasn't slept for days, lost $20,000 gambling, is agitated, and has pressured speech. Diagnosis? Treatment?	Acute mania. Start a mood stabilizer (e.g., lithium)
After a minor fender bender, a man wears a neck brace and requests permanent disability.	Malingering
A nurse presents with severe hypoglycemia; blood analysis reveals no elevation in C peptide.	Factitious disorder (Munchausen syndrome)
A patient continues to use cocaine after being in jail, losing his job, and not paying child support.	Substance abuse
A violent patient has vertical and horizontal nystagmus.	Phencyclidine hydrochloride (PCP) intoxication
A woman who was abused as a child frequently feels outside of or detached from her body.	Depersonalization disorder
A man has repeated, intense urges to rub his body against unsuspecting passengers on a bus.	Frotteurism (a paraphilia)
A schizophrenic patient takes haloperidol for one year and develops uncontrollable tongue movements. Diagnosis? Treatment?	Tardive dyskinesia. ↓ or discontinue haloperidol and consider another antipsychotic (e.g., risperidone, clozapine)
A man unexpectedly flies across the country, takes a new name, and has no memory of his prior life.	Dissociative fugue

PULMONARY

Risk factors for DVT.	Stasis, endothelial injury and hypercoagulability (Virchow's triad)
Criteria for exudative effusion.	Pleural/serum protein > 0.5; pleural/serum LDH > 0.6
Causes of exudative effusion.	Think of leaky capillaries. Malignancy, TB, bacterial or viral infection, pulmonary embolism with infarct, and pancreatitis

Causes of transudative effusion.	Think of intact capillaries. CHF, liver or kidney disease, and protein-losing enteropathy
Normalizing P_{CO_2} in a patient having an asthma exacerbation may indicate?	Fatigue and impending respiratory failure
Dyspnea, lateral hilar lymphodenopathy on CXR, noncaseating granulomas, increased ACE, and hypercalcemia.	Sarcoidosis
PFT showing $\downarrow FEV_1/FVC$.	Obstructive pulmonary disease (e.g., asthma)
PFT showing $\uparrow FEV_1/FVC$.	Restrictive pulmonary disease
Honeycomb pattern on CXR. Diagnosis? Treatment?	Diffuse interstitial pulmonary fibrosis. Supportive care. Steroids may help
Treatment for SVC syndrome.	Radiation
Treatment for mild, persistent asthma.	Inhaled β-agonists and inhaled corticosteroids
Acid-base disorder in pulmonary embolism.	Hypoxia and hypocarbia
Non–small cell lung cancer (NSCLC) associated with hypercalcemia.	Squamous cell carcinoma
Lung cancer associated with SIADH.	Small cell lung cancer (SCLC)
Lung cancer highly related to cigarette exposure.	SCLC
A tall white male presents with acute shortness of breath. Diagnosis? Treatment?	Spontaneous pneumothorax. Spontaneous regression. Supplemental O_2 may be helpful
Treatment of tension pneumothorax.	Immediate needle thoracostomy
Characteristics favoring carcinoma in an isolated pulmonary nodule.	Age > 45–50 years; lesions new or larger in comparison to old films; absence of calcification or irregular calcification; size > 2 cm; irregular margins
Hypoxemia and pulmonary edema with normal pulmonary capillary wedge pressure.	ARDS
$\uparrow$ risk of what infection with silicosis?	*Mycobacterium tuberculosis*
Causes of hypoxemia.	Right-to-left shunt, hypoventilation, low inspired O_2 tension, diffusion defect, V/Q mismatch
Classic CXR findings for pulmonary edema.	Cardiomegaly, prominent pulmonary vessels, Kerley B lines, "bat's-wing" appearance of hilar shadows, and perivascular and peribronchial cuffing

Renal tubular acidosis (RTA) associated with abnormal H^+ secretion and nephrolithiasis.	Type I (distal) RTA
RTA associated with abnormal HCO_3^- and rickets.	Type II (proximal) RTA
RTA associated with aldosterone defect.	Type IV (distal) RTA
"Doughy skin."	Hypernatremia
Differential of hypervolemic hyponatremia.	Cirrhosis, CHF, nephritic syndrome
Chvostek's and Trousseau's signs.	Hypocalcemia
The most common causes of hypercalcemia.	Malignancy and hyperparathyroidism
T-wave flattening and U waves.	Hypokalemia
Peaked T waves and widened QRS.	Hyperkalemia
First-line treatment for moderate hypercalcemia.	IV hydration and loop diuretics (furosemide)
Type of ARF in a patient with $Fe_{Na} < 1\%$.	Prerenal
A 49-year-old male presents with acute-onset flank pain and hematuria.	Nephrolithiasis
The most common type of nephrolithiasis.	Calcium oxalate
A 20-year-old man presents with a palpable flank mass and hematuria. Ultrasound shows bilateral enlarged kidneys with cysts. Associated brain anomaly?	Cerebral berry aneurysms (AD PCKD)
Hematuria, hypertension, and oliguria.	Nephritic syndrome
Proteinuria, hypoalbuminemia, hyperlipidemia, hyperlipiduria, edema.	Nephrotic syndrome
The most common form of nephritic syndrome.	Membranous glomerulonephritis
The most common form of glomerulonephritis.	IgA nephropathy (Berger's disease)
Glomerulonephritis with deafness.	Alport's syndrome
Glomerulonephritis with hemoptysis.	Wegener's granulomatosis and Goodpasture's syndrome
Presence of red cell casts in urine sediment.	Glomerulonephritis/nephritic syndrome
Eosinophils in urine sediment.	Allergic interstitial nephritis
Waxy casts in urine sediment and Maltese crosses (seen with lipiduria).	Nephrotic syndrome

HIGH-YIELD FACTS

RAPID REVIEW

Drowsiness, asterixis, nausea, and a pericardial friction rub.	Uremic syndrome seen in patients with renal failure
A 55-year-old man is diagnosed with prostate cancer. Treatment options?	Wait, surgical resection, radiation and/or androgen suppression
Low urine specific gravity in the presence of high serum osmolality.	DI
Treatment of SIADH?	Fluid restriction, demeclocycline
Hematuria, flank pain, and palpable flank mass.	Renal cell carcinoma (RCC)
Testicular cancer associated with β-hCG, AFP.	Choriocarcinoma
The most common type of testicular cancer.	Seminoma—a type of germ cell tumor
The most common histology of bladder cancer.	Transitional cell carcinoma
Complication of overly rapid correction of hyponatremia.	Central pontine myelinolysis
Salicylate ingestion → in what type of acid-base disorder?	Anion gap acidosis and 1° respiratory alkalosis due to central respiratory stimulation
Acid-base disturbance commonly seen in pregnant women.	Respiratory alkalosis
Three systemic diseases → nephrotic syndrome.	DM, SLE, and amyloidosis
Elevated erythropoietin level, elevated hematocrit, and normal O_2 saturation suggest?	RCC or other erythropoietin-producing tumor; evaluate with CT scan
A 55-year-old man presents with irritative and obstructive urinary symptoms. Treatment options?	Likely BPH. Options include no treatment, terazosin, finasteride, or surgical intervention (TURP)

SELECTED TOPICS IN EMERGENCY MEDICINE

Class of drugs that may cause syndrome of muscle rigidity, hyperthermia, autonomic instability, and extrapyramidal symptoms.	Antipsychotics (neuroleptic malignant syndrome)
Side effects of corticosteroids.	Acute mania, immunosuppression, thin skin, osteoporosis, easy bruising, myopathies
Treatment for DTs.	Benzodiazepines
Treatment for acetaminophen overdose.	N-acetylcysteine
Treatment for opioid overdose.	Naloxone
Treatment for benzodiazepine overdose.	Flumazenil
Treatment for neuroleptic malignant syndrome.	Dantrolene or bromocriptine

Clinical Images

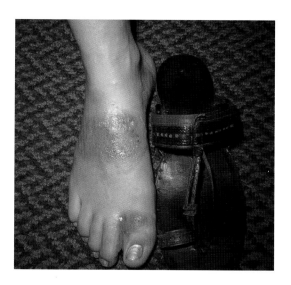

Contact dermatitis. Erythematous papules, vesicles, and serous weeping localized to areas of contact with the offending agent are characteristic. (Reproduced, with permission, from Hurwitz RM, *Pathology of the Skin: Atlas of Clinical–Pathological Correlation,* 1st ed. Stamford, CT: Appleton & Lange, 1991: p. 3, Fig. 1–5.)

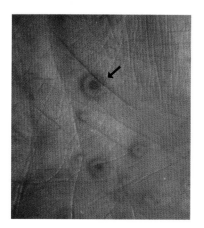

Erythema multiforme. The classic target lesion has a dull red center, pale zone, and darker outer ring (arrow). This acute self-limited reaction may occur with infection, antibiotic use, exposure to radiation or chemicals, or malignancy. (Reproduced, with permission, from Bondi EE, *Dermatology: Diagnosis and Therapy,* 1st ed., Stamford, CT: Appleton & Lange, 1991: p. 392, Fig. 19.)

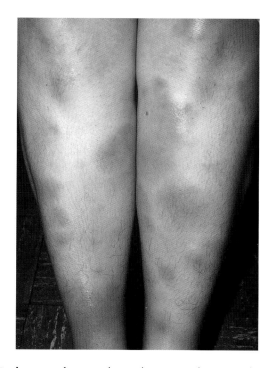

Erythema nodosum. The erythematous plaques and nodules are commonly located on pretibial areas. Lesions are painful and indurated and heal spontaneously without ulceration. (Reproduced, with permission, from Hurwitz RM, *Pathology of the Skin: Atlas of Clinical–Pathological Correlation,* 1st ed., Stamford, CT: Appleton & Lange, 1991: p. 132, Fig. 10–1A.)

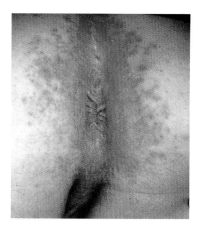

Candidial intertrigo. Erythematous areas surrounded by satellite pustules are restricted to warm, moist intertriginous areas. (Reproduced, with permission, from Bondi EE, *Dermatology: Diagnosis and Therapy,* 1st ed., Stamford, CT: Appleton & Lange, 1991: p. 390, Fig. 11.)

1

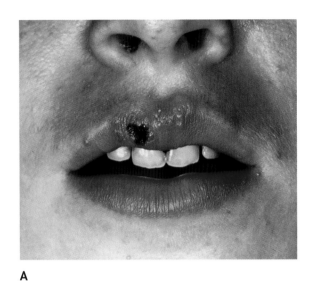

A

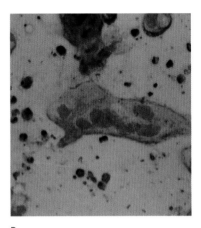

B

Herpes simplex. (A) Primary infection. Grouped vesicles on an erythematous base on the patient's lips and oral mucosa may progress to pustules before resolving. (B) Tzanck smear. The multinucleated giant cells from vesicular fluid provide a presumptive diagnosis of HSV infection. However, the Tzanck smear cannot distinguished between HSV and VZV infection. (Reproduced, with permission, from Hurwitz RM, *Pathology of the Skin: Atlas of Clinical–Pathological Correlation*, 1st ed., Stamford, CT: Appleton & Lange, 1991: p. 145, Fig. 11–9 and Bondi EE, *Dermatology: Diagnosis and Therapy*, 1st ed., Stamford, CT: Appleton & Lange, 1991: p. 396, Fig. 47.)

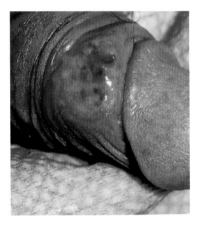

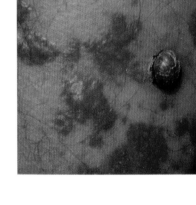

Primary syphilis. The chancre, which appears at the site of infection, is an ulcerated papule with a smooth, clean base; raised, indurated borders; and scant discharge. (Reproduced, with permission, from Bondi EE, *Dermatology: Diagnosis and Therapy,* 1st ed., Stamford, CT: Appleton & Lange, 1991: p. 394, Fig. 33.)

Kaposi's sarcoma. Manifests as red to purple nodules and surrounding pink to red macules. The latter appear most often in immunosuppressed patients. (Reproduced, with permission, from Bondi EE, *Dermatology: Diagnosis and Therapy,* 1st ed., Stamford, CT: Appleton & Lange, 1991: p. 393, Fig. 25.)

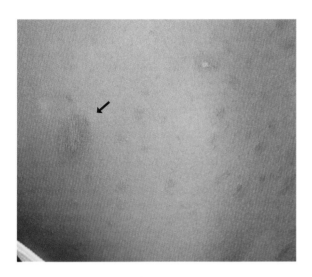

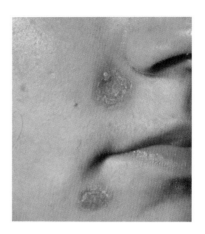

Pityriasis rosea. The round to oval erythematous plaques are often covered with a fine white scale ("cigarette paper") and are often found on the trunk ("Christmas tree distribution") and proximal extremities. The plaques are often preceded by a larger herald patch (arrow). (Reproduced, courtesy of the Yale Department of Dermatology.)

Impetigo. Dried pustules with superficial golden-brown crust are most commonly found around the nose and mouth. (Reproduced, with permission, from Bondi EE, *Dermatology: Diagnosis and Therapy,* 1st ed., Stamford, CT: Appleton & Lange, 1991: p. 390, Fig. 12.)

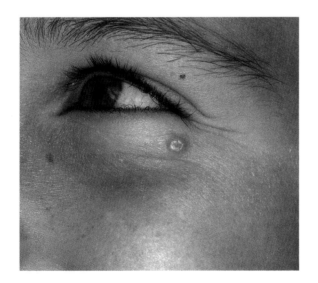

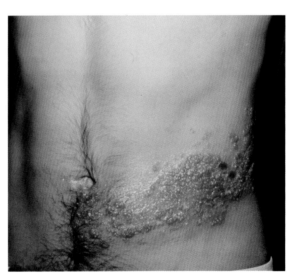

Molluscum contagiosum. The dome-shaped, fleshy, umbilicated papule on the child's eyelid is characteristic. (Reproduced, with permission, from Hurwitz RM, *Pathology of the Skin: Atlas of Clinical–Pathological Correlation,* 1st ed., Stamford, CT: Appleton & Lange, 1991: p. 149, Fig. 11–19.)

Herpes zoster. The unilateral dermatomal distribution of the grouped vesicles on an erythematous base is characteristic. (Reproduced, courtesy of the Yale Department of Dermatology.)

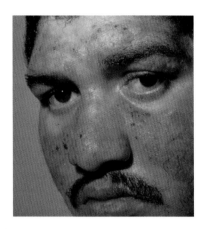

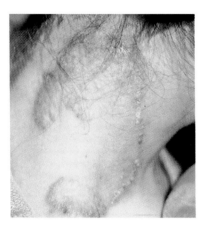

Malar rash of systemic lupus erythematosus. The malar rash is a red to purple continuous plaque extending across the bridge of the nose and to both cheeks. (Reproduced, with permission, from Bondi EE, *Dermatology: Diagnosis and Therapy,* 1st ed., Stamford, CT: Appleton & Lange, 1991: p. 395, Fig. 38.)

Tinea corporis. Ring-shaped, erythematous, scaling macules with central clearing are characteristic. (Reproduced, with permission, from Bondi EE, *Dermatology: Diagnosis and Therapy,* 1st ed., Stamford, CT: Appleton & Lange, 1991: p. 389, Fig. 4.)

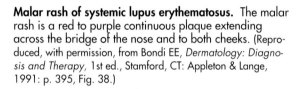

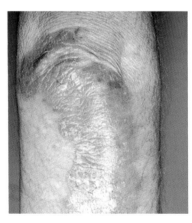

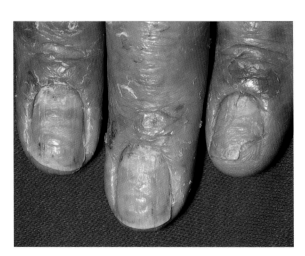

A

B

Psoriasis. (A) Skin changes. The classic sharply demarcated dark red plaques with silvery scales are commonly located on extensor surfaces (e.g., elbows, knees). (B) Nail changes. Note the pitting, onycholysis, and oil spots. (Reproduced, with permission, from Bondi EE, *Dermatology: Diagnosis and Therapy,* 1st ed., Stamford, CT: Appleton & Lange, 1991: p. 389, Fig. 1 and Hurwitz RM, *Pathology of the Skin: Atlas of Clinical–Pathological Correlation,* 1st ed., Stamford, CT: Appleton & Lange, 1991: p. 15, Fig. 1–55.)

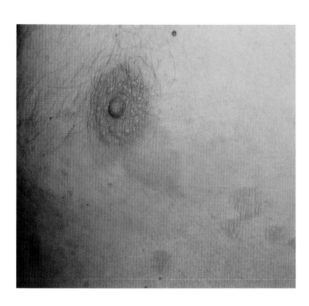

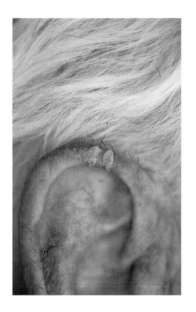

Tinea versicolor. These pinkish scaling macules commonly appear on the chest and back. Lesions may also be lightly pigmented or hypopigmented depending on the patient's skin color and sun exposure. (Reproduced, courtesy of the Yale Department of Dermatology.)

Actinic keratosis. The discrete patch has an erythematous base and rough white scaling. Actinic keratosis is a premalignant lesion that may progress to squamous cell carcinoma. It is most commonly found in sun-exposed areas. (Reproduced, with permission, from Hurwitz RM, *Pathology of the Skin: Atlas of Clinical–Pathological Correlation,* 1st ed., Stamford, CT: Appleton & Lange, 1991: p. 354, Fig. 31–3.)

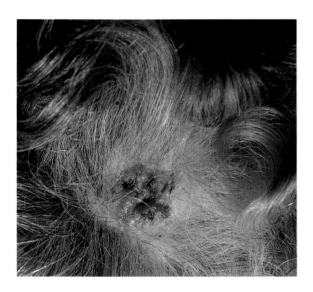

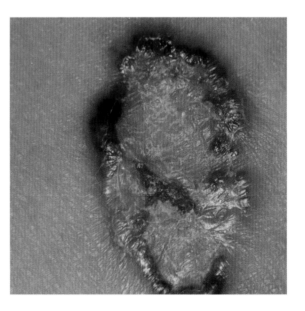

Squamous cell carcinoma. Note the crusting and ulceration of this erythematous plaque. Most lesions are exophytic nodules with erosion or ulceration. (Reproduced, with permission, from Hurwitz RM, *Pathology of the Skin: Atlas of Clinical–Pathological Correlation,* 1st ed., Stamford, CT: Appleton & Lange, 1991: p. 360, Fig. 31–20.)

Basal cell carcinoma. Note the pearly, translucent surface (often covered with fine telangectasias), rolled border, and central ulceration. (Reproduced, courtesy of the Yale Department of Dermatology.)

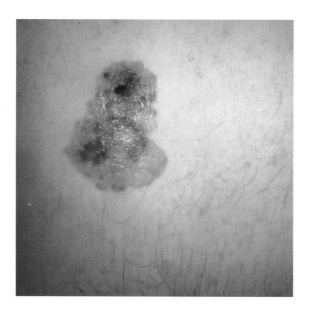

Melanoma. Note the **a**symmetry, **b**order irregularity, **c**olor variation, and large **d**iameter of this plaque. (Reproduced, with permission, from Hurwitz RM, *Pathology of the Skin: Atlas of Clinical–Pathological Correlation,* 1st ed., Stamford, CT: Appleton & Lange, 1991: p. 432, Fig. 36–8.)

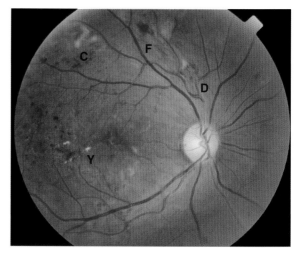

Nonproliferative diabetic retinopathy. Flame hemorrhages (F), dot-blot hemorrhages (D), cotton-wool spots (C), and yellow exudate (Y) result from small vessel damage and occlusion. (Reproduced, courtesy of the Washington University Department of Ophthalmology.)

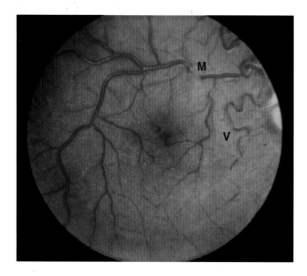

Hypertensive retinopathy. Note the tortuous retinal veins (V) and venous microaneurysms (M). Other findings include hemorrhages, retinal infarcts, detachment of the retina, and disk edema. (Reproduced, courtesy of the Washington University Department of Ophthalmology.)

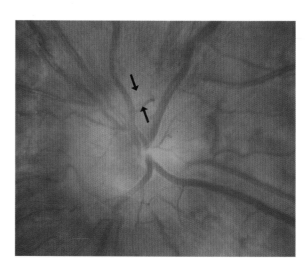

Papilledema. Look for blurred disk margins due to edema of the optic disk (arrows). (Reproduced, courtesy of the Washington University Department of Ophthalmology.)

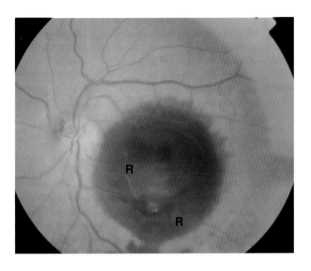

Subretinal hemorrhage. Note the preretinal blood and overlying retinal vessels (R). Subretinal hemorrhages may be seen in any condition with abnormal vessel proliferation (e.g., diabetes, hypertension) or in trauma. (Reproduced, courtesy of the Washington University Department of Ophthalmology.)

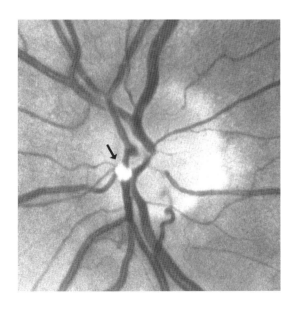

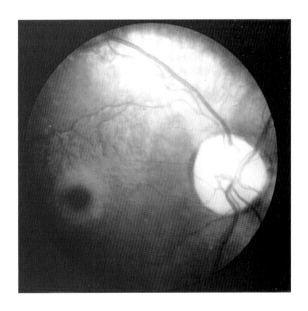

Cholesterol emboli. Cholesterol emboli (Hollenhorst plaque; arrow) usually arise in atherosclerotic carotid arteries and often lodge at the bifurcation of retinal arteries. (Reproduced, with permission, from Vaughan D, *General Ophthalmology,* 14th ed., Stamford, CT: Appleton & Lange, 1995: p. 299, Fig. 15–6.)

Tay–Sachs. Cherry-red spot. The red spot in the macula may be seen in Tay–Sachs disease, Niemann–Pick disease, central retinal artery occlusion, and methanol toxicity. (Reproduced, with permission, from Vaughan D, *General Ophthalmology,* 14th ed., Stamford, CT: Appleton & Lange, 1995: p. 293, Fig. 14–29.)

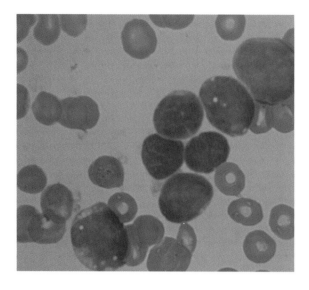

Acute lymphoblastic leukemia. Peripheral blood smear reveals numerous large, uniform lymphoblasts with fine granular cytoplasm and faint nucleoli. (Reproduced, courtesy of Dr. Peter McPhedran, Yale Department of Hematology.)

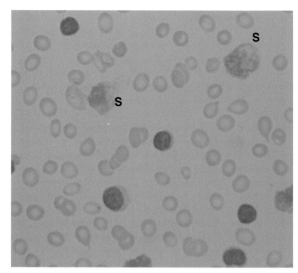

Chronic lymphocytic leukemia. The numerous, small, mature lymphocytes and smudge cells (S; fragile malignant lymphocytes are disrupted during blood smear preparation) are characteristic. (Reproduced, courtesy of Dr. Peter McPhedran, Yale Department of Hematology.)

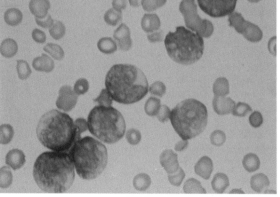
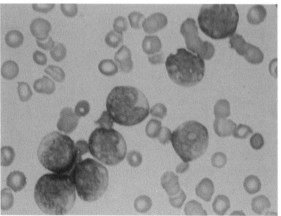

Acute myelocytic leukemia. Large, uniform myeloblasts with notched nuclei and prominent nucleoli are characteristic. (Reproduced, courtesy of Dr. Peter McPhedran, Yale Department of Hematology.)

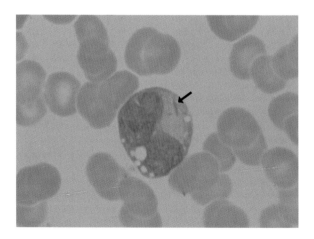

Auer rod in acute myelocytic leukemia. The red rod-shaped structure (arrow) in the cytoplasm of the myeloblast is pathognomonic. (Reproduced, courtesy of Dr. Peter McPhedran, Yale Department of Hematology.)

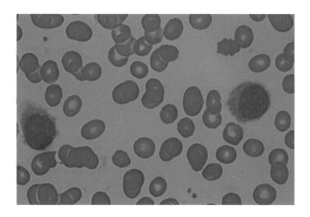

Hairy cell leukemia. Note the hairlike cytoplasmic projections from neoplastic lymphocytes. (Reproduced, courtesy of Dr. Peter McPhedran, Yale Department of Hematology.)

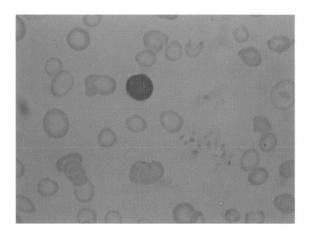

Iron deficiency anemia. Note the microcytic, hypochromic red blood cells ("doughnut cells") with enlarged areas of central pallor. (Reproduced, courtesy of Dr. Peter McPhedran, Yale Department of Hematology.)

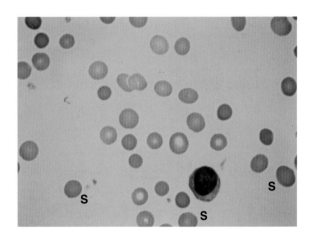

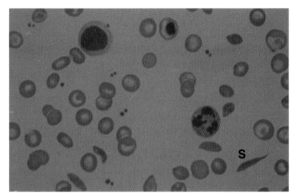

Spherocytes. These RBCs (S) lack areas of central pallor. Spherocytes are seen in autoimmune hemolysis and hereditary spherocytosis. (Reproduced, courtesy of Dr. Peter McPhedran, Yale Department of Hematology.)

Sickle cells. Sickle-shaped RBCs (S) may appear during infection, dehydration, or hypoxia. Anisocytosis, poikilocytosis, target cells, and nucleated RBCs are also seen in sickle cell disease. (Reproduced, courtesy of Dr. Peter McPhedran, Yale Department of Hematology.)

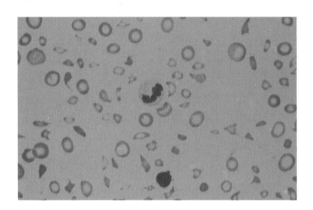

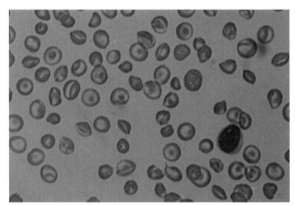

Schistocytes. These fragmented red blood cells may be seen in microangiopathic hemolytic anemia and mechanical hemolysis. (Reproduced, courtesy of Dr. Peter McPhedran, Yale Department of Hematology.)

Target cells. The dense zone of hemoglobin in the RBC center is characteristic. Target cells are seen in hemoglobin C or S disease and thalassemia, or they may be an artifact. (Reproduced, courtesy of Dr. Peter McPhedran, Yale Department of Hematology.)

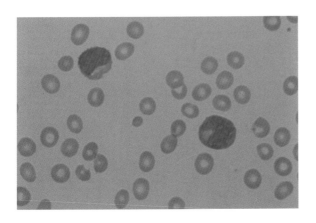

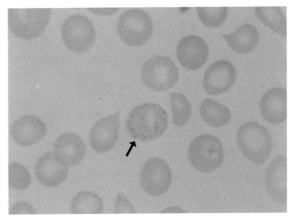

Mononucleosis. These lymphocytes, with enlarged nuclei and prominent nucleoli, are seen in EBV and CMV infections. (Reproduced, courtesy of Dr. Peter McPhedran, Yale Department of Hematology.)

Basophilic stippling. The basophilic granules (arrow) within the red blood cells are a nonspecific finding that may suggest megaloblastic anemia, lead poisoning, or a benign condition. (Reproduced, courtesy of Dr. Peter McPhedran, Yale Department of Hematology.)

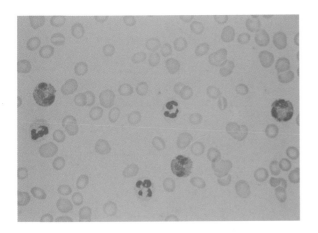

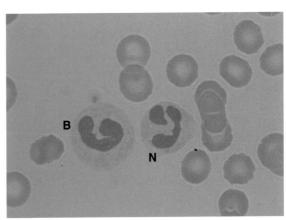

Eosinophilia. Eosinophils have red-staining cytoplasmic granules. Eosinophilia may be seen in allergic reactions, parasitic infections, collagen vascular diseases, malignancies such as Hodgkin's disease, and adrenal insufficiency. (Reproduced, courtesy of Dr. Peter McPhedran, Yale Department of Hematology.)

Neutrophil (N) and band (B). The more immature band form has a U-shaped rather than a segmented nucleus. (Reproduced, courtesy of Dr. Peter McPhedran, Yale Department of Hematology.)

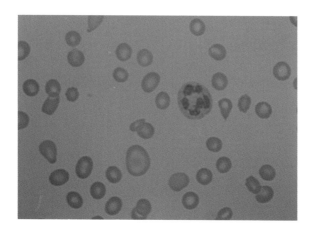

Hypersegmentation. The nucleus of this hypersegmented neutrophil has six lobes (six or more nuclear lobes are required). This is a characteristic finding of megaloblastic anemia. (Reproduced, courtesy of Dr. Peter McPhedran, Yale Department of Hematology.)

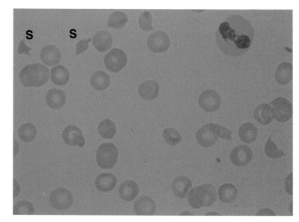

Thrombotic thrombocytopenic purpura (TTP). Note the schistocytes (S) and paucity of platelets. TTP is characterized by microangiopathic hemolytic anemia, thrombocytopenia, fever, neurologic abnormalities, and renal failure. (Reproduced, courtesy of Dr. Peter McPhedran, Yale Department of Hematology.)

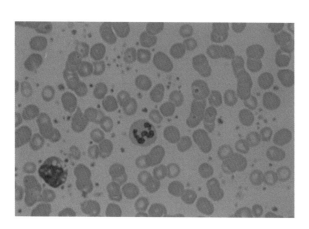

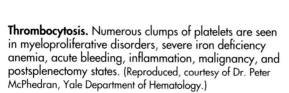

Thrombocytosis. Numerous clumps of platelets are seen in myeloproliferative disorders, severe iron deficiency anemia, acute bleeding, inflammation, malignancy, and postsplenectomy states. (Reproduced, courtesy of Dr. Peter McPhedran, Yale Department of Hematology.)

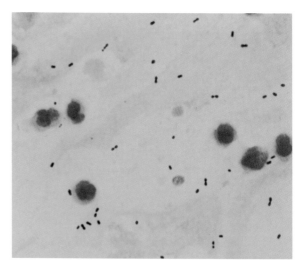

Streptococcus pneumoniae. This is a sputum sample from a patient with pneumonia. Note the characteristic lancet-shaped gram-positive diplococci. (Reproduced, courtesy of Vinnie Piscitelli, Yale Microbiology Lab.)

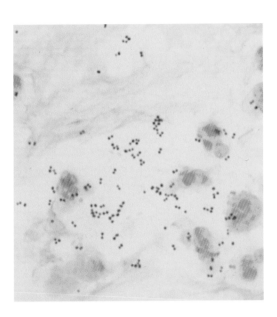

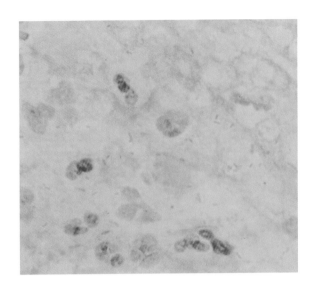

Staphylococcus aureus. These clusters of gram-positive cocci were isolated from the sputum of a patient with pneumonia. (Reproduced, courtesy of Vinnie Piscitelli, Yale Microbiology Lab.)

Pseudomonas aeruginosa. This sputum sample from a patient with pneumonia revealed gram-negative rods. The large number of neutrophils and relative paucity of epithelial cells indicate that this sample is not contaminated with oropharyngeal flora. (Reproduced, courtesy of Vinnie Piscitelli, Yale Microbiology Lab.)

HIGH-YIELD FACTS

Clinical Images

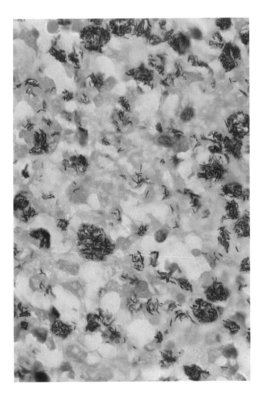

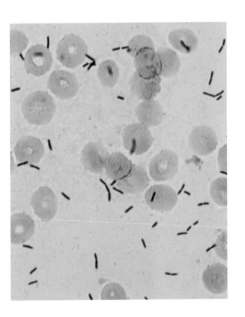

Listeria. These numerous rod-shaped bacilli were isolated from the blood of a patient with *Listeria* meningitis. (Reproduced, courtesy of Vinnie Piscitelli, Yale Microbiology Lab.)

Tuberculosis (AFB smear). Note the red color of the tubercle bacilli an acid-fast staining of a sputum sample ("red snappers"). (Reproduced, with permission, from Milikowski C, *Color Atlas of Basic Histopathology,* 1st ed., Stamford, CT: Appleton & Lange, 1997: p. 193, Fig. 9–10.)

13

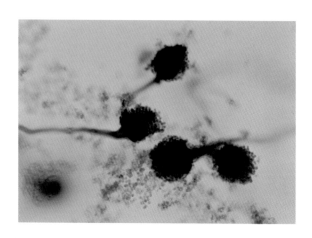

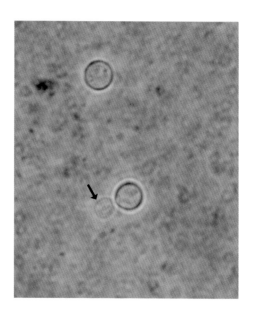

Aspergillosis. Note the characteristic appearance of *Aspergillus* spores in radiating columns. (Reproduced, courtesy of Vinnie Piscitelli, Yale Microbiology Lab.)

Cryptococcus. Note the budding yeast (arrow) and wide capsule of cryptococcus isolated from CSF. (Reproduced, courtesy of Vinnie Piscitelli, Yale Microbiology Lab.)

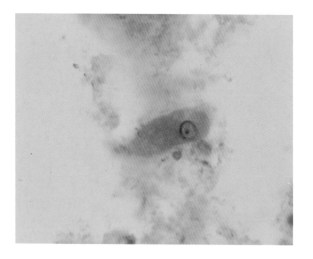

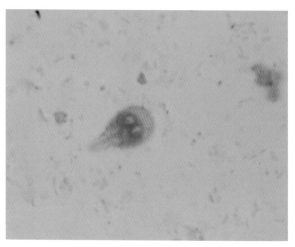

Entamoeba. *Entamoeba* cysts have large nuclei. This is a sample from diarrheal stool. (Reproduced, courtesy of Vinnie Piscitelli, Yale Microbiology Lab.)

Giardia trophozoite in stool. The trophozoite exhibits a classic pear shape with two nuclei imparting an owl's-eye appearance. (Reproduced, courtesy of Vinnie Piscitelli, Yale Microbiology Lab.)

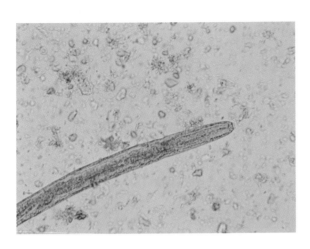

Strongyloides. These filarial larva were found in the stool of a patient watery diarrhea. (Reproduced, courtesy of Vinnie Piscitelli, Yale Microbiology Lab.)

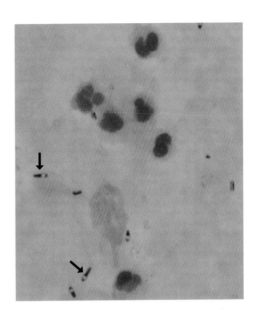

***Clostridium* wound infection.** The lucency at the end of each gram-positive bacillus is the terminal spore (arrow). This sample was isolated from an infected wound site. (Reproduced, courtesy of Vinnie Piscitelli, Yale Microbiology Lab.)

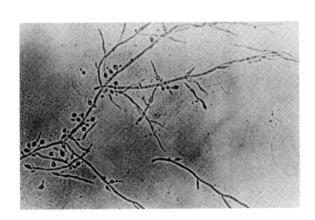

Candidal vaginitis. Branched and budding *Candida albicans* are evident on KOH preparation of vaginal discharge. (Reproduced, with permission, from DeCherney A, *Current Obstetrics and Gynecology Diagnosis and Treatment,* 8th ed., Stamford, CT: Appleton & Lange, 1994: p. 692, Fig. 34–4.)

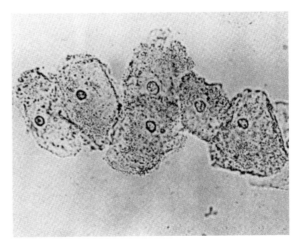

Gardnerella vaginalis. Saline wet mount of vaginal fluid reveals granulations on vaginal epithelial cells ("clue cells") due to adherence of *G. vaginalis* organisms to the cell surface. (Reproduced, with permission, from DeCherney A, *Current Obstetrics and Gynecology Diagnosis and Treatment,* 8th ed., Stamford, CT: Appleton and Lange, 1994: p. 692, Fig. 34–2.)

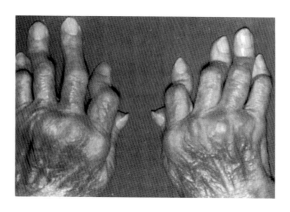

Rheumatoid arthritis. The swan-neck deformities of the digits and severe involvement of the proximal interphalangeal joints are characteristic. (Reproduced, with permission, from Chandrasoma P, *Concise Pathology,* 3rd ed., Stamford, CT: Appleton & Lange, 1998: p. 978, Fig. 68–2.)

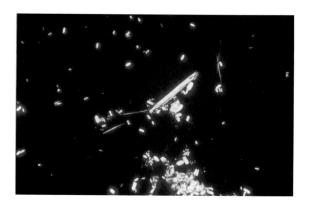

Gout. Negatively birefringent crystals. (Reproduced, with permission, from Milikowshi C, *Color Atlas of Basic Histopathology,* 1st ed., Stamford, CT: Appleton & Lange, 1997: p. 546.)

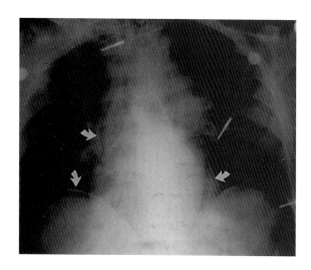

Pneumomediastinum. The lucency outlining the left heart border on chest x-ray suggests air in the mediastinum. (Reproduced, with permission, from Goldfrank LR, *Toxic Emergencies,* 6th ed., Stamford, CT: Appleton & Lange, 1998: p. 285, Fig. 8–2A.)

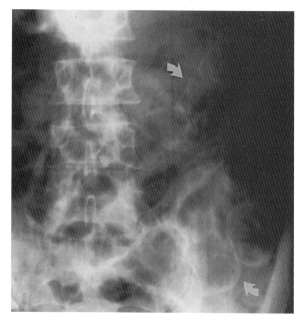

Pneumoperitoneum. The lucency outlining small bowel on abdominal x-ray indicated the abnormal presence of air. (Reproduced, with permission, from Goldfrank LR, *Toxic Emergencies,* 6th ed., Stamford, CT: Appleton & Lange, 1998: p. 285, Fig. 8–2B.)

Treatment for malignant hypertension.	Nitroprusside
Treatment of AF.	Rate control, rhythm conversion, and anticoagulation
Treatment of supraventricular tachycardia (SVT).	Rate control with carotid massasge or other vagal stimulation
Causes of drug-induced SLE.	INH, penicillamine, hydralazine, procainamide
Macrocytic, megaloblastic anemia with neurologic symptoms.	B_{12} deficiency
Macrocytic, megaloblastic anemia without neurologic symptoms.	Folate deficiency
A burn patient presents with cherry-red flushed skin and coma. Sao_2 is normal, but carboxyhemoglobin is elevated. Treatment?	Treat CO poisoning with 100% O_2 or with hyperbaric O_2 if severe poisoning or pregnant
Blood in the urethral meatus or high-riding prostate.	Bladder rupture or urethral injury
Test to rule out urethral injury.	Retrograde cystourethrogram
Radiographic evidence of aortic disruption or dissection.	Widened mediastinum (> 8 cm), loss of aortic knob, pleural cap, tracheal deviation to the right, depression of left main stem bronchus
Radiographic indications for surgery in patients with acute abdomen.	Free air under the diaphragm, extravasation of contrast, severe bowl distention, space-occupying lesion (CT), mesenteric occlusion (angiography)
The most common organism in burn-related infections.	*Pseudomonas*
Method of calculating fluid repletion in burn patients.	Parkland formula
Acceptable urine output in a trauma patient.	50 cc/hour
Acceptable urine output in a stable patient.	30 cc/hour
Cannon "a" waves.	Third-degree heart block
Signs of neurogenic shock.	Hypotension and bradycardia
Signs of ↑ ICP (Cushing's triad).	Hypertension, bradycardia, and abnormal respirations
↓ CO, ↓ pulmonary capillary wedge pressure (PCWP), ↑ peripheral vascular resistance (PVR).	Hypovolemic shock
↓ CO, ↑ PCWP, ↑ PVR.	Cardiogenic shock
↑ CO, ↓ PCWP, ↓ PVR.	Septic or anaphylactic shock

Treatment of septic shock.	Fluids and antibiotics
Treatment of cardiogenic shock.	Identify cause; pressors (e.g., dobutamine)
Treatment of hypovolemic shock.	Identify cause; fluid and blood repletion
Treatment of anaphylactic shock.	Diphenhydramine or epinephrine 1:1000
Supportive treatment for ARDS.	Continuous positive airway pressure
Signs of air embolism.	A patient with chest trauma who was previously stable suddenly dies
Trauma series.	AP chest, AP/lateral C-spine, AP pelvis

SECTION 3

Top-Rated Review Resources

This section is a database of recommended clinical science review books, sample examination books, and commercial review courses marketed to medical students studying for the USMLE Step 2. For each book, we list the **Title** of the book, the **First Author** (or editor), the **Current Publisher,** the **Copyright Year,** the **Edition,** the **Number of Pages,** the **ISBN Code,** the **Approximate List Price,** the **Format** of the book, and the **Number of Test Questions.** Most entries also include Summary Comments that describe their style and utility for studying. Finally, each book receives a **Rating.** The books are sorted into a comprehensive section as well as into sections corresponding to the seven clinical disciplines (internal medicine, neurology, OB/GYN, pediatrics, preventive medicine, psychiatry, and surgery).Within each section, books are arranged first by Rating, then by Author, and finally by Title.

For this fifth edition of *First Aid for the USMLE Step 2 CK,* the database of review books has been completely revised, with in-depth summary comments on more than 100 books and software. A letter rating scale with ten different grades reflects the detailed student evaluations. Each book receives a rating as follows:

A+	Excellent for boards review.
A A–	Very good for boards review; choose among the group.
B+ B B–	Good, but use only after exhausting better sources.

The **Rating** is meant to reflect the overall usefulness of the book in preparing for the USMLE Step 2 examination. This is based on a number of factors, including:

- The cost of the book
- The readability of the text
- The appropriateness and accuracy of the book
- The quality and number of sample questions
- The quality of written answers to sample questions
- The quality and appropriateness of the illustrations (e.g., graphs, diagrams, photographs)
- The length of the text (longer is not necessarily better)
- The quality and number of other books available in the same discipline
- The importance of the discipline on the USMLE Step 2 examination

Please note that **the rating does not reflect the quality of the book for purposes other than reviewing for the USMLE Step 2 examination.** Many books with low ratings are well written and informative but are not ideal for boards preparation. We have also avoided listing or commenting on the wide variety of general textbooks available in the clinical sciences.

Evaluations are based on the cumulative results of formal and informal surveys of hundreds of medical students from medical schools across the country. The summary comments and overall ratings represent a consensus opinion, but there may have been a large range of opinions or limited student feedback on any particular book.

Please note that the data listed are subject to change because:

- Publishers' prices change frequently.
- Individual bookstores often charge an additional markup.
- New editions come out frequently, and the quality of updating varies.
- The same book may be reissued through another publisher.

We actively encourage medical students and faculty to submit their opinions and ratings of these clinical science review books so that we may update our database (see "How to Contribute," p. xiii). In addition, we ask that publishers and authors submit review copies of clinical science review books, including new editions and books not included in our database, for evaluation. We also solicit reviews of new books or suggestions for alternate modes of study that may be useful in preparing for the examination, such as flash cards, computer-based tutorials, commercial review courses, and Internet Web sites.

DISCLAIMER/CONFLICT OF INTEREST STATEMENT

No material in this book, including the ratings, reflects the opinion or influence of the publisher. All errors and omissions will gladly be corrected if brought to the attention of the authors through the publisher. Please note that the *Underground Clinical Vignette* series are publications by the authors of this book.

A   ***Boards & Wards***   *$34.95*   Review

AYALA

Blackwell, 2003, 2nd ed., 363 pages, ISBN 1405103418

Concise book in outline format, packed with key information across the various fields of medicine. **Pros:** Very high yield. Nice use of tables and charts. Good for quick study and last-minute review. Can be used during clinical rotations as well as in preparation for Step 2. **Cons:** Small print. Not tremendously detailed, but covers many topics. Requires more in-depth books for further explanation. **Summary:** Good, comprehensive review, although it lacks some detail.

A   ***USMLE Step 2 Mock Exam***   *$29.95*   Test/750 q

BROCHERT

Elsevier, 2004, 2nd ed., 348 pages, ISBN 1560536101

Consists of 750 vignette-style questions in 15 test blocks. **Pros:** Questions are case based and offer a good approximation of real boards questions. Questions cover high-yield topics, and explanations are terse but adequate. Many questions also include images and associated laboratory findings. **Cons:** Explanations may not be adequate for those who require an in-depth review of certain topics. **Summary:** Excellent vignette-type questions in mock exam format.

A⁻   ***USMLE Step 2 Secrets***   *$34.95*   Review

BROCHERT

Elsevier, 2004, 2nd ed., 296 pages, ISBN 156053608X

Typical Secrets-series format, with questions and answers organized by specialty. **Pros:** Concise review of many high-yield topics. Good use of clinical images, including patient photos, blood smears, and radiographs. Gives clinical pearls that help differentiate and diagnose common clinical presentations. **Cons:** No clinical vignettes; simply lists questions that might be posed on the wards. Does not follow Step 2 format. Expensive. Content overlaps with that of other books by Brochert. **Summary:** Overall, good content for self-quizzing and study, but does not substitute for a formal review or practice tests. Portable book that stresses relevant topics in a quick, easy format.

B+

Underground Clinical Vignettes: Nine-Volume Set   *$143.95*   Review
BHUSHAN
Blackwell, 2005, 3rd ed., 942 pages, ISBN 140510418X
Nine-volume set containing clinical case scenarios of the various specialties, including OB/GYN, neurology, internal medicine, surgery, emergency medicine, psychiatry, and pediatrics, along with an extensive color atlas supplement. **Pros:** Well organized by focus points: pathogenesis, epidemiology, management, complications, and associated diseases. Recently revised and updated. **Cons:** Not comprehensive; use as a supplement to review. **Summary:** Organized and easy-to-read clinical vignettes. Excellent as a supplement to studying, but not sufficient by itself. More economical to purchase the nine-volume set than individual volumes.

B+

Crush the Boards Step 2   *$32.95*   Review
BROCHERT
Elsevier, 2002, 2nd ed., 200 pages, ISBN 1560535423
Comprehensive review of many high-yield topics, organized by specialty. **Pros:** Good emphasis on key points. Conversational style is easy to read. Good use of charts and diagrams. Covers surgical topics in more depth than similar books. **Cons:** Not comprehensive. No practice questions or vignettes. Not enough detail to be used alone for Step 2 preparation. **Summary:** An excellent review of key points and frequently tested topics. Should probably be supplemented with other review material and practice tests.

B+

A&L's Review for the USMLE Step 2   *$39.95*   Test/1060 q
CHAN
McGraw-Hill, 2002, 4th ed., 372 pages, ISBN 007137728X
Review questions organized by specialty along with two comprehensive practice exams. **Pros:** Overall question content is good, with broad coverage of high-yield topics. Well illustrated. **Cons:** Vignettes are brief, with short explanations. Some questions are too detailed and do not reflect the level of actual Step 2 questions. **Summary:** Good overall review questions on high-yield topics make it well suited to focused specialty review. Good buy for the number of questions.

NMS Review for USMLE Step 2

IBSEN

$42.95   Test/900 q

Lippincott Williams & Wilkins, 1999, 2nd ed., 470 pages, ISBN 0683302833

Comprehensive review book in question-and-answer format. **Pros:** Clear, concise, and broad coverage of high-yield topics, presented in a format similar to that of the actual Step 2 exam. Complete explanations. **Cons:** Questions are more detailed than needed for the boards. Lacks illustrations or images. Needs updating. **Summary:** Good source of Step 2–style questions with appropriate format and content, but questions may focus on details not emphasized on the actual exam.

Cracking the Boards

MARIANI

$29.95   Review

Princeton Review, 2000, 2nd ed., 544 pages, ISBN 0375761640

Clinical vignette review organized by specialty with more than 400 vignette-style questions. **Pros:** Well organized, with a uniform format throughout the book and numerous charts. Appropriate emphasis on treatment. Questions reflect the style of the Step 2 exam and present classic clinical cases. **Cons:** Few images. **Summary:** Useful review that follows the emphasis of Step 2 on clinical vignettes.

Medical Boards Step 2 Made Ridiculously Simple

CARL

$29.95   Review

MedMaster, 2003, 2nd ed., 384 pages, ISBN 0940780623

General review of topics for the Step 2 exam. Outline format with tables and brief discussions. **Pros:** Quick review. Useful in areas that might otherwise be overlooked—e.g., ophthalmology, dermatology, and ENT. Helpful for last-minute review. **Cons:** The table format of the book does not provide substantive details but aids in the memorization of lists. **Summary:** Highlights most high-yield topics, but should not be used alone for review.

Rx: Prescription for the Boards USMLE Step 2

FEIBUSCH

$34.95   Review

Lippincott Williams & Wilkins, 2002, 3rd ed., 512 pages, ISBN 0781734002

Text review based on the widely used USMLE content outline. **Pros:** Covers high-yield core and specialty topics. Well-designed format. **Cons:** Not enough detail for each topic. Provides a framework for studying, but cannot be used alone. Lacks tables and diagrams to facilitate studying. Facts outlining the next step in management are often not discussed. **Summary:** Good book for Step 2 review, but cannot be used as the sole resource for study.

Advanced Life Support for the USMLE Step 2

$24.95 Review

FLYNN

Lippincott Williams & Wilkins, 1999, 2nd ed., 142 pages, ISBN 0781719763

Brief outline format with high-yield topics described in tables or illustrations. **Pros:** Quick, easy read. Emphasis is on high-yield facts. Amusing cartoons highlight key concepts and excellent mnemonics. Great for last-minute review. **Cons:** Not adequate for in-depth review. **Summary:** Worthwhile review for the days right before the exam.

A&L's Practice Tests: USMLE Step 2

$39.95 Test/900 q

GOLDBERG

McGraw-Hill, 2002, 2nd ed., 253 pages, ISBN 0071377409

Comprehensive test questions. **Pros:** Great source of high-yield questions covering all topics. Many questions include radiographs and photographs of pathology. Adequate explanations. **Cons:** Some questions are not vignette style and do not reflect boards format. **Summary:** Good compilation of test questions that focus on high-yield material, but some questions still do not reflect boards style. Can be used as an extra resource for more practice questions.

Classic Presentations and Rapid Review for USMLE Step 2

$25.00 Review

O'CONNELL

J&S, 1999, 1st ed., 215 pages, ISBN 1888308052

Light overview organized by specialty, with emphasis on "classic" presentations of commonly seen conditions. Presented in bullet-point format. **Pros:** Good for last-minute studying. **Cons:** Neither comprehensive nor consistent in the material provided on each topic. Information is not overly detailed. No clinical images, ECGs, or clinical case examples. **Summary:** Quick and superficial review.

Insider's Guide to the USMLE Step 2

$44.95 Review/450 q

STANG

Elsevier, 2000, 1st ed., 426 pages, ISBN 0721682790

Contains case-based questions with explanations and includes suggested review topics. **Pros:** "Pop quizzes" after each section encourage retention. Practice test has detailed explanations to answers. **Cons:** Sparse information; may serve as a study guide rather than a review book. Some topics are not relevant to the boards. Questions do not reflect the vignette format on Step 2. **Summary:** A well-organized but not overly detailed comprehensive review. Some content is irrelevant to Step 2.

A

Kaplanmedical.com
KAPLAN

$149–$499

Compilation of online programs for Step 2 review, including a large test bank. **Pros:** Questions can be arranged by topic or randomly to simulate the real exam. Tests are timed to simulate boards conditions. Extensive number of questions in vignette format. Content level of questions reflects the boards test. Explanations are thorough. Allows students to identify strong and weak points. **Cons:** Very expensive. Online lectures can be difficult to watch for extensive periods of time. **Summary:** A good source of questions with thorough explanations, but the price may be prohibitive for many.

A

USMLEWorld.com
USMLEWorld

$90–$175

Test bank with over 2000 questions. Similar to the Kaplan test bank as described above. **Pros:** Well-written questions with explanations. Cheaper than Kaplan. **Cons:** Some questions are overly picky. **Summary:** A good source of questions that is cheaper than Kaplan.

B

USMLEasy.com
McGraw-Hill

$99–$199

Comprehensive test bank with over 3300 questions and explanations. Similar in style to the Kaplan question bank described above. **Pros:** Large number of questions. Mimics the CBT format. Cheaper than Kaplan. **Cons:** Awkward "enhanced" format and Web design. Questions can be more obscure than those appearing on the actual exam. **Summary:** A fair source of questions that may be good for supplemental review.

REVIEW RESOURCES

ONLINE REVIEW

Step-Up to Medicine
AGABEGI
Lippincott Williams & Wilkins, 2004, 1st ed., 516 pages, ISBN 0781747872

$34.95   Review

Comprehensive review of commonly tested diseases and topics in internal medicine organized in an outline format. Includes a color atlas and an appendix on interpreting x-rays, ECGs, and physical exam findings. **Pros:** Very comprehensive, with informative tables and diagrams to help synthesize information. Includes occasional clinical vignettes that correlate with the topic being discussed. Quick facts to remember are included in the margins of each page. **Cons:** Very lengthy. Geared more toward clerkship preparation than Step 2 review. **Summary:** Good book packed with useful information for the wards, but may be too lengthy and detailed for Step 2.

Blueprints Clinical Cases in Medicine
GANDHI
Blackwell, 2002, 1st ed., 160 pages, ISBN 0632046031

$20.95   Test/200 q

Compendium of vignette-type cases arranged by symptom followed by related questions and answers. **Pros:** Excellent companion to the Blueprints series. Focuses on high-yield cases. Easy to read with nice illustrations and review of management. **Cons:** Not comprehensive; use as a supplement for review. Better suited to clerkship preparation than to Step 2. **Summary:** Organized and easy-to-read supplement. Adds clinical correlates to the Blueprints series. Best if used with the Blueprints text.

High-Yield Internal Medicine
NIRULA
Lippincott Williams & Wilkins, 2003, 2nd ed., 223 pages, ISBN 0781742420

$24.95   Review

Core review of internal medicine in outline format. **Pros:** Focus is on high-yield diseases and symptoms. Quick and easy read. **Cons:** Not comprehensive. Some mistakes in formulas. Needs more illustrations. No index. **Summary:** Good, fast review presented in a format that allows for quick and repetitive readings. Use as a supplement, not as a primary study source.

First Aid for the Medicine Clerkship
STEAD
McGraw-Hill, 2001, 1st ed., 300 pages, ISBN 0071364218

$29.95   Review

High-yield review of symptoms and diseases. **Pros:** Comprehensive review; well organized by symptoms with good illustrations, scenarios, diagrams, algorithms, and mnemonics. **Cons:** May not be suited to the reader who prefers information arranged in text form. May be too basic for certain topics. **Summary:** Excellent, concise review of medicine.

B+

PreTest Medicine
$24.95   Test/500 q

BERK

McGraw-Hill, 2003, 10th ed., 190 pages, ISBN 007140287X

Question-and-answer format organized by medical subspecialty. **Pros:** Organization by subspecialty helps pinpoint weak areas. Good number of vignette-style questions, with detailed explanations. **Cons:** Many questions are more detailed than needed for the boards and are geared more toward the shelf exam. Few illustrations. **Summary:** Solid source of challenging review questions.

B+

Underground Clinical Vignettes: Emergency Medicine
$17.95   Review

BHUSHAN

Blackwell, 2005, 3rd ed., 120 pages, ISBN 1405104198

Clinical vignette review of emergency medicine topics. **Pros:** Recently revised and updated. Well organized by focus points: pathogenesis, epidemiology, management, complications, and associated diseases. Well illustrated, and includes high-yield "minicases" and links to the UCV Clinical/Basic Color Atlas. **Cons:** Not comprehensive; use as a supplement. **Summary:** Organized and easy-to-read supplement to studying.

B+

Underground Clinical Vignettes: Internal Medicine, Vols. I and II
$17.95 each   Review

BHUSHAN

Blackwell, 2005, 3rd ed., ISBN 1405104201, 140510421X

Clinical vignette review of common topics in internal medicine. **Pros:** Recently revised and updated. Well organized by focus points: pathogenesis, epidemiology, management, complications, and associated diseases. Vignettes mirror the boards-style presentation of questions. **Cons:** Not comprehensive; use as a supplement. **Summary:** Organized and easy-to-read supplement to studying.

B+

Platinum Vignettes: Internal Medicine
$23.95   Review

BROCHERT

Elsevier, 2002, 1st ed., 102 pages, ISBN 1560535318

Clinical vignette review of common topics in internal medicine. **Pros:** Well-written cases similar to boards-type vignettes. Well illustrated. Discussion is organized by pathophysiology, diagnosis and treatment, and more high-yield facts. **Cons:** Expensive for amount of material. Not comprehensive; use as a supplement. **Summary:** Organized and easy-to-read supplement to studying.

B+ ***Platinum Vignettes: Internal Medicine Subspecialties***   ***$23.95***   Review
BROCHERT
Elsevier, 2002, 1st ed., 105 pages, ISBN 1560535377
Clinical vignette review of common topics in the internal medicine subspecialties. **Pros:** Information is taught through the presentation of common clinical cases. Explanations are organized by pathophysiology, diagnosis and treatment, and more high-yield facts. **Cons:** Expensive for amount of material. Not comprehensive; use as a supplement. **Summary:** Organized and easy-to-read supplement to studying.

B+ ***A&L's Review of Internal Medicine***   ***$34.95***   Test/1100+ q
GOLDLIST
McGraw-Hill, 2002, 3rd ed., 276 pages, ISBN 007138524X
General review with questions and answers divided by subspecialty. **Pros:** Well-written vignette questions reflect the boards format. Representative of the content of the boards. Complete explanations. Well illustrated. **Cons:** Questions are shorter, and some nonvignette questions are more straightforward than those on the exam. **Summary:** Good source of questions that accurately reflect the multistep nature of boards questions.

B+ ***PreTest Preventive Medicine and Public Health***   ***$24.95***   Test/500 q
RATELLE
McGraw-Hill, 2000, 9th ed., 238 pages, ISBN 0071359621
Question-and-answer review of epidemiology, biostatistics, and preventive medicine. **Pros:** Majority of test questions appropriately simulate boards content and difficulty. Good explanations. **Cons:** Some questions contain too many calculations. The biostatistics chapter is too detailed. Few vignettes. **Summary:** Good question-and-answer review for a low-yield topic.

B+ ***Blueprints in Medicine***   ***$35.95***   Review/89 q
YOUNG
Blackwell, 2003, 3rd ed., 368 pages, ISBN 1405103353
Text review of internal medicine organized by common diseases and common symptoms. Question-and-answer section with explanations. **Pros:** Well-organized, concise review. Easy reading. Differential diagnoses for symptoms are helpful. Good charts and diagrams. **Cons:** Few illustrations. Has some superfluous details; some areas are too broad and simplistic to be useful for testing purposes. **Summary:** Good primary boards review for internal medicine, although poorly illustrated.

Medical Secrets

ZOLLO

$36.95   Review

Elsevier, 2004, 4th ed., 480 pages, ISBN 1560533870

Question-and-answer style typical of the Secrets series. **Pros:** Covers a great deal of clinically relevant information. Concise answers are given with pearls, tips, and memory aids. **Cons:** Too lengthy and detailed for USMLE review. **Summary:** May be most appropriate for wards use. Not a focused review.

B

Medicine Recall

BERGIN

$32.95   Review

Lippincott Williams & Wilkins, 2003, 2nd ed., 1035 pages, ISBN 0781736765

Standard Recall-series question-and-answer format, organized by medical specialty. **Pros:** Addresses a broad range of high-yield clinical topics. Good format for self-quizzing. Appropriate level of detail. **Cons:** No vignettes and no images; requires significant time commitment. Style simulates questions asked on rounds, not those on Step 2. **Summary:** Style may be more conducive to wards than to boards preparation. Use as a supplement to other resources.

B

In A Page Emergency Medicine

CATERINO

$31.95   Review

Blackwell, 2003, 1st ed., 316 pages, ISBN 1405103574

Collection of short, one-page summaries of 250 medical emergencies discussed in terms of etiology, differential diagnosis, presentation, diagnostic tests, treatment, and disposition. **Pros:** Concise and high yield. Covers a wide variety of emergencies seen in the ER. **Cons:** Text is crowded and somewhat confusing. No images or diagrams. **Summary:** Good for use during the emergency medicine clerkship, but may not be appropriate for Step 2 review.

B

Internal Medicine Pearls

HEFFNER

$41.95   Review

Elsevier, 2001, 2nd ed., 249 pages, ISBN 1560534044

Detailed clinical vignettes with laboratory and radiographic findings followed by a discussion of clinically important pearls. **Pros:** High-quality, realistic vignettes. Questions focus on decision making and management. **Cons:** Selected topics; not comprehensive. Discussions may be too detailed for purposes of review. Miscellaneous details. **Summary:** Good, clinically focused supplement for review.

In A Page Medicine
KAHAN

$31.95   Review

Blackwell, 2003, 1st ed., 275 pages, ISBN 1405103256

One-page reviews of 211 diseases discussed by etiology, epidemiology, signs/symptoms, differential diagnosis, diagnostic tests, treatment, and prognosis. **Pros:** Fast and concise review of high-yield information on common diseases. **Cons:** Text is crowded onto one page without any images or diagrams. **Summary:** Useful for quick study on the wards, but may not be comprehensive enough for Step 2.

Blueprints Clinical Cases in Family Medicine
LESKO

$20.95   Test/200 q

Blackwell, 2002, 1st ed., 152 pages, ISBN 0632046546

Compendium of vignette-type cases arranged by symptom followed by related questions and answers. **Pros:** Excellent companion to the Blueprints series. Focuses on high-yield cases. Easy to read with nice illustrations and review of management. **Cons:** Not comprehensive; use as a supplement for review. **Summary:** Organized and easy-to-read supplement. Adds clinical correlates to the Blueprints series. Best if used with the Blueprints text.

Blueprints Q & A Step 2 Medicine
SHINAR

$17.95   Test/200 q

Blackwell, 2004, 2nd ed., 153 pages, ISBN 1405103892

Two hundred vignette-style questions. **Pros:** Nice companion to the Blueprints series. Focuses on high-yield topics. Explanations are easy to follow. **Cons:** Not comprehensive; use as a supplement for review. Expensive; includes few questions given the cost of the book. **Summary:** Organized and easy-to-read supplement. Adds clinical correlates to the Blueprints series.

First Aid for the Emergency Medical Clerkship
STEAD

$29.95   Review

McGraw-Hill, 2001, 1st ed., 470 pages, ISBN 0071364269

High-yield review of symptoms and diseases. **Pros:** Comprehensive review; well organized by symptoms with good illustrations, scenarios, diagrams, algorithms, and mnemonics. **Cons:** May not be suited to the reader who prefers information arranged in text form. **Summary:** Excellent review of emergency medicine and nice presentation of high-yield topics for Step 2 preparation, but not intended for boards review.

B+

PreTest Neurology
$24.95   Test/500 q

ANSCHEL

McGraw-Hill, 2003, 5th ed., 340 pages, ISBN 0071411380

Question-and-answer review of neurology. **Pros:** Thorough coverage of neurology topics with a good number of clinical vignettes. Good emphasis on common topics, and thorough explanation of answers. Good practice for interpreting common head CTs/MRIs that might be tested. **Cons:** Some questions may be more detailed than needed for the boards. **Summary:** Good source of test questions for rapid review of neurology.

B+

Underground Clinical Vignettes: Neurology
$17.95   Review

BHUSHAN

Blackwell, 2005, 3rd ed., 112 pages, ISBN 1405109228

Clinical vignette review of high-yield topics in neurology. **Pros:** Recently revised and updated. Well organized by focus points: pathogenesis, epidemiology, management, complications, and associated diseases. Well illustrated, and includes "minicases," links to a color atlas supplement, and updated treatments. **Cons:** Not comprehensive; use as a supplement to review. **Summary:** Organized and easy-to-read supplement to studying. Lengthy for dedicated review of neurology.

B+

Blueprints in Neurology
$32.95   Review

DRISLANE

Blackwell, 2002, 1st ed., 232 pages, ISBN 0632045396

Review of neurology by disease and symptom with a brief exam. **Pros:** Reviews high-yield topics and is easy to follow. Good use of tables, images, and diagrams. Questions in the exam are similar to those found on both the shelf exam and Step 2. **Cons:** Lengthy. **Summary:** Excellent review of high-yield material for the wards and Step 2.

B

Blueprints Clinical Cases in Neurology
$20.95   Review

JOSHI

Blackwell, 2002, 1st ed., 152 pages, ISBN 0632046139

Compendium of vignette-type cases organized by symptom followed by related question and answers. **Pros:** Excellent companion to the Blueprints subspecialty series. Focuses on high-yield cases. Easy to read, with nice illustrations and review of management. **Cons:** Not comprehensive; use as a supplement. Few illustrations. **Summary:** Organized and easy to read. Adds clinical correlates to the Blueprints series.

REVIEW RESOURCES

NEUROLOGY

Neurology Recall

MILLER

Lippincott Williams & Wilkins, 2003, 2nd ed., 377 pages, ISBN 0781745888

Brief question-and-answer format. **Pros:** Many important facts are reviewed; useful for self-quizzing. **Cons:** Not a comprehensive review. Lengthy and lacks illustrations. Concepts are not integrated. **Summary:** Good for review of some high-yield concepts, but not a stand-alone resource for this topic.

Neurology Secrets

ROLAK

Elsevier, 2001, 3rd ed., 438 pages, ISBN 1560534656

Secrets-series question-and-answer format. **Pros:** Concise review of many high-yield topics. Good use of clinical images. Quick question-and-answer approach. **Cons:** No clinical vignettes; instead offers lists of questions that might be posed on the wards. Does not have a structured format and leaves out important information. Relatively expensive and lengthy. Not a reference book. **Summary:** Overall, good content for self-quizzing and study, but does not substitute for a formal review or practice tests. More appropriate for clerkship than for boards review.

Neurology Pearls

WACLAWIK

Elsevier, 2000, 1st ed., 228 pages, ISBN 1560532610

Detailed clinical vignettes, including laboratory and test results and radiographic findings, followed by a discussion of diagnosis and emphasis on important pearls. **Pros:** High-quality vignettes on many important neurologic conditions. **Cons:** Requires significant time investment. **Summary:** Challenging clinical scenarios to supplement a more structured topic review.

Underground Clinical Vignettes: OB/GYN   **_$17.95_**   Review
BHUSHAN
Blackwell, 2005, 3rd ed., 120 pages, ISBN 1405104236
Clinical vignette review of frequently tested diseases in obstetrics and gynecology. **Pros:** Recently revised and updated. Well organized by focus points: pathogenesis, epidemiology, management, complications, and associated diseases. Well illustrated. Easy read and stresses high-yield facts. **Cons:** Not comprehensive; use as a supplement. **Summary:** Well-organized and easy-to-read practice vignettes.

Platinum Vignettes: Obstetrics and Gynecology   **_$23.95_**   Review
BROCHERT
Elsevier, 2002, 1st ed., 102 pages, ISBN 1560535326
Clinical vignette review of common topics in obstetrics and gynecology. **Pros:** Well-written cases are similar to boards-type vignettes. Discussion is organized by pathophysiology, diagnosis and treatment, and more high-yield facts. **Cons:** Expensive for amount of material. Not comprehensive; use as a supplement. Few illustrations. **Summary:** Organized and easy-to-read supplement to studying.

Blueprints in Obstetrics and Gynecology   **_$35.95_**   Review/149 q
CAUGHEY
Blackwell, 2003, 3rd ed., 352 pages, ISBN 1405103310
Text review with tables and illustrations. Includes a short exam with explanations. **Pros:** Strong emphasis on high-yield topics with concise text, clear diagrams, and many classic illustrations. Easy read. Appropriate for both clinical clerkship and Step 2 preparation. **Cons:** Some topics are overly detailed, while some are not detailed enough. **Summary:** Overall, a good choice for boards and wards preparation.

Blueprints Clinical Cases in Obstetrics and Gynecology   **_$20.95_**   Test/200 q
CAUGHEY
Blackwell, 2002, 1st ed., 139 pages, ISBN 0632046112
Compendium of vignette-type cases arranged by symptom followed by related questions and answers. **Pros:** Excellent companion to the Blueprints series. Focuses on high-yield cases. Easy to read, with nice illustrations and review of management. **Cons:** Not comprehensive; use as a supplement. **Summary:** Organized and easy-to-read supplement. Adds clinical correlates to the Blueprints series.

A⁻

NMS Obstetrics and Gynecology
SIDDIGHI

$36.95   Review/500 q

Lippincott Williams & Wilkins, 2004, 5th ed., 512 pages, ISBN
0781726794

Detailed outline of OB/GYN with few tables and diagrams. **Pros:**
Comprehensive review for both wards and boards. Final exam is relatively good, with complete explanations. **Cons:** Dense and lengthy
OB/GYN review. Many questions do not reflect the boards format.
Lacks illustrations. **Summary:** Complete review with questions and
discussion. Too ambitious for exam preparation alone; more helpful if
used throughout clerkship.

B⁺

High-Yield Obstetrics and Gynecology
SAKALA

$24.95   Review

Lippincott Williams & Wilkins, 2001, 192 pages, ISBN
0781723949

Review of high-yield topics in outline format. Clinical scenarios at
the end of each chapter highlight key points. **Pros:** Easy read with
good discussion of high-yield topics. **Cons:** Lacks depth. No practice
questions. **Summary:** A quick but superficial review.

B⁺

First Aid for the OB/GYN Clerkship
STEAD

$29.95   Review

McGraw-Hill, 2001, 1st ed., 280 pages, ISBN 0071364234

High-yield review of symptoms and diseases. **Pros:** Comprehensive review with nice diagrams, images, charts, algorithms, and mnemonics.
Cons: Lengthy review. **Summary:** Excellent review of OB/GYN, but
lengthy for boards review.

B

Obstetrics and Gynecology Secrets
BADER

$36.95   Review

Elsevier, 2004, 3rd ed., 432 pages, ISBN 1560534753

Secrets-series question-and-answer format, organized by topic within
OB/GYN. **Pros:** Good coverage of many high-yield, clinically relevant
topics. **Cons:** Detailed; not useful for rapid review. No vignettes; few
illustrations and images. **Summary:** Good clinical context, but does
not serve as a formal topic review. Better for use during clerkship than
for Step 2 preparation.

BRS Obstetrics and Gynecology

$32.95   Review/500 q

SAKALA

Lippincott Williams & Wilkins, 2000, 2nd ed., 443 pages, ISBN 0683307436

General review text with questions at the end of the chapters and a comprehensive exam at the end of the book. **Pros:** Appropriate content for boards and wards study. New edition offers more detail on pregnancy complications and a new STD chapter. **Cons:** Some sections are overly detailed with few diagrams. Questions offer few clinical vignettes. **Summary:** Appropriate content review, but more helpful for wards than for boards.

Case Files: Obstetrics and Gynecology Review

$29.95   Review

TOY

McGraw-Hill, 2002, 1st ed., 488 pages, ISBN 0071402845

Review of OB/GYN in case format with questions and answers following each vignette. **Pros:** Cases reflect high-yield topics and are arranged in an easy-to-follow format. **Cons:** Some topics are either not covered or given only brief treatment. Few diagrams and images. Lengthy and time-consuming for one topic. Explanations are terse. **Summary:** Comprehensive review with emphasis on vignette-style case presentation, but some areas are not very detailed.

Blueprints Q & A Step 2 Obstetrics & Gynecology

$17.95   Test/200 q

TRAN

Blackwell, 2002, 1st ed., 153 pages, ISBN 0632045949

One hundred vignette-style questions. **Pros:** Nice companion to the Blueprints series. Focuses on high-yield topics. Explanations are easy to follow. **Cons:** Not comprehensive; use as a supplement for review. Sparse images. Some questions are esoteric and not boards-like. **Summary:** Organized and easy-to-read supplement. Adds clinical correlates to the Blueprints series.

PreTest Obstetrics and Gynecology

$24.95   Test/500 q

WYLEN

McGraw-Hill, 2003, 10th ed., 240 pages, ISBN 0071411399

Question-and-answer review with detailed explanations for OB/GYN. **Pros:** Organization by subtopic may be useful for studying weak areas. Good content emphasis. Generally well illustrated. **Cons:** Some questions are too difficult or detailed. Vignette-based questions are short and simplistic compared to Step 2 content. **Summary:** Decent source of questions to supplement topic study, especially for addressing specific areas of weakness.

Obstetrics and Gynecology Recall

$32.95   Review/350 q

BOURGEOIS

Lippincott Williams & Wilkins, 2004, 2nd ed., 582 pages, ISBN
0781748798

Recall-series question-and-answer style. **Pros:** Two-column format
makes it useful for self-quizzing. Reviews many high-yield concepts
and facts. **Cons:** Questions emphasize individual facts but do not integrate concepts. No vignettes or images. Spotty coverage of some topics. **Summary:** Useful for review of selected concepts, but not a comprehensive source for USMLE preparation. More appropriate for
clerkship than for boards.

A&L's Review of Obstetrics and Gynecology

$34.95   Test/1600+ q

VONTVER

McGraw-Hill, 2003, 7th ed., 300 pages, ISBN 0071386491

Detailed review of OB/GYN in question-and-answer format. **Pros:** Includes some high-yield sections such as clinical endocrinology. Offers
many questions. **Cons:** Overall emphasis is not appropriate for Step 2
preparation. At times redundant. May be more appropriate for specialty preparation. **Summary:** Far more detailed than required for
Step 2.

A⁻

Underground Clinical Vignettes: Pediatrics   **$17.95**   Review
BHUSHAN
Blackwell, 2005, 3rd ed., 120 pages, ISBN 1405104236
Clinical vignette review of frequently tested topics in pediatrics. **Pros:** Recently revised and updated. Well organized by focus points: pathogenesis, epidemiology, management, complications, and associated diseases. Well illustrated, and the new edition includes "minicases" to broaden subject material and present more high-yield information. **Cons:** Not comprehensive; use as a supplement to text review. **Summary:** Well organized and easy to read, but meant as a supplement for review.

A⁻

Platinum Vignettes: Pediatrics   **$23.95**   Review
BROCHERT
Elsevier, 2002, 1st ed., 100 pages, ISBN 1560535334
Clinical vignette review of common topics in pediatrics. **Pros:** Well-written cases are similar to boards-type vignettes. Well illustrated. Discussion is organized by pathophysiology, diagnosis and treatment, and more high-yield facts. **Cons:** Expensive for amount of material. Not comprehensive; use as a supplement. **Summary:** Organized and easy-to-read supplement to studying.

B⁺

Blueprints Clinical Cases in Pediatrics   **$20.95**   Test/200 q
LONDHE
Blackwell, 2002, 1st ed., 148 pages, ISBN 0632046058
Compendium of vignette-type cases arranged by symptom followed by related questions and answers. **Pros:** Excellent companion to the Blueprints series. Focuses on high-yield cases. Easy to read with nice illustrations and review of management. **Cons:** Not comprehensive; use as a supplement for review. **Summary:** Organized and easy-to-read supplement. Adds clinical correlates to the Blueprints series.

B⁺

Blueprints in Pediatrics   **$35.95**   Review/268 q
MARINO
Blackwell, 2003, 2nd ed., 320 pages, ISBN 1405103337
Text review of pediatrics with tables and diagrams. Includes a question-and-answer section with explanations. **Pros:** Appropriate focus on high-yield topics. **Cons:** Relatively dense text with few illustrations. Overly detailed. **Summary:** Good for a more comprehensive review.

Pediatrics: Review for USMLE Step 2
PAULSON
$25.00   Test/545 q

F. A. Davis, 2000, 1st ed., 276 pages, ISBN 080360761X

Test booklet with many clinical vignettes covering a broad range of topics within pediatrics. **Pros:** Organized by topic; informative answer explanations. Not too dense for last-minute review. **Cons:** Few images; includes non-boards-type questions ("except" and K-type answers). **Summary:** Good content review; does not replicate boards style.

A&L's Review of Pediatrics
VIESSMAN
$34.95   Test/1000+ q

McGraw-Hill, 2004, 6th ed., 250 pages, ISBN 0838503039

Question-and-answer review of pediatrics with detailed explanations. **Pros:** Questions focus on boards-relevant content. The last chapter includes excellent vignette-based questions. Thorough, well-written explanations. Nice primer on test-taking strategies. **Cons:** Non-vignette-based questions are shorter and more straightforward than those on Step 2. Some questions may be too detailed for Step 2 preparation. Poorly illustrated. **Summary:** Excellent, concise review with appropriate content and good discussions, but the majority of questions do not reflect Step 2 style.

PreTest Pediatrics
YETMAN
$24.95   Test/500 q

McGraw-Hill, 2003, 10th ed., 345 pages, ISBN 0071398724

Question-and-answer review with detailed discussion. **Pros:** Organization by organ system is useful for pinpointing weaknesses. Strong, thorough explanations. Fair number of vignette-style questions. Well illustrated. **Cons:** Some questions are too detailed or emphasize low-yield topics. **Summary:** Good source of questions and review for pediatrics. Appropriate content with good illustrations, although not entirely in Step 2 format.

Blueprints Q & A Step 2 Pediatrics
CLEMENT
$17.95   Test/100 q

Blackwell, 2004, 2nd ed., 240 pages, ISBN 1405103914

Two hundred vignette-style questions. **Pros:** Nice companion to the Blueprints series. Focuses on high-yield topics. Explanations are easy to follow. **Cons:** Not comprehensive; use as a supplement for review. Sparse images. Some questions are esoteric and not boards-like. **Summary:** Organized and easy-to-read supplement. Adds clinical correlates to the Blueprints series.

B-   *NMS Pediatrics*   *$34.95*   Review/166+ q

DWORKIN

Lippincott Williams & Wilkins, 2001, 4th ed., 768 pages, ISBN 078173850

General review of pediatrics in outline format. Includes questions at the end of each chapter. **Pros:** Thorough, detailed review of pediatrics. Boldfacing highlights key points. Case studies and a comprehensive exam (also provided on CD-ROM) at the end of the book are helpful. Good discussion. **Cons:** Dense, lengthy text. Lacks good illustrations of any kind. **Summary:** Thorough review, but more appropriate for clerkships than for Step 2 review.

B   *In A Page Pediatrics*   *$31.95*   Review

KAHAN

Blackwell, 2003, 1st ed., 294 pages, ISBN 1405103264

One-page reviews of 228 diseases/topics discussed by etiology, epidemiology, signs/symptoms, differential diagnosis, diagnostic tests, treatment, and prognosis. **Pros:** Fast and concise review of high-yield information on common diseases. **Cons:** Text is crowded onto one page, without any images or diagrams. Includes low-yield topics. **Summary:** Useful for quick study on the wards, but too time intensive for Step 2 review.

B-   *Pediatrics Recall*   *$32.95*   Review

McGAHREN

Lippincott Williams & Wilkins, 2002, 2nd ed., 461 pages, ISBN 0781726115

Concise question-and-answer format typical of the Recall series. **Pros:** Two-column format makes self-quizzing easy. Emphasizes diagnosis and management. **Cons:** Requires time commitment. Not all topics are covered thoroughly. No vignettes. **Summary:** Useful material, but does not provide a systematic review or substitute for practice tests.

B-   *Pediatric Secrets*   *$36.95*   Review

POLIN

Elsevier, 2001, 3rd ed., 731 pages, ISBN 1560534567

Question-and-answer format typical of the Secrets series, organized by pediatric subspecialty. **Pros:** Thorough discussion of a wide variety of clinical topics. **Cons:** Detailed content geared toward the wards; requires a large time investment. No images or illustrations. **Summary:** Too detailed for USMLE review. Better suited to clerkship.

REVIEW RESOURCES

PEDIATRICS

Underground Clinical Vignettes: Psychiatry

$17.95   Review

BHUSHAN

Blackwell, 2005, 3rd ed., 128 pages, ISBN 1405104252

Clinical vignette review of frequently tested topics in psychiatry. **Pros:** Well organized by focus points: pathogenesis, epidemiology, management, and associated diseases. Well illustrated, and includes "mini-cases" that present high-yield information. **Cons:** Not comprehensive; use as a supplement. **Summary:** Organized and easy-to-read practice vignettes.

Platinum Vignettes: Psychiatry

$23.95   Review

BROCHERT

Elsevier, 2002, 1st ed., 102 pages, ISBN 1560535342

Clinical vignette review of common topics in psychiatry. **Pros:** Well-written cases are similar to boards-type vignettes. Well illustrated. Discussion is organized by pathophysiology, diagnosis and treatment, and more high-yield facts. **Cons:** Not comprehensive; use as a supplement. **Summary:** Organized and easy-to-read supplement to studying.

Blueprints Clinical Cases in Psychiatry

$20.95   Test/200 q

HOBLYN

Blackwell, 2002, 1st ed., 152 pages, ISBN 0632046090

Compendium of vignette-type cases arranged by symptom followed by related questions and answers. **Pros:** Excellent companion to the Blueprints series. Focuses on high-yield cases. Easy to read with nice illustrations and review of management. **Cons:** Not comprehensive; use as a supplement for review. **Summary:** Organized and easy-to-read supplement. Adds clinical correlates to the Blueprints series.

Blueprints in Psychiatry

$26.95   Review/74 q

MURPHY

Blackwell, 2000, 2nd ed., 128 pages, ISBN 0632044888

Brief text review of psychiatry with DSM-IV criteria. Includes a brief question-and-answer section at the end of the book. **Pros:** Clear, concise review of psychiatry with helpful tables. Good coverage of high-yield topics, including the pharmacology section. Quick read. **Cons:** Relatively expensive, and some areas are not detailed enough. **Summary:** Rapid review with appropriate coverage of high-yield topics.

High-Yield Psychiatry

FADEM

Lippincott Williams & Wilkins, 2003, 2nd ed., 150 pages, ISBN 078174684

Brief outline-format review of psychiatry. **Pros:** Quick read with clinical vignettes scattered throughout. Concise tables. **Cons:** Not enough detail for in-depth review. **Summary:** Excellent, quick review of psychiatry, but may lack depth. Similar to *High-Yield Behavioral Sciences* by the same author.

$24.95   Review

Psychiatry

MORGAN

Biotest, 2002, 1st ed., 280 pages, ISBN 1893720101

Thorough review of psychiatry in outline format with questions. **Pros:** Many high-yield tables; questions are included at the end of each chapter with a reference to the text or explanations. **Cons:** Few illustrations, dense and lengthy, and lacking in vignette-style questions. **Summary:** Fairly comprehensive review of psychiatry with an emphasis on high-yield topics, but many questions do not reflect Step 2 style.

$25.95   Review/500q

A&L's Review of Psychiatry

ORANSKY

McGraw-Hill, 2002, 7th ed., 304 pages, ISBN 0071402535

General review of psychiatry with questions and answers. **Pros:** Includes 114 vignette-style questions appropriate for boards review. Appropriate content emphasis; thorough explanations. The new edition features updated treatment and management sections. **Cons:** Questions are shorter and more straightforward than those of the boards. **Summary:** Decent boards review for psychiatry, but does not reflect boards format.

$34.95   Test/900+ q

PreTest Psychiatry

PAN

McGraw-Hill, 2003, 10th ed., 288 pages, ISBN 0071389199

Question-and-answer review of topics in psychiatry. **Pros:** Questions are well written and organized. Most questions have appropriate content level. Good explanations. **Cons:** Too few vignette-type questions. Some questions are too detailed. **Summary:** Good source of questions and review for psychiatry, although the format may not reflect the actual test.

$24.95   Test/500 q

REVIEW RESOURCES

PSYCHIATRY

NMS Psychiatry

SCULLY

Lippincott Williams & Wilkins, 2001, 4th ed., 339 pages, ISBN 0683307916

General review of topics in outline format with questions at the end of each chapter and a comprehensive final exam. **Pros:** Well-written text with concise disease discussions. Includes an expanded pharmacology section. Questions test appropriate content and have complete explanations, and the new edition offers more vignette-style questions. Good companion text for clerkship. **Cons:** Not enough vignette-style questions. Lengthy for purposes of boards review. **Summary:** Detailed review that requires time commitment. Good single choice for clerkship study and boards review.

$34.95   Review/500 q

First Aid for the Psychiatry Clerkship

STEAD

McGraw-Hill, 2005, 2nd ed., 184 pages, ISBN 0071448721

High-yield review of symptoms and diseases. **Pros:** Comprehensive review that includes DSM-IV criteria with nice mnemonics and scenarios. Includes high-yield tear-out cards. **Cons:** May not appeal to readers who prefer information in text format. **Summary:** Good review of high-yield topics in psychiatry, but better suited for the wards than to the Step 2 exam.

$34.95   Review

Blueprints Q & A Step 2 Psychiatry

CLEMENT

Blackwell, 2004, 2nd ed., 240 pages, ISBN 1405103914

Two hundred vignette-style questions. **Pros:** Nice companion to the Blueprints series. Focuses on high-yield topics. Explanations are easy to follow. **Cons:** Not comprehensive; use as a supplement for review. Sparse images. Some questions are esoteric and not boards-like. **Summary:** Organized and easy-to-read supplement. Adds clinical correlates to the Blueprints series.

$17.95   Test/200 q

Psychiatry Made Ridiculously Simple

GOOD

MedMaster, 2005, 4th ed., 98 pages, ISBN 0940780682

Part of the "Made Ridiculously Simple" series. **Pros:** Comprehensive, fast read with nice tables and entertaining illustrations to highlight key points. **Cons:** Some areas are not detailed enough; other areas are too verbose. Not boards oriented. **Summary:** Good, fast review, but more helpful for clerkship than for boards.

$13.95   Review

REVIEW RESOURCES

PSYCHIATRY

B

BRS Psychiatry

SHANER

$32.95   Review/400 q

Lippincott Williams & Wilkins, 2004, 2nd ed., 419 pages, ISBN
0683307665

Comprehensive review of psychiatry in outline format. Vignette-style
questions follow each chapter. **Pros:** Thorough, systematic review of
clinical psychiatry. Clear, concise definitions are provided. Includes a
good pharmacology section. **Cons:** Great deal of information for single-topic review. **Summary:** Good material, but requires a large time
investment; not for last-minute review of all topics.

B−

Psychiatry Recall

FADEM

$32.95   Review

Lippincott Williams & Wilkins, 2004, 2nd ed., 210 pages, ISBN
078174511X

Quick question-and-answer format of the Recall series. **Pros:** Two-
column format is conducive to self-quizzing. Covers many high-yield
facts and concepts necessary for the USMLE. **Cons:** Lacks vignettes,
so does not substitute for practice tests. **Summary:** Requires time
commitment. Some topics are glossed over. Use as a supplement to
other resources.

B−

Psychiatric Secrets

JACOBSON

$36.95   Review

Lippincott Williams & Wilkins, 2001, 2nd ed., 536 pages, ISBN
1560534184

Question-and-discussion format of the Secrets series, organized by
topic. **Pros:** Clear explanations of important concepts in psychiatry.
Good wards reading. **Cons:** Too detailed and lengthy for review purposes. Lacks vignettes. **Summary:** Requires significant time to read;
not for rapid, focused review.

B−

Saint-Frances Guide to Psychiatry

MCCARTHY

$28.95   Review

Lippincott Williams & Wilkins, 2000, 3rd ed., 279 pages, ISBN
0683306618

Comprehensive text review of psychiatry. **Pros:** Thorough; outline format is easy to read and follow. Portable. Clinical correlates stress key
points. **Cons:** Lengthy. Some areas have superfluous information. Not
geared toward the boards. **Summary:** Nice review of psychiatry with
helpful correlates that emphasize key points, but may be more helpful
for clerkship than for boards.

A−

Underground Clinical Vignettes: Surgery
BHUSHAN

$17.95   Review

Blackwell, 2005, 3rd ed., 178 pages, ISBN 1405104260

Clinical vignette review of frequently tested surgical topics. **Pros:** Recently revised and updated. Well organized by focus points: pathogenesis, epidemiology, management, complications, and associated diseases. Well illustrated and includes "minicases" that present high-yield information. **Cons:** Not comprehensive; use as a supplement to review. **Summary:** Well-organized and easy-to-read practice vignettes.

B+

Surgical Recall
BLACKBOURNE

$34.95   Review

Lippincott Williams & Wilkins, 2002, 3rd ed., 745 pages, ISBN 0781729734

Question-and-answer format, as with other Recall-series books. **Pros:** Questions emphasize important, high-yield clinical concepts. Columns allow self-testing. Fast review. Good preparation for "pimping" on rounds. **Cons:** Not boards-type questions. Poorly organized. Spotty coverage of some topics. **Summary:** Useful adjunct to a more organized topic review. More appropriate for clerkship than for boards review.

B+

Platinum Vignettes: Surgery and Trauma
BROCHERT

$23.95   Review

Elsevier, 2002, 1st ed., 102 pages, ISBN 1560535350

Clinical vignette review of common topics in surgery and trauma medicine. **Pros:** Well-written cases similar to boards-type vignettes. Well illustrated. Discussion is organized by pathophysiology, diagnosis and treatment, and more high-yield facts. **Cons:** Expensive for amount of material. Not comprehensive; use as a supplement. **Summary:** Organized and easy-to-read supplement to studying.

B+

Platinum Vignettes: Surgical Subspecialties
BROCHERT

$23.95   Review

Elsevier, 2002, 1st ed., 105 pages, ISBN 1560535385

Clinical vignette review of common topics in internal medicine. **Pros:** Well-written cases similar to boards-type vignettes. Well illustrated. Discussion is organized by pathophysiology, diagnosis and treatment, and more high-yield facts. **Cons:** Expensive for amount of material. Not comprehensive; use as a supplement. **Summary:** Organized and easy-to-read supplement to studying.

REVIEW RESOURCES

SURGERY

PreTest Surgery $24.95   Test/500 q
GELLER
McGraw-Hill, 2003, 10th ed., 356 pages, ISBN 0071412999
Review of topics in general surgery in question-and-answer format.
Pros: Predominantly case based. Well organized by subspecialty.
Cons: Many questions are too detailed or esoteric and do not reflect
boards style. Some explanations are overly detailed. **Summary:** Thorough review, but questions may be beyond the level needed for Step 2
preparation.

 Blueprints in Surgery $29.95   Review/62 q
KARP
Blackwell, 2003, 3rd ed., 320 pages, ISBN 1405103329
Short text review of general surgery with tables and diagrams. Brief
question-and-answer section is included. **Pros:** Well organized. Easy
to read with strong focus on high-yield topics. Clear diagrams. **Cons:**
Some sections are overly detailed (e.g., anatomy). Some information
is simplistic. Few illustrations. **Summary:** Concise review of surgery
with appropriate emphasis on high-yield topics.

A&L's Review of Surgery $34.95   Test/1000+ q
WAPNICK
McGraw-Hill, 2002, 320 pages, ISBN 0071378146
General review of surgery with questions and answers. **Pros:** Good
clinical emphasis. Many vignette-style questions. Explanations are
thorough. **Cons:** Some questions are too short, and style does not reflect that of the Step 2 exam. Questions are highly variable in difficulty. Few illustrations. **Summary:** Good content for the exam, but
some questions are picky.

NMS Surgery $34.95   Review/350 q
JARRELL
Lippincott Williams & Wilkins, 2000, 4th ed., 699 pages, ISBN
0683306154
Outline review of general surgery and surgical subspecialties. **Pros:**
Well organized and thorough. Vignette-style questions are included
after each chapter with good explanations. **Cons:** Dense, detailed
text. Few tables or illustrations. **Summary:** Comprehensive surgery review, but very time-consuming. More appropriate for clerkship than
for boards review.

SURGERY

In A Page Surgery
KAHAN

$31.95   Review

Blackwell, 2003, 1st ed., 206 pages, ISBN 1405103655

One-page reviews of 154 diseases/topics discussed by etiology, epidemiology, signs/symptoms, differential diagnosis, diagnostic tests, treatment, and prognosis. **Pros:** Fast and concise review of high-yield information on common diseases. **Cons:** Text is crowded onto one page, without any images or diagrams. Includes low-yield topics. **Summary:** Useful for quick study on the wards, but too time intensive for Step 2 review.

Blueprints Clinical Cases in Surgery
LI

$20.95   Test/200 q

Blackwell Science, 2002, 1st ed., 152 pages, ISBN 0632046074

Compendium of vignette-type cases arranged by symptom followed by related questions and answers. **Pros:** Excellent companion to the Blueprints series. Focuses on high-yield cases. Easy to read with nice illustrations and review of management. **Cons:** Not comprehensive; use as a supplement for review. **Summary:** Organized and easy-to-read supplement. Adds clinical correlates to the Blueprints series.

Blueprints Q & A Step 2 Surgery
NELSON

$17.95   Test/200 q

Blackwell, 2004, 2nd ed., 169 pages, ISBN 1405103930

Two hundred vignette-style questions. **Pros:** Nice companion to the Blueprints series. Focuses on high-yield topics. Explanations are easy to follow. **Cons:** Not comprehensive; use as a supplement for review. Sparse images. Some questions are esoteric and not boards-like. Expensive, and includes few questions given the cost of the book. **Summary:** Organized and easy-to-read supplement. Adds clinical correlates to the Blueprints series.

High-Yield Surgery
NIRULA

$24.95   Review

Lippincott Williams & Wilkins, 2000, 1st ed., 150 pages, ISBN 068330691X

Outline review of most common general surgery topics. **Pros:** Concise; useful for quick topic review. Well organized. **Cons:** Information can be superficial. Some topics are omitted. No practice questions. **Summary:** Lean text for rapid review.

BRS General Surgery

$29.95   Review/375 q

CRABTREE

Lippincott Williams & Wilkins, 2000, 1st ed., 564 pages, ISBN 0683306367

Comprehensive review in outline format, organized by topic or organ. **Pros:** Appropriate clinical emphasis for boards and wards. Includes vignette-style review questions at the end of each chapter. **Cons:** Lengthy for single-topic review. Some information is not specific enough to be useful. Few images or illustrations. **Summary:** Overall, a strong review resource. Requires time commitment, so may not be suited to rapid review.

BRS Surgical Specialties

$32.95   Review/150 q

CRABTREE

Lippincott Williams & Wilkins, 2000, 1st ed., 262 pages, ISBN 0781727715

Focused review of topics in the surgical subspecialties in outline format. **Pros:** Good emphasis for boards and wards. Good use of illustrations. Vignette-style review questions. **Cons:** Some information may be redundant from review of other topics, and some information may be beyond the scope of the Step 2 exam. **Summary:** For the advanced surgery student.

Abernathy's Surgical Secrets

$36.95   Review

HARKEN

Elsevier, 2003, 5th ed., 381 pages, ISBN 1560535865

Question-and-answer Secrets-series format. **Pros:** Discussions are up to date and thorough. **Cons:** Too detailed for the purposes of the USMLE, yet not comprehensive. **Summary:** Not a well-organized review. Better suited to clerkship than to boards preparation.

Pocket Surgery

$29.95   Review

MOSCA

Blackwell Science, 2002, 1st, 144 pages, ISBN 0781735793

Review of high-yield surgical material in outline format. **Pros:** Fast, easy read. Portable. Highlights high-yield information in "fact boxes." **Cons:** Some material is not detailed enough. No illustrations. **Summary:** Good for rapid review during clerkship. Does not contain enough detailed information to be used as a single study source for the boards.

Dermatology for Boards and Wards

AYALA

$20.95   Review

Blackwell Science, 2001, 1st ed., 96 pages, 0632045728

Brief book with pictures of dermatologic findings **Pros:** Brief, with pictures of high-yield topics. **Cons:** Minimal explanations. **Summary:** Short book with pictures of high-yield dermatologic diagnoses and findings.

First Aid for the International Medical Graduate

CHANDLER

$29.95   Review

McGraw-Hill, 2002, 1st ed., 295 pages, ISBN 0071385320

High-yield review for the IMG on how to pass the USMLE boards and adapt to medical culture in the United States. **Pros:** Comprehensive, well-organized review. **Cons:** Some readers may need to obtain additional information from other sources. **Summary:** Excellent review of material for the IMG. Best used as a primer for boards review.

The IMG's Guide to Mastering the USMLE & Residency

CHANDLER

$29.95   Test/500 q

McGraw-Hill, 2000, 1st ed., 310 pages, ISBN 0071347240

Comprehensive guide for IMGs that navigates the complicated process of training in the United States. Includes information on visas, USMLE and TOEFL exams, the Step 2 CS exam, and applying to residencies, with emphasis on overcoming the many obstacles that IMGs face along the way. Also provides practical advice on establishing a home in the United States, residency survival skills, and finding a job.

REVIEW RESOURCES

MISCELLANEOUS

Commercial preparation courses can be helpful for some students, but these courses are expensive and require significant time commitment. They are usually effective in organizing study material for students who feel overwhelmed by the volume of material. Note that multiweek courses may be quite intense and may thus leave limited time for independent study. Also note that some commercial courses are designed for first-time test takers while others focus on students who are repeating the examination. In addition, some courses focus on IMGs who want to take all three Steps in a limited amount of time. Student experience and satisfaction with review courses are highly variable. We suggest that you discuss options with recent graduates of the review courses you are considering. Course content and structure can change rapidly. Some student opinions can be found in discussion groups on the World Wide Web. Below is contact information for some Step 2 commercial review courses.

Falcon Physician Reviews
1431 Greenway Drive, #800
Irving, TX 75038
(214) 632-5466
info@falconreviews.com
www.falconreviews.com

Kaplan Medical
700 South Flower Street
Los Angeles, CA 90017
(800) KAP-TEST (800-527-8378)
www.kaptest.com

Northwestern Medical Review
P.O. Box 22174
East Lansing, MI 48909-2174
(866) MedPass (866-633-7277)
registrar@northwesternmedicalreview.com
http://northwesternmedicalreview.com

Postgraduate Medical Review Education (PMRE)
1909 Taylor Street, Suite 305
Hollywood, FL 33020
(800) 323-6430
sales@pmre.com
www.pmre.com

Youel's Prep, Inc.
P.O. Box 4605
West Palm Beach, FL 33402
(800) 645-3985
Fax: (561) 366-8628
info@youelsprep.com
www.youelsprep.com

APPENDIX

Abbreviations and Symbols

Abbreviation	Meaning
A-a	alveolar-arterial (oxygen gradient)
ABG	arterial blood gas
ABI	ankle-brachial index
ABVD	Adriamycin (doxorubicin), bleomycin, vinblastine, dacarbazine
ACA	anterior cerebral artery
ACC	American College of Cardiology
ACE	angiotensin-converting enzyme
ACEI	angiotensin-converting enzyme inhibitor
ACh	acetylcholine
ACLS	advanced cardiac life support
ACTH	adrenocorticotropic hormone
AD	Alzheimer's disease
ADA	American Diabetes Association
ADH	antidiuretic hormone
ADHD	attention-deficit hyperactivity disorder
AF	atrial fibrillation
AFI	amniotic fluid index
AFP	α-fetoprotein
AHA	American Heart Association
AIDS	acquired immunodeficiency virus
ALL	acute lymphocytic leukemia
ALS	amyotrophic lateral sclerosis
ALT	alanine aminotransferase
AMA	American Medical Association
AML	acute myelogenous leukemia
ANA	antinuclear antibody
ANCA	antineutrophil cytoplasmic antibody
AOA	American Osteopathic Association
AP	anteroposterior
aPTT	activated partial thromboplastin time
AR	attributable risk
ARB	angiotensin receptor blocker
ARC	Appalachian Regional Commission
ARDS	acute respiratory distress syndrome
ARF	acute renal failure
5-ASA	5-aminosalicylic acid

Abbreviation	Meaning
ASA	acetylsalicylic acid
ASCUS	atypical squamous cells of undetermined significance
ASD	atrial septal defect
ASO	antistreptolysin O
AST	aspartate aminotransferase
ATN	acute tubular necrosis
AV	atrioventricular
AVM	arteriovenous malformation
AVN	avascular necrosis
AVNRT	atrioventricular nodal reentry tachycardia
AXR	abdominal x-ray
AZT	azidothymidine (zidovudine)
BID	twice a day
BMI	body mass index
BP	blood pressure
BPH	benign prostatic hyperplasia
bpm	beat per minute
BPP	biophysical profile
BPPV	benign paroxysmal positional vertigo
BSA	body surface area
BT	bleeding time
BUN	blood urea nitrogen
CABG	coronary artery bypass graft
CAD	coronary artery disease
CaEDTA	calcium disodium edetate
CALLA	common ALL antigen
CBC	complete blood count
CBT	cognitive-behavioral therapy, computer-based testing
CCS	computer-based case simulations
CD	cluster of differentiation
CEA	carcinoembryonic antigen
CF	cystic fibrosis
cGMP	cyclic guanosine monophosphate
CHF	congestive heart failure
CHOP	cytoxan, Adriamycin (doxorubicin), Oncovin (vincristine), prednisone
CIN	candidate identification number, cervical intraepithelial neoplasia

Abbreviation	Meaning
CK	creatine kinase, Clinical Knowledge
CK-MB	creatine kinase, MB fraction
CLL	chronic lymphocytic leukemia
CML	chronic myelogenous leukemia
CMP	cytidine monophosphate
CMV	cytomegalovirus
CN	cranial nerve
CNS	central nervous system
COGME	Council on Graduate Medical Education
COMT	catechol-O-methyltransferase
COPD	chronic obstructive pulmonary disease
CPAP	continuous positive airway pressure
CPK	creatine phosphokinase
CRP	C-reactive protein
CS	Clinical Skills
CSF	cerebrospinal fluid
CST	contraction stress test
CT	computed tomography
CXR	chest x-ray
D&C	dilation and curettage
DCIS	ductal carcinoma in situ
DDAVP	1-deamino (8-D-arginine) vasopressin
DES	diethylstilbestrol
DEXA	dual-energy x-ray absorptiometry
DHEAS	dehydroepiandrosterone sulfate
DHS	Department of Homeland Security
DI	diabetes insipidus
DIC	disseminated intravascular coagulation
DIP	distal interphalangeal (joint)
DKA	diabetic ketoacidosis
DL_{CO}	diffusing capacity of carbon monoxide
DM	diabetes mellitus
DMARD	disease-modifying antirheumatic drug
DMD	Duchenne muscular dystrophy
DNA	deoxyribonucleic acid
DNase	deoxyribonuclease
DNI	do not intubate
DNR	do not resuscitate
DPOA	durable power of attorney
DRE	digital rectal examination
DS	double strength
DSM	Diagnostic and Statistical Manual (of Mental Disorders)
DTaP	diphtheria, tetanus, acellular pertussis (vaccine)
DTR	deep tendon reflex
DTs	delirium tremens
DVT	deep venous thrombosis
EBV	Epstein-Barr virus
ECFMG	Educational Commission for Foreign Medical Graduates

Abbreviation	Meaning
ECG	electrocardiography
ECT	electroconvulsive therapy
ED	erectile dysfunction
EEG	electroencephalography
EF	ejection fraction
EGD	esophagogastroduodenoscopy
ELISA	enzyme-linked immunosorbent assay
EMG	electromyography
ENT	ears, nose, and throat
EPS	extrapyramidal symptom(s)
ER	emergency room, estrogen receptor
ERAS	Electronic Residency Application Service
ERCP	endoscopic retrograde cholangiopancreatography
ESR	erythrocyte sedimentation rate
ESWL	extracorporeal shock-wave lithotripsy
ETEC	enterotoxic E. coli
EtOH	ethanol
FAP	familial adenomatous polyposis
FAST	focused abdominal sonography for trauma
Fe_{Na}	fractional excretion of sodium
FEV_1	forced expiratory volume in one second
FFP	fresh frozen plasma
FiO_2	fraction of inspired oxygen
FNA	fine-needle aspiration
FOBT	fecal occult blood test
FSH	follicle-stimulating hormone
FSMB	Federation of State Medical Boards
FTA-ABS	fluorescent treponemal antibody absorption (test)
FTT	failure to thrive
5-FU	5-fluorouracil
FUO	fever of unknown origin
FVC	forced vital capacity
G6PD	glucose-6-phosphate dehydrogenase
GA	gestational age
GAS	group A streptococcus
GBM	glomerular basement membrane
GBS	group B streptococcus, Guillain-Barré syndrome
GC	gonorrhea and chlamydia (screen)
G-CSF	granulocyte colony-stimulating factor
GERD	gastroesophageal reflux disease
GFR	glomerular filtration rate
GGT	gamma-glutamyl transferase
GH	growth hormone
GI	gastrointestinal
GNR	gram-negative rod
GnRH	gonadotropin-releasing hormone
GTD	gestational trophoblastic disease
GU	genitourinary

Abbreviation	Meaning
GVHD	graft-versus-host disease
H&P	history and physical
HAV	hepatitis A virus
Hb	hemoglobin
HbA$_{1C}$	hemoglobin A$_{1C}$
HBcAb	hepatitis B core antibody
HbO$_2$	hyperbaric oxygen
HBsAb	hepatitis B surface antibody
HBsAg	hepatitis B surface antigen
HBV	hepatitis B virus
hCG	human chorionic gonadotropin
HCTZ	hydrochlorothiazide
HCV	hepatitis C virus
HDL	high-density lipoprotein
HDV	hepatitis D virus
HHNK	hyperosmolar hyperglycemic nonketotic (coma)
HHS	Health and Human Services
HHV	human herpesvirus
Hib	Haemophilus influenzae type B (vaccine)
HIDA	hepato-iminodiacetic acid (scan)
HIV	human immunodeficiency virus
HLA	human leukocyte antigen
HMG-CoA	hydroxymethylglutaryl coenzyme A
HNPCC	hereditary nonpolyposis colorectal cancer
hpf	high-power field
HPL	human placental lactogen
HPSAs	Health Professional Shortage Areas
HPV	human papillomavirus
HRT	hormone replacement therapy
HSV	herpes simplex virus
HUS	hemolytic-uremic syndrome
HVA	homovanillic acid
IBD	inflammatory bowel disease
IBS	irritable bowel syndrome
ICD	implantable cardiac defibrillator
ICP	intracranial pressure
ICU	intensive care unit
I/E	inspiratory/expiratory (ratio)
IFN	interferon
IFN-α	α-interferon
Ig	immunoglobulin
IGF	insulin-like growth factor
IHSS	idiopathic hypertrophic subaortic stenosis
IM	intramuscular
IMED	International Medical Education Directory
IMG	international medical graduate
INH	isoniazid
INR	International Normalized Ratio
I/O	input/output

Abbreviation	Meaning
IPV	inactivated polio vaccine
IR	incidence rate
ITP	idiopathic thrombocytopenic purpura
IUD	intrauterine device
IUGR	intrauterine growth rate
IV	intravenous
IVC	inferior vena cava
IVF	in vitro fertilization
IVIG	intravenous immunoglobulin
IVP	intravenous pyelography
JNC-7	Joint National Committee on Prevention, Detection, Evaluation, and Treatment of High Blood Pressure
JRA	juvenile rheumatoid arthritis
JVD	jugular venous distention
JVP	jugular venous pressure
KOH	potassium hydroxide
KUB	kidney, ureter, bladder
LBBB	left bundle branch block
LBP	low back pain
LCL	lateral collateral ligament
LDH	lactate dehydrogenase
LDL	low-density lipoprotein
LEEP	loop electrosurgical excision procedure
LES	lower esophageal sphincter
LFT	liver function test
LH	luteinizing hormone
LLQ	left lower quadrant
LMN	lower motor neuron
LMP	last menstrual period
LMWH	low-molecular-weight heparin
LP	lumbar puncture
LR	lactated Ringer's
LVEDP	left ventricular end-diastolic pressure
LVH	left ventricular hypertrophy
MAC	membrane attack complex, *Mycobacterium avium* complex
MAOI	monoamine oxidase inhibitor
MCA	middle cerebral artery
MCHC	mean corpuscular hemoglobin concentration
MCL	medial collateral ligament
MCP	metacarpophalangeal (joint)
MCV	mean corpuscular volume
MDE	major depressive episode
MEN	multiple endocrine neoplasia
MgSO$_4$	magnesium sulfate
MGUS	monoclonal gammopathy of undetermined significance
MHC	major histocompatibility complex
MHPSAs	Mental Health Professional Shortage Areas

Abbreviation	Meaning
MI	myocardial infarction
MIBG	metaiodobenzylguanidine
MMR	measles, mumps, rubella (vaccine)
MoM	multiple of the median
MRA	magnetic resonance angiography
MRI	magnetic resonance imaging
MS	multiple sclerosis
MSAFP	maternal serum α-fetoprotein
MTP	metatarsophalangeal (joint)
MUA/Ps	Medically Underserved Areas and Populations
MuSK	muscle-specific kinase
MVA	motor vehicle accident
NaHCO$_3$	sodium bicarbonate
NBME	National Board of Medical Examiners
NF	neurofibromatosis
NG	nasogastric
NKH	nonketotic hyperglycemia
NPO	nil per os (nothing by mouth)
NPV	negative predictive value
NS	normal saline
NSAID	nonsteroidal anti-inflammatory drug
NSCLC	non–small cell lung cancer
NST	nonstress test
NYHA	New York Heart Association
O&P	ova and parasites
OCD	obsessive-compulsive disorder
OCP	oral contraceptive pill
OR	odds ratio, operating room
ORIF	open reduction and internal fixation
PaCO$_2$	partial pressure of carbon dioxide in arterial blood
PaO$_2$	partial pressure of oxygen in arterial blood
PAS	periodic acid–Schiff
PCA	posterior cerebral artery
PCKD	polycystic kidney disease
PCL	posterior cruciate ligament
PCO$_2$	partial pressure of carbon dioxide
PCOS	polycystic ovarian syndrome
PCP	phencyclidine hydrochloride, *Pneumocystis carinii* pneumonia
PCR	polymerase chain reaction
PCWP	pulmonary capillary wedge pressure
PDA	patent ductus arteriosus
PDE	phosphodiesterase
PEA	pulseless electrical activity
PEEP	positive end-expiratory pressure
PFT	pulmonary function test
PG	prostaglandin
PID	pelvic inflammatory disease
PIP	proximal interphalangeal (joint)
PIV	parainfluenza virus

Abbreviation	Meaning
PMI	point of maximal impulse
PML	promyelocytic leukemia
PMN	polymorphonuclear (leukocyte)
PO	per os (by mouth)
PO$_2$	partial pressure of oxygen
POC	product of conception
P$_{PA}$	pulmonary arterial pressure
PPD	purified protein derivative (of tuberculin)
PPI	proton pump inhibitor
PPV	pneumococcal polysaccharide vaccine, positive predictive value
PR	progesterone receptor
PROM	premature rupture of membranes
PSA	prostate-specific antigen
PT	prothrombin time
PTCA	percutaneous transluminal coronary angioplasty
PTH	parathyroid hormone
PTHrP	parathyroid hormone–related protein
PTSD	post-traumatic stress disorder
PTT	partial thromboplastin time
PUD	peptic ulcer disease
PUVA	psoralen plus ultraviolet A
PVC	premature ventricular contraction
PVR	peripheral vascular resistance
QD	once a day
QID	four times a day
RA	rheumatoid arthritis
RAIU	radioactive iodine uptake
RBBB	right bundle branch block
RBC	red blood cell
RCT	randomized controlled trial
RDS	respiratory distress syndrome
RDW	red cell distribution width
RF	rheumatoid factor
RLQ	right lower quadrant
RNA	ribonucleic acid
ROM	range of motion, rupture of membranes
RPR	rapid plasma reagin
RR	relative risk, respiratory rate
RSV	respiratory syncytial virus
RTA	renal tubular acidosis
RUQ	right upper quadrant
RVH	right ventricular hypertrophy
SA	sinoatrial
SAAG	serum-ascites albumin gradient
SAB	spontaneous abortion
SAH	subarachnoid hemorrhage
SaO$_2$	oxygen saturation in arterial blood
SBO	small bowel obstruction
SCLC	small cell lung cancer

Abbreviation	Meaning
SCPE	slipped capital femoral epiphysis
SD	standard deviation
SES	socioeconomic status
SEVIS	Student and Exchange Visitor Information System
SEVP	Student and Exchange Visitor Program
SIADH	syndrome of inappropriate secretion of antidiuretic hormone
SIL	squamous intraepithelial lesion
SIRS	systemic inflammatory response syndrome
SJS	Stevens-Johnson syndrome
SLE	systemic lupus erythematosus
SPEP	serum protein electrophoresis
SQ	subcutaneous
SRPs	sponsoring residency programs
SS	single strength
SSRI	selective serotonin reuptake inhibitor
STD	sexually transmitted disease
SVT	supraventricular tachycardia
T_3	triiodothyronine
T3RU	T_3 resin uptake
T_4	thyroxine
TA	temporal arteritis
TAH/BSO	total abdominal hysterectomy and bilateral salpingo-oophorectomy
TB	tuberculosis
TBG	thyroxine-binding globulin
3TC	dideoxythiacytidine (lamivudine)
TCA	tricyclic antidepressant
TdT	terminal deoxynucleotidyl transferase
TEE	transesophageal echocardiography
TEF	tracheoesophageal fistula
TEN	toxic epidermal necrolysis
TENS	transcutaneous electrical nerve stimulation
TFT	thyroid function test
TIA	transient ischemic attack
TIBC	total iron-binding capacity
TID	three times a day

Abbreviation	Meaning
TIPS	transjugular intrahepatic portosystemic shunt
TLC	total lung capacity
TMNG	toxic multinodular goiter
TMP-SMX	trimethoprim-sulfamethoxazole
TNF	tumor necrosis factor
TNM	tumor, node, metastasis (staging)
TOEFL	Test of English as a Foreign Language
tPA	tissue plasminogen activator
TPN	total parenteral nutrition
TPO	thyroid peroxidase
TSH	thyroid-stimulating hormone
TSS	toxic shock syndrome
TSST	toxic shock syndrome toxin
TTP	thrombotic thrombocytopenic purpura
TURP	transurethral resection of the prostate
TV	tidal volume
UA	urinalysis
UMN	upper motor neuron
U_{Na}	urinary sodium
UPEP	urine protein electrophoresis
URI	upper respiratory infection
USDA	United States Department of Agriculture
USIA	United States Information Agency
USMLE	United States Medical Licensing Examination
UTI	urinary tract infection
UV	ultraviolet
VDRL	Venereal Disease Research Laboratory
VIN	vulvar intraepithelial neoplasia
VLDL	very low density lipoprotein
VMA	vanillylmandelic acid
V/Q	ventilation-perfusion (ratio)
vWD	von Willebrand's disease
vWF	von Willebrand's factor
VZV	varicella-zoster virus
WHO	World Health Organization

NOTES

INDEX

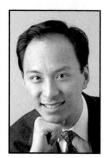
Tao Le, MD

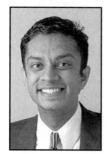
Vikas Bhushan, MD

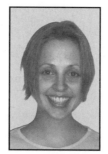
Kerry Dierberg, MPH

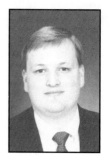
Robert Grow, MD

Tao Le, MD

Dr. Le has led multiple medical education projects over the past 13 years. As a medical student, he was editor-in-chief of the University of California, San Francisco *Synapse,* a university newspaper with a weekly circulation of 9000. Subsequently, he authored *First Aid for the Wards* and *First Aid for the Match* and led the most recent revision of *First Aid for the USMLE Step 2.* At Yale, he was a regular guest lecturer on the USMLE review courses and an adviser to the Yale University School of Medicine curriculum committee. Dr. Le earned his medical degree from the University of California, San Francisco in 1996 and completed his residency training and board certification in internal medicine at Yale–New Haven Hospital. He subsequently went on to cofound Medsn and served as its Chief Medical Officer. Dr. Le conducted research in asthma education as a fellow in allergy and clinical immunology at the Johns Hopkins Asthma and Allergy Center. He is currently Assistant Professor of Pediatrics at the University of Louisvillle.

Vikas Bhushan, MD

Dr. Bhushan is a world-renowned author, publisher, entrepreneur, and board-certified diagnostic radiologist who resides in Los Angeles, California. Dr. Bhushan conceived and authored the original *First Aid for the USMLE Step 1* in 1992, which, after 11 consecutive editions, has become the most popular medical review book in the world. Following this, he coauthored three additional *First Aid* books as well as developed the highly acclaimed 17-title *Underground Clinical Vignettes* series. He completed his training in diagnostic radiology at the University of California, Los Angeles. Dr. Bhushan has more than 13 years of entrepreneurial experience and started two successful software and publishing companies prior to cofounding Medsn. He has worked directly with dozens of medical school faculty, colleagues, and consultants and corresponded with thousands of medical students from around the world. Dr. Bhushan earned his bachelor's degree in biochemistry from the University of California, Berkeley, and his MD with thesis from the University of California, San Francisco.

Kerry Dierberg, MPH

Ms. Dierberg is currently a fourth-year medical student at Johns Hopkins School of Medicine. She completed her undergraduate degree at Washington University in St. Louis, Missouri, and then worked for a nongovernmental organization in Kenya before starting her medical education. Kerry recently completed a master's degree in public health at the Johns Hopkins Bloomberg School of Public Health. She plans to pursue a career in the field of infectious disease.

Robert Grow, MD

Dr. Grow is currently a resident in emergency medicine at the Mayo Clinic in Rochester, Minnesota. He completed his undergraduate education at Brigham Young University, a master's degree in biotechnology at Georgetown University, and medical school training at the Johns Hopkins University School of Medicine in Baltimore, Maryland. His interests include disaster medicine, bioterrorism and biosecurity, and medical education.

ABOUT THE AUTHORS

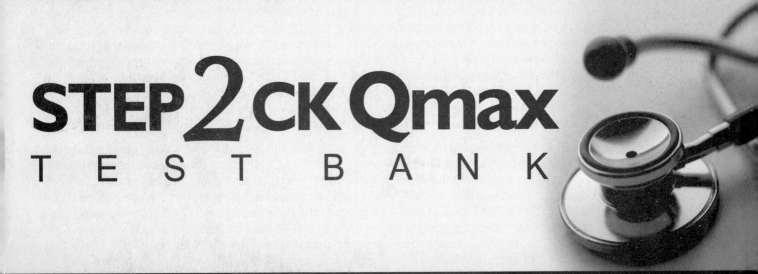